THE PRINCIPLES OF HOMŒOPATHY

AN INTRODUCTION
TO THE
PRINCIPLES AND PRACTICE
OF
HOMŒOPATHY

By

CHARLES E. WHEELER
M.D., B.S., B.Sc.(Lond.)

Consulting Physician to the London Homœopathic Hospital, Past
President British Homœopathic Society, Author of "Knaves or
Fools ?", "The Case for Homœopathy," Honyman Gillespie
Lecturer on Materia Medica at the London Homœopathic Hospital.

THIRD EDITION

revised throughout by the Author with the assistance of J. DOUGLAS
KENYON, M.B., Ch.B., L.R.C.P., B.Sc.(Vict.), Physician London
Homœopathic Hospital, FRANCIS H. BODMAN, M.D., Ch.B.
(Bristol), Physician Bristol Homœopathic Hospital.

" Nasce per quello, a guisa di rampollo,
Appiè del vero il dubbio : ed è natùra,
Ch'al sommo pinge noi di collo in collo."
Dante

THE C. W. DANIEL CO., LTD.
1 CHURCH PATH,
SAFFRON WALDEN, ESSEX,
ENGLAND

Third Edition 1948
Second Impression September 1971
Third Impression January 1978
Fourth Impression September 1982

ISBN 0 85032 062 3

Reproduced and printed in Great Britain by
The Eastern Press Limited, Reading, Berkshire

PREFACE TO THIRD EDITION

THERE has been no need for much alteration in the body of the work. A few things have been omitted which seemed uncertain, at any rate with our present knowledge.

The main feature of this third edition is the addition of several studies of remedies, making a small enlargment of the material on which to base those clinical experiments which alone can determine the value of the therapeutic rule of practice.

Homœopathy has for so long been cold shouldered (to put it mildly) by the profession that it is inevitable that a busy practitioner should hesitate to undertake the study which homœopathy undoubtedly demands before it can be judged fairly. For such physicians it may be difficult to undertake an investigation at a teaching centre for the six months or so that is needed. For them there is, however, the possibility of testing the rule in their daily work in the following way. *Let them first understand the basic principles*, then get a clear vision of the symptomatology of a few drugs, which experience has shown to be frequently needed from the resemblance of their symptoms to those met with in cases of disease. Then if the drug so indicated is given, that is a test so far of the truth of the rule of homœopathy.

For such tests clearly it is desirable to describe as clearly as we can a number of drugs, not too many to confuse a beginner, but sufficient to meet a proportion of the cases which a practitioner will encounter. Rightly, he will test first on cases that fail to respond to the methods he has hitherto used.

This is as it should be since homœopathy claims to be an *addition* to existing therapeutic resources and whenever a physician has already such aids as he trusts, he will not look beyond them.

It is in the hope that we may supply means of assistance to a greater number of cases that we have added a few more drug studies to those of the earlier edition.

I wish to put on record the fact that in the additions and the general preparation of this volume for the Press, Dr. Kenyon has done most of the real work, and to him I am more than grateful.

I have another debt to acknowledge. The revision of the proofs and the assistance in the preparation of the Repertory has been lightened by the co-operation of Dr. B. C. Sekar.

C. E. WHEELER.

CONTENTS

PAGE

PREFACE TO THIRD EDITION v

THE PRINCIPLES OF HOMŒOPATHY . . . 1

(a) DEFINITION OF GENERAL CONSIDERATIONS . 1

(b) THE STRUCTURE OF THE HOMŒOPATHIC MATERIA
MEDICA 8

(c) HOMŒOPATHIC PHARMACY, POTENTISATION,
DOSAGE 13

(d) THE CHOICE AND MODE OF ADMINISTRATION OF
THE REMEDY 26

MATERIA MEDICA 45

ACONITE 45

ANACARDIUM 54

ANTIMONIUM TARTARICUM 62

APIS 69

ARGENTUM METALLICUM 75

ARSENICUM ALBUM 86

BAPTISIA 104

BELLADONNA 110

BRYONIA 121

CALCAREA CARBONICA 128

CHAMOMILLA 138

CHINA 143

CIMICIFUGA RACEMOSA 152

COCA 155

FERRUM 168

FERRUM PHOSPHORICUM 173

GELSEMIUM 176

IGNATIA 181

PAGE

IPECACUANHA 186

KALI CARBONICUM 192

LACHESIS 200

LUETICUM 209

LYCOPODIUM 218

MANGANUM 227

MEDORRHINUM 231

MERCURY 236

NATRUM MURIATICUM 245

NUX VOMICA 251

PHOSPHORUS 260

PLATINUM 271

PULSATILLA 276

RHUS TOXICODENDRON 282

SEPIA 287

SILICA 297

SULPHUR 303

THUJA 319

TUBERCULINUM 328

VERATRUM ALBUM 349

THERAPEUTIC INDEX AND REPERTORY . . 353

GENERAL INDEX 367

THE PRINCIPLES OF HOMŒOPATHY

DEFINITION OF GENERAL CONSIDERATIONS

FOR more than a hundred years the world of medicine has wrangled over the value of homœopathy. At any single moment the verdict of the great majority would have been given against it and to a hasty observation this fact might appear conclusive. But dispassionate examination of medical history reveals first that hardly any advance in the science and art of healing has escaped violent and virulent opposition ; and second that very, very few of those who condemn homœopathy have a knowledge even of its principles, to say nothing of its practice. Wherefore it is clear that in the court of science their testimony, however voluble and dogmatic, is vain. Hahnemann and his followers make certain definite statements concerning the use of drugs for the relief of diseases : they claim to base their statements upon clinical experiments many times repeated. Clearly at the judgment bar of science, only experiments equally careful, equally numerous, but leading to opposite conclusions can be accepted as countervailing material. The question in brief is a practical one. Are the statements of the homœopathist justified ? How but by experiment can they be tested ?

Nevertheless, the road of experiment is toilsome : the mental labour demanded of physicians does not diminish, but increases as the years bring new knowledge and except a man feel reasonably sure that he will gain some reward, he may be forgiven if he hesitates to climb the hill (for it is long and steep) that leads to conviction. Any who feel disposed to use their energy elsewhere can well be forgiven, provided that they own that of this pathway they are ignorant, and place no barriers of prejudice and contempt to impede those minded to try it. But it is a commonplace among physicians to deplore both the too frequent failures of drugs and the lack of much clear guidance in their use. Homœopathy at least offers a promise and a few may be willing to give it a trial. They cannot begin without a clear knowledge of its meaning

1

and purpose and may be encouraged by any theoretical considerations seeming to suggest a confidence that its promise will not be wholly vain. To define homœopathy and suggest that it is not an unreasonable conception of the relation of drugs to diseases is the purpose of this chapter.

Diseases are known to us by the symptoms which they produce, using the word symptoms here (and throughout this volume) to denote the objective signs (physical signs) observable by the physician by means of his instruments of precision and by his unaided senses, as well as the subjective experiences of the patient. Without the presence of symptoms it can hardly be said that an individual is diseased. It may be possible to cultivate specific germs from a surface or secretion of his body, it may even be desirable to deal with the condition that may thus make him a " carrier " of disease, but treatment is then a matter of public rather than of private health. The man is a possible source of danger to others but not himself an obvious patient. The symptoms of diseases, as observed, fall into a variety of categories more or less well defined, enabling the physician to construct a nomenclature of disorders : but side by side with the relatively constant features in a symptom-complex which allow it to be classed as a pneumonia, a colitis or whatever, are invariably found symptoms less constant, varying from case to case with individual " constitution," so that no one case, even of a well-defined disease, exactly resembles another any more than any two individuals are ever absolutely identical.

Just as the so-called " natural " diseases present themselves as symptom-complexes capable of individual differentiation as well as of general grouping into classes, so when drugs are administered to healthy persons, characteristic symptom-complexes are produced with certain general resemblances and definite individual differences, so that from every agent capable of affecting the human body can be elicited a summary of its effects on the body until the picture, e.g., of phosphorus poisoning, can become as clear a mental image as the picture of pneumonia.

The initial and all-important generalisation of Hahnemann was based on the fact (observed from the days of Hippocrates by individuals, though never before Hahnemann made the basis of practice *) *that when the symptom-complex of any case of disease is compared with the symptom-complexes produced by drugs, there will almost always be found a resemblance, often extraordinarily close, between the disease-picture and the picture of the effects of some drug on healthy persons.* This relationship is a fact that becomes increasingly clear the more knowledge is accumulated of the effects of drugs, and the failure of the physician to recognise it is due to the prevailing ignorance of the symptoms which drugs can cause on the healthy. But any physician who will master the symptoms producible by (say) arsenic, phosphorus, nux vomica, etc., on the healthy will not need to look long or far before he finds a case of disease which will recall the effects of one of these drugs to his mind, often with a parallelism of detail almost startling.

The fundamental generalisation, the bedrock of homœopathy, is that the most successful drug for any given occasion will be the drug whose own symptomatology presents the clearest and closest resemblance to the symptom-complex of the sick person in question. Briefly, " Likes should be treated with likes " ; the *simillimum*, the most-resembling drug, should be preferred. Whenever this rule is followed (even unconsciously) homœopathy is practised.

Hahnemann was put on the track of this generalisation by an experiment when he discovered that cinchona bark, the great remedy for ague, could produce upon himself symptoms (even some of the lesser ones) of an attack of ague. From this initial experiment he worked in two directions for the rest of his life, and only after years of labour did he reach absolute convictions which thereafter he extended and amplified. His two paths of knowledge were the less important one of research into past records to discover accidental confirmations of the likelihood of cures by " similar " remedies (and he found many), and the much more important road of direct experiment. First, drugs had to be tested, " proved," on the healthy, then as their symptomatology became defined they were given to " similar " cases of disease and their effects noted. No words, nothing but direct investigation, can give any conception of the magnitude of Hahnemann's labours, but his ceaseless toil both confirmed his belief in his great generalisa-

* Unless perhaps by Paracelsus. See below.

tion and made easier the tests of those who care to follow him. Homœopathy rests on experiment. By experiment alone can it be tested, by experiment alone confirmed or confuted. This then is what homœopathy is, a rule of practice for the administration of drugs.* It demands a knowledge of the effects of drugs upon the healthy which can only be fully obtained by experiment, correlating and extending the results of accidental poisonings and observations on the sick (the so-called clinical symptoms) ; and this knowledge the Homœopathic Materia Medica seeks to supply. When this knowledge is used to select for any case of disease a similar (the most similar) remedy, then an experiment is made in homœopathy. Practical experience from Hahnemann onwards adds the recommendation to give the remedy in a small (not necessarily an infinitesimal) dose. But the dose, of which more will be said in a later chapter, is secondary to the choice of the remedy. It is this choice that stamps a treatment as homœopathic.

It will now be realised that the practice of homœopathy is concerned alone with the administration of remedies. It is a branch of therapeutics, a specialism if the name be preferred, and the study of it is an addition to the resources of the physician, not an impediment to the use of any other treatment justifiably prized. The value and need of surgery, the refinement of diagnosis, the study of pathology, the application of diet and exercises and physical stimuli, all that the years have given of worth, are as much the prized possession of the believer in homœopathy as of his unbelieving colleague. Even with regard to other uses of drugs than their homœopathic application, the homœopathist is free to employ any that he requires. If he uses little morphia and aspirin, purgatives with care and local applications with some reluctance, his relative denial of their efficacy is based on the possession of a guide that generally relieves him of the need for these remedies. If the symptoms point clearly to a *simillimum* that agent will seldom fail to relieve pain or put constipation or skin disease in the way of recovery, perhaps more slowly but generally more surely and permanently than the (apparently) readier methods of treat-

* And for that matter of other (physical) agents.

ment. But if through lack of knowledge or of skill (for it is not easy to practise homœopathy finely) he is at a loss, he is free and ready to turn to the more orthodox resources, being (it is to be hoped) a physician before he is a homœopathist. Only, the more skilled the believer in homœopathy the less often he has need of these other uses of drugs and in his caution in the use of them he has the countenance and support of great teachers of medicine themselves.

There is one aspect of the orthodox uses of drugs which deserves a word or two. Over and over again the homœopathist finds drugs recommended by non-homœopathic authority for conditions to which they are similar. In many instances the similarity is unrecognised from ignorance of the drug " provings " and the symptoms so elicited ; but in some cases (e.g., cantharides for nephritis, opium for constipation, etc.) it might be thought that a suspicion at least of homœopathicity would cross the minds of those who recommend them. Comment has been made by others than homœopathists on the resemblance of symptoms of emetine poisoning to those of the dysentery for whose cure it is given. The late Dr. Dyce Brown collected some seventy examples of this unconscious " homœopathising." The number of these illustrations of the truth of the Hahnemannian generalisation is usually unrecognised. If it were recognised, the possibility that these scattered instances could be gathered under one formula might surely strike even the unobservant, and the success of vaccine therapy comes to strengthen the possibility that " like " may be a remedy for " like " : for if it is not homœopathy to make remedies for diseases out of the agents which are held to be the causes of these diseases it is difficult to find a better word. It will be argued perhaps that the response in anti-body production to the stimulus of a vaccine is a phenomenon observed and brought to usefulness with no thought of homœopathy. This is true, but the fact increases the significance of the observations. It is, of course, not thereby *proved* that a drug that can produce similar symptoms to a disease will be a remedy for that disease, but it makes the possibility of such a relationship more credible, and surely therefore increases the urgency of such tests as alone can establish or deny the Hahnemannian claim. Vaccine therapy does not prove the. truth of homœopathy, but does it not make it less paradoxical and incite to independent research ?

Thus historically it must be admitted that while the truth of homœopathy must rest on experiment, widespread and satisfactory testing has been hitherto denied and thus a road promising much of value to the physician has remained unexplored. The few who have been led along it rarely retrace their steps or fail to praise it and this fact should be a further inducement to research. But general biological considerations, apart from clinical experience, can make a case for experiment in this matter. Disease is ultimately an affair of the reactions of protoplasm, and in the response of protoplasm to stimuli we should find, if anywhere, material for generalisations upon disease and treatment. Now these responses of protoplasm have been well investigated, and appear to follow a constant rule generally summarised as Arndt's Law.* The simple statement of this rule is that small stimuli encourage life activity, medium to strong stimuli tend to impede it, and very strong stimuli to stop or destroy it. Thus strong solutions of arsenious acid will destroy the yeast cell,† less strong impede its fermentative activity, but very dilute solutions will encourage its activity, at any rate for a time.

Considering only the behaviour of protoplasm, we should be led to argue that since in disease the cells specially attacked are the cells specially in need of a stimulus (since their life activities are threatened), that stimulus will be found in a small dose of the agent which in large dose can damage or destroy precisely these particular cells. How can the special relationships of drugs to cells be known ? How but by a testing of drugs upon the healthy ? Drugs given to persons in health will influence certain cells and tissues according to their individual " affinities " : when by symptoms thus produced we know that a drug can damage this or that set of cells, then we can use a small dose of the same drug to stimulate the same set of cells if oppressed by disease. In other words,

* Law in a biological sense (and medicine is a biological study) implies no eternal binding force, but merely that hitherto in experience certain results follow certain causes in a definite predicable sequence.

† It is a commonplace of all Materia Medica that the first effects of a drug should often be opposite to its last effects, e.g., camphor will be aphrodisiac at first and later anaphrodisiac.

the responses of protoplasm to stimuli would justify the recommendations :

(a) Test drugs on the healthy and note the symptoms.

(b) When treating disease, look for a drug which has produced similar symptoms on the healthy, for only thus can there be any confidence that it will influence the tissues affected.

(c) Give a small dose.

This summary is sufficiently close to the Hahnemannian generalisation to encourage the testing of it, yet it is reached by arguments from non-clinical experience.

Finally it is significant to note how the generalisation of Hahnemann has been both anticipated and independently reached subsequently by other observers. Hippocrates noted that drugs could sometimes cure " similar " diseases, though he made no rule of practice from the observation. Paracelsus wrapped his teaching in such obscurity that it is rash to dogmatise upon it, but if I interpret him rightly he believed that " Like to like " was the sound rule of prescription : his suggestion of naming diseases by the drugs which would relieve them seems to mean that it was from similarity that he selected them. John Hunter conceived from the resemblance of the symptoms of chronic mercury poisoning to those of syphilis and the undoubted power of the drug to relieve that disease, that " similarity " might be a clue to the best uses of remedies. And since Hahnemann, the great Trousseau (for all his hatred of homœopathy) suggested a principle of " substitution therapy " which led in practice to the use of " similar " medicines. Dr. Reith (more or less forgotten now) and Professor Hugo Schulz (more recently) deduced, independently of one another and of any knowledge of homœopathy, from biological considerations such as have been outlined above, a system of therapeutics which closely resembles that of homœopathy. Both of these men came quickly to realise where their clues had led them and made fullest acknowledgment of Hahnemann's precedence in the field. Professor Schulz will be often quoted in this volume and his independent work is the most important addition to homœopathic literature which has been made from any source not avowedly deriving from Hahnemann. Homœopathy therefore is a principle of drug therapeutics : it teaches that drugs must be tested on the healthy and chosen for diseases by their similarity of symptoms : the closer the similarity between drug symptoms and disease symptoms the greater the chance of permanent and speedy relief. It claims to be justifiable on general grounds, but can derive final validity only from clinical experiment. Subsequent chapters must ·deal with the supply of material for such experiments and the best method and manner in which to make them.*

THE STRUCTURE OF THE HOMŒOPATHIC MATERIA MEDICA

Hahnemann called the Materia Medica which owed (and still owes) its conception, initiation, and the most valuable part of its structure to his devotion and genius, by the name " Pure," whereby he meant to indicate that it should be experimental, rather than conjectural, recording the effects of drugs upon the healthy and little or nothing else. In the main his followers have retained his ideal and the extension of his work has followed, for the greater part, on the lines laid down by him. When a homœopathist desires to study a drug, hitherto unknown as a remedy, he must begin by getting it " proved " by as many persons of both sexes as possible. Preferably they should be thoroughly healthy, old enough to

* It is not unusual to recommend a method of treatment by statistics whenever comparison is possible. Homœopathy has no reason to fear the test of figures, and has indeed largely profited by such tests, but its followers are well aware of the many fallacies that may lurk in records of cases, similarly named but perhaps differing widely in many respects, and their limited control of public institutions (fever hospitals, asylums, etc.) deprives them of the opportunity of simple comparisons year by year. But they can fairly urge that the personal experience of their converts has a value that may be called statistical. Every physician in Europe who adopts homœopathy is trained in all the wisdom of orthodoxy, has his own clinical experience of its value and has seen the practice in detail of the masters of its art. If he faces the contempt and obloquy of avowed homœopathy (much less than of old, but not negligible even to-day)—and no man lightly severs himself from professional fellowship—it can only be because he believes that through homœopathy he obtains better results. Yet in attaining these results his general knowledge remains the same, and the power of his personality is unchanged. The only new factor in his practice is his new therapeutic learning and it is only fair to attribute to it the gain for whose sake he is ready to face the smile of contempt and perhaps the cold shoulder of ostracism. He undertakes new and hard labour for no obvious gain except greater power to heal the sick : before he is dubbed merely credulous, his critics should repeat his experiments, and the price he is willing to pay should attest the sincerity of his belief in the worth of his prize.

report their subjective symptoms intelligently, but young enough to have sensitive tissues unpoisoned by errors of diet or drugging and undamaged by the results of physical indulgence. For many remedies this ideal has been tolerably well attained, and their pathogeneses, sifted through many clinical experiences, can be set forth with confidence as veritable drug pictures. Many other remedies have been proved with less completeness, but still sufficiently to make them available for use, and of others again we have but little knowledge : these last await their true place in the Materia Medica.

But although the deliberate systematic testing of medicines upon the healthy must remain by far the most important source of our Materia Medica, there remain other springs not by any means to be despised. The first of these is the knowledge derived from poisoning by drugs, accidental or intentional. Hereby are revealed the gross effects of overwhelming doses and here frequently it is possible by post-mortem examinations to judge something of the massive pathological changes produced by these agents. This knowledge has definite value, but is of less worth for the prescriber's purposes than the observations of the provers. It is universally admitted that it is in the earliest stage that diseases are most amenable to treatment and in this stage the symptoms of the conflict between disease and life are more likely to be subjective and indirect than significant of the gross tissue changes that may be about to follow. The aim of the homœopathist is to discover the *simillimum* for the disease while it expresses itself in such preliminary symptoms, and this he is more likely to find among drug pictures gradually built up by administration of small doses during a considerable time than in the overwhelming effects of large quantities. Many tissues once destroyed can by no means be reintegrated and to delay treatment till the spinal sclerosis or interstitial nephritis is unmistakable is to leave little but palliation possible for the physician.

The often (mistakenly) derided interest of the homœopathist in symptoms therefore finds its justification as an attempt to cure diseases while they are still curable. It need hardly be added that the disappearance of symptoms which *may* have been the first signs of tissue changes impending does not for a moment warrant the claim that these tissue changes would inevitably have followed the neglect of our remedies and that the cases are therefore to be classed as " cures " of sclerosis or nephritis, or whatever it may be. That would be an assumption quite unwarrantable in any given instance. For that matter, though the recovery of any isolated case may raise a reasonable presumption that treatment has been effective, it can never establish its effectiveness as a fact beyond cavil. Only by prolonged experience over many years and comparison of many cases can homœopathists have any confidence that their treatment of preliminary symptoms does sometimes ward off serious disease ; but this experience has been gained and these comparisons made, and the desirability of attempting this task may be taken as established for those who have studied the subject. In any case the need of the patient for relief is obvious and homœopathy offers a way of choosing a remedy which has claims to relieve not only fugitive symptoms, but those that may be forerunners of graver troubles and there for the moment the matter may rest. It suffices to indicate the reason for the preference of the deliberate proving over the poisoning as a guide to the remedy. When the tissue change is established the pathological relation of drug to disease is an invaluable guide to a remedy which may cure an acute recoverable tissue-effect of illness (e.g., pneumonia) or relieve or palliate a chronic and irrecoverable one.

Similar advantages and disadvantages belong to drug experiments upon animals. They are not to be despised, but they have a special defect of their own in that the bodies of animals cannot be expected always to react to stimuli as do the bodies of human beings. He who would for instance make the effect of belladonna on the rabbit the sole guide to its use on patients might well be led into error. All this material, therefore, homœopathy uses gratefully enough as regards any hints of possible action, but with considerable caution. Seeing that in practice a drug is to be given to human beings, it is to the effects of the drug upon men and women that the physician looks with most confidence for guidance. The veterinary practitioner naturally finds a special value in animal " provings."

Over and above provings, poisonings, experiments on animals, there remains clinical experience. This is of value in two ways.

In the first place, it will strike the inquirer at once that symptoms (especially subjective symptoms) set down by provers may not be drug effects at all. Imagination, stimulated by attention and expectation, is capable of producing the most definite phenomena. How shall the true drug effects be distinguished from the false ? In the first instance homœopathy relies on the acumen of the supervisor of the proving. By cross-examining his subjects and using all his knowledge of their capabilities and qualities, he can often from the first throw out or query symptoms unlikely to have been produced by the drug. Further, the multiplication of provers is a great help, for obviously symptoms reported independently by two or three or more, are less likely to be spurious than those which appear only in the record of one. Care, however, must be exercised in applying this test, for among several provers one or two will be more susceptible to the drug and may well obtain genuine symptoms of its action which the others miss. There are records of the infinity of pains and patient labour which Hahnemann devoted to the verification of symptoms, and given a trained, alert, sceptical but not prejudiced mind, even one or two provings will yield fruits of value. Nevertheless, without a doubt some imaginary symptoms will pass the first sieve.

But now comes the final testing, the application to the actual case. If a belief in the truth of the homœopathic generalisation exists in the physician (and it is not too much to say that it can safely be founded on clinical experiments which admit the use of no doubtful symptoms), then this belief can be further used to test the provings. If any recorded symptom proves a valid guide to the choice of a remedy (as vouched for by the disappearance of the symptom after administration of the drug), then that counts in favour of the truth of that symptom of the proving. It must be premised, of course, that the symptom under trial shall be accompanied by others warranting the choice of the remedy as the *simillimum* and that the tests must be repeated in several instances. But granting these conditions, it is fair to say that the symptom that consistently justifies itself as a guide to the curative remedy deserves to be accepted as a genuine drug symptom and may be henceforth held in honour. Similarly, symptoms which consistently fail as guides can be discarded. In this way clinical experience " proves " the provings.

But it has another value. Two phenomena can be frequently observed in the course of practice with remedies. First, the appearance of new symptoms in the patient following the administration of a drug ; second, the disappearance of symptoms (under treatment) which are unrepresented in the provings of the agent employed. In either case the remedy *may* be responsible for the phenomenon.

The appearance of new symptoms in the course of disease under treatment demands the most detached, unprejudiced consideration before a conclusion is drawn, and any conclusion can be no more at first than tentative and lightly held. The power of disease to give rise to unusual symptoms is as boundless as are the variations in human constitutions and the first assumption with regard to a newly appearing symptom, however strange, must be that it is probably due to the disorder and not to the drug administered. Nevertheless, if the new symptom is observed to have close connection with the remedial agent, rising and falling in intensity with the nearness to or remoteness from the times of administration, if it is accompanied by other symptoms known to be characteristic of the drug, the *possibility* may be considered that it is a drug-produced symptom which thereupon becomes a candidate for inclusion in the pathogenesis of the remedy. The pretensions of the candidates need the most cautious testing. If future experience shows that the new symptom not only repeatedly arises in association with other symptoms of the medicine but that, in other cases, it also disappears after the administration of the drug, then by degrees a reasonable degree of conviction can be attained, and the symptom placed among the others of the drug-picture as a trustworthy guide to the use of the remedy.

The disappearance of symptoms under treatment, however, is a more fruitful field for observation. Suppose a remedy is chosen on the ground of its resemblance to the symptoms of a case, but suppose (as often happens) that the resemblance, though fairly close, has one or more notable gaps, the disease presenting a marked symptom or two for which no parallel can be found in the proving. Suppose, nevertheless, that no closer *simillimum* can be found and that the drug is given. If now it proves successful it will probably remove not only the symptoms that were known to appear in its pathogenesis, but also the ones unrecorded. In such a case it is not unreasonable to adopt, as a working hypothesis, the theory that the symptoms removed may be valuable indications of the remedy and to include them in the pathogenesis temporarily until further clinical experience has justified their permanent retention there or condemned them.

By these means clinical symptoms are often obtained of permanent value and for practical purposes if a symptom has repeatedly shown itself a trustworthy guide to the choice of a remedy, there is no reason why it should be ignored because it has never happened to appear in any proving. Largely by clinical experience a large store of information has also accumulated as to the general characteristics of patients in regard to their susceptibilities to various drugs. This knowledge is very valuable, as will be realised in the course of this work, and it is owed to a combination of clinical observation and application of provings where it is far from easy to apportion the respective values of the contributions.

The Homœopathic Materia Medica, therefore, is drawn from all these sources. In the drug studies that follow, the intention of the writer is to incorporate only such material as can be regarded as trustworthy, but no space will be given to details of discrimination as to the particular fountain from which this or that symptom has flowed. If it justifies itself as a sure ground for a prescription its value is assured.

HOMŒOPATHIC PHARMACY, POTENTISATION, DOSAGE

The preparation of remedies for use according to the principle of homœopathy is simple in method, but demands the greatest care and conscientiousness in practice. Here the physician is necessarily dependent upon the chemist, and no considerations of expense should be allowed to stand in the way of procuring the best prepared tinctures and potencies. In any case, the drug bills of homœopathy will always be incomparably smaller than those of " orthodox " medicine.

When Hahnemann began to test the truth of his great generalisation, he used remedies in dosage not very far removed from that of his former practice. He seems never to have favoured the massive doses of most of his contemporaries, and using a single remedy at a time, in no great quantity, his new method must have seemed to him in no way to err on the side of excess. Nevertheless, experience soon taught him that his dosage was unnecessarily large, for frequently, although his patients were ultimately relieved, the first effect of his medicines was an aggravation of symptoms, not to be wondered at seeing that the drug had powers similar to those of the disease, but nevertheless undesirable. In the endeavour to avoid this preliminary aggravation of symptoms, he began to reduce his doses and speedily found that most drugs, given " homœopathically," seemed effective in quantities of a smallness hitherto inconceivable. He therefore systematised his pharmacy and the practice of homœopathy as received from Hahnemann is as follows.

From medicinal plants tinctures are prepared in the way customary with all druggists, with the proviso that homœopathists desire the fresh plant to be used if possible and generally the whole of it, from root to flower. The flowering season is the time appointed for collecting plants. The very strongest possible tincture is made in this way, and is named the Mother Tincture : it is symbolised in writing prescriptions by the Greek letter ϕ or θ. The successive dilutions or " potencies," as they are called, are made from this on either the centesimal scale (Hahnemann's own) or the decimal. In the first series, potency number 1 (potencies are prescribed by number, 1, 6, 12, 30, etc.) consists of 1 drop of the tincture to 99 drops of the neutral fluid, usually spirits of wine, with a small quantity of water. A drop of number 1, with a further 99 drops of the medium is the second potency : a drop of this and 99 drops of the medium make the third, and so on, as far as the physician desires. Each successive potency should receive the most thorough succussion and agitation so as to distribute the tincture fully and evenly through the whole mass of the diluting medium.

In the second (decimal) series, the steps are made by tens instead of by hundreds. Thus the first decimal ($1x$ potency) consists of 1 drop of tincture and 9 drops of spirits of wine, suitably shaken up together ; then a drop of this $1x$ and 9 further drops of alcohol and water gives the second decimal or $2x$, and so on, to $3x$, $4x$, as far as may be desired. In actual quantity of tincture present, therefore, the $2x$ equals the first centesimal (written simply 1, or sometimes 1c), the $6x$ equals the third centesimal (3 or 3c), the $30x$ equals the 15c and so on, but the number on the decimal scale involves a greater number of succussions for its preparation than its parallel in the centesimal scale. Generally speaking, potencies from the tincture to the third centesimal (or $6x$) are classified as " low " ; from 3 to 12 ($6x$ to $24x$) as " medium," and from 12 or 15 upwards as high, ranging to very high potencies.

For mineral substances the principle of preparation is similar. Each potency is reckoned to contain a corresponding proportion of the pure substance : thus $1x$ would imply a strength of one in ten of the pure mineral, $3x$ would imply the presence of one in a thousand. If the substance is soluble in alcohol, alcohol and water is used as the medium for making potencies. If the mineral is insoluble in alcohol but soluble in water, then distilled water is used for the lower potencies at any rate, though a proportion of alcohol is added when the higher are reached. Such drugs as phosphorus require special treatment.

If the substance is insoluble in the familiar sense of the word (e.g., gold, lead, silica, etc.), it is prepared by prolonged trituration with sugar of milk, but the proportions are graduated as before, so that a $2x$ trituration (or the first centesimal) implies 1 part of the substance with 99 of sugar of milk. After the $6x$, however, the further potencies can be made with alcohol and water, for prolonged trituration appears to produce a physical change converting these insoluble substances into the colloidal state. In this condition they can be suspended in a fluid medium indefinitely and the suspensions behave for medicinal purposes like solutions. Observation and experiment enabled Hahnemann to assure himself of this fact, although he could not give the physical explanation of it, since in his day " colloids " were unknown. Hardly any statement of his has been held up to a greater ridicule than this assertion that solutions could be made of insoluble substances. Now, however, time has done him right ; if not technically solutions, these preparations can be treated as solutions from a pharmaceutical standpoint. The whole episode demonstrates once again the close observation of Hahnemann and his trust in careful experiment, and also the folly of reckless denials of the results of experiment, when the denials are based not on countervailing tests, but on prejudice and preconceived ideas.

The foregoing pages are in no sense a full account of homœopathic pharmacy, for there are individual peculiarities of certain drugs which demand special pharmaceutical treatment. Details can be found in the official Homœopathic Pharmacopœias of Europe and America. But the main outlines of the general method of preparation should now be clear. The aim is to obtain a series of preparations wherein the actual quantity of the drug becomes less and less. These preparations are known as potencies and the process of making them as potentisation and their value and spheres of usefulness remain to be considered.

Since the central homœopathic generalisation concerns only the choice of the remedy, homœopathy can be practised without recourse to potencies at all. Experience will quickly teach the advisability of the small dose, but much good homœopathic work has been done, and can be done, with tinctures and easily demonstrable quantities of drugs and the instinct of most beginners is to stay in this more familiar region. But the feeling that prompts this tendency is really a legacy from the dark ages of medicine, a relic of the conception of a drug as an agent of power independent of the body mechanism, power to give strength from itself (" tonic "), power to combat disease directly as in the days when a " hot " disorder was countered by a " cold " remedy. Now it is known that, except possibly for certain remedies to be considered in a moment, this conception is a false one. Whatever resistance is made to a disease, or attempt at repair of damage to tissues, is made by a definite and usually specific body mechanism and to-day we catch many glimpses of the nature and mode of action of these mechanisms. The physician can help or hinder these natural processes by drugs, but since the drug, if it acts at all, will act by influencing a pre-existing mechanism, the only quantity of it required is that quantity that will set in motion a machinery temporarily disused, or speed up one insufficiently used, or control one racing wastefully. Such glimpses as we can catch of these protoplasmic processes always suggest a comparison with the work of enzymes as agents, and it is notorious that enzyme action demands the presence of only a small, even an infinitesimal quantity. In so far, then, as drugs can either replace enzymes or stimulate their production, there is no a priori reason (rather the contrary) for expecting large quantities to be necessary, and clearly since a drug may be, and generally is, a foreign substance, the less of it that can be used to produce an effect the better ; any surplus can be but an impediment to the processes of life.

An analogy (used with caution, as all analogies should be) may serve to illustrate the position. The tissues have a daily income and expenditure of energy, as individuals in society have an income and expenditure of money. But as the luckier among men have reserves of wealth (say a deposit, as well as a current, banking account), so have all the tissues reserves of energy. The power to deal with disease lies finally with one or more of these reserves, but just as money on deposit cannot be obtained without certain formalities, so sometimes tissue reserves are used slowly and ineffectively Conceivably the drug sometimes sets free these reserves or modifies the speed with which they can be used and to do this it is unnecessary to invoke large quantities of drugs, or at least the quantity required becomes a legitimate subject for experiment.

Of late years the minds of physicians have turned (following Ehrlich) to the thought of " great sterilisers " for parasitic diseases, agents to destroy invaders directly, independently of any forces of the body. The conception of such drugs is a striking one, but few would maintain that any substance at present available fulfils these requirements exactly. There is none that has not some effect on tissues, whatever its power over the parasites ; therefore, as yet, tissue reactions must be considered in handling these agents. If, however, the ideal be ever attained and it become possible to destroy pathogenic bacteria without affecting the body of the host, such " sterilising " agents will be gratefully used by the homœopathist as readily as by any of his colleagues.   But till this goal is reached there remain one or two points of interest.

In the first place, when the effects of these drugs are examined a striking common characteristic appears.   The principal agents believed to act as parasiticides are quinine in malaria, mercury and arsenic in syphilis, emetine in dysentery.   There is not one of them that has not the power to produce on the body symptoms similar to those of the disease for which it is held to be specific.   That is to say, there is a certain definite homœopathy about all of them.   But this fact inevitably suggests that, since the drug makes the body react in a way similar to the reaction to the disease (and since in each case the body reaction is probably an expression of body resistance), so the curative action of the drug is probably not direct action upon the parasite but indirect, exerted by encouraging the normal mechanisms of resistance.   The drug is administered and the parasites are found to be dead (in favourable cases), but this result would equally follow an indirect or a direct action, and is no proof that only the latter has been involved. *Some* direct action there would almost certainly be after intravenous injections, but it is noteworthy that good results appear to follow concentrations of the drugs in the body fluids lower than those that are alone effective in test tubes, and this again suggests an action indirect and not immediate. But if the effect is not directly exerted on the parasites (when considerable doses would seem desirable), it may be that large doses are unnecessary and that the body resistance can be stimulated with smaller quantities.

A second consideration with regard to parasiticidal remedies is that vaccines designed for just such emergencies are acknowledged to have an indirect action, and that it is not at all inconceivable that there should be drugs capable of setting in motion or stimulating a mechanism even as the vaccine is believed to do.   There are experiments (homœopathic and non-homœopathic) that support this view.   But vaccines have to be given with caution and drugs (if such there be) capable of a " vaccine " reaction should similarly be given in relatively small doses.

Finally, therefore, it can hardly be contested that dosage

is a matter for experiment. Hahnemann believed, and nearly all his followers come to believe, that drugs are effective in very small quantities, and only experiment can decide for or against them. Let it at once be granted that the most patient and sceptical observation is required of multitudes of cases before the relation of drug to recovery can be claimed as cause and effect. Nevertheless, most physicians are inclined to think that the relation can be established sometimes if not often, in spite of all the baffling possibilities of spontaneous recovery and cure by mental suggestion. The same kind of evidence as that which suffices to convince the physician that drugs can ever have values, must serve also to convince him as to the desirable dosage of them. There is no logical reason why experience which would convince for the worth of a tincture should not convince for the worth of a potency. It is simply a question of enough evidence : prejudice has no voice in the decision.

It is of interest to point out that since Sir Almroth Wright's classical discoveries of opsonins and their estimation, a dosage of tuberculin at least has come into vogue that is almost as immeasurable, except by its clinical effects, as a drug-potency. Doses of one ten-thousandth of a milligramme and much less are held to be effective.* The judgment for their efficacy is given mainly on clinical evidence and if the non-homœopathist may invoke it for one drug, homœopathists may follow suit for many, provided only that they are tireless in experiment and cautious in conclusion. Of course, there is always the evidence of increased anti-body formation when these substances can be estimated, but this resource is also open to the homœopathist, and in an increasing number of instances (to which reference will be made under the various drug headings) it has given most striking results. For the ordinary practitioner these tests are not freely available and he has to decide by the clinical evidence ; but when all is said this is the court of final appeal. The laboratory findings must be checked by the clinical results as well as the results by the findings, and it would profit the practitioner little to have favourable

* Since this was written there has been a general tendency to use vaccines in smaller doses. The experience of Dr. Warren Crowe with streptococcal injections for arthritis illustrates the way in which experience touches the desirability of both lesser amounts and longer intervals between doses.

laboratory reports if his patient failed to improve. Every possible extension of laboratory experiment is desirable, but we do well to remember also that the laboratory was made for the patient, not the patient for the laboratory. The value, therefore, of the infinitesimal doses of homœopathy rests on evidence, and there is no lack of it or lack of opportunity for any inquirer to supply more. But it remains yet to investigate the historical fact of the general preference of homœopathists in practice for the potencies. Nearly all inquirers follow Hahnemann's own road, using first ordinary (if small) material doses. Yet, like Hahnemann, they are generally led on by experience to the use of potencies and even (frequently) of very high ones, and this in spite of the fact that they know that these preparations may be a subject of derision to colleagues, who for all their ignorance of the subject are nevertheless not wantonly to be flouted. This trend of experience is of itself evidence of the value of potencies, for no man lightly widens the gulf between himself and his fellow physicians. But it is worth while to pursue the matter further.

Hahnemann began, it seems, to make dilutions of tinctures in the attempt to avoid the aggravations of symptoms which, he found, often preceded a cure by the similar remedy ; but he speedily discovered that this avoidance of aggravation by no means always resulted. It is the common experience of many observers to find a preliminary aggravation of symptoms follow the administration of the *simillimum* in any form (even more frequently with high potencies), and within limits, it has come to be regarded as a valuable indication for a good prognosis, corresponding to the "negative phase" of Sir Almroth Wright's early opsonic investigations. But although Hahnemann did not succeed in avoiding "aggravations," he found other virtues in his very small doses which led him to call them potencies and in these later conclusions again most of his followers confirm him. He found that in many cases (probably a large majority) the use of the potency gave swifter and profounder results which endured more permanently, and he concluded that his pharmaceutical methods in some way (or ways) changed the energy of the drug, making it more effective for his purposes. It is because his followers have had

similar experiences that they generally add to their first
experiment in the heresy of the homœopathic generalisation,
the almost greater heresy of using the infinitesimal dose.
Now it is clear that no theoretical conclusions can decide
the matter, and every man who desires a scientific opinion
must experiment for himself, but it may be of interest to
speculate a little upon the possible nature of potentisation.
The ground must to some extent be cleared by remembrance
of facts universally acknowledged. No man now believes
that a drug acts simply by virtue of its mass. Large doses of
Epsom salts and so forth, or the hypertonic injections of Dr.
Leonard Rogers, are attempts to use a physical action of a
particular kind ; ordinary drug actions are not conceived in
this way. The increased drug power of grey powder over that
of metallic mercury is a simple instance of the value of sub-
division. Add the well-known facts of ionisation in solutions
(which increases up to a point with progressive dilution), add
the assumption of the colloidal state by substances under
prolonged trituration and the extraordinary powers of colloidal
" solutions," and it is not easy to deny that the earlier stages
of homœopathic pharmacy may well be justified as procedures
likely to increase the power of drugs. Incidentally also it
must be remembered that a diseased tissue is (generally at
least) a tissue more sensitive to stimuli. The stable equilibrium
of health may be unaffected by quantities that are readily
capable of influencing the unstable equilibrium of disease.
The whole conception of the *simillimum* is that it shall be an
agent to attack the most diseased tissues principally, and the
smallest dose that can affect them effectively is large enough.
This consideration can be set side by side with that of the
possibly increased activity, as stimuli, of drugs prepared by
the pharmacy of homœopathy, and reasons for choosing the
lower to medium potencies are thus suggested and experiment
confirms them.

But experiment does more than this. It asserts a value,
and tends to assert an increasing value, for potencies rising
beyond the power of ionisation or of chemical activity to
explain. Long before the thirtieth centesimal is reached any
explanations of effectiveness based on atomic structure as at
present conceived become difficult. Yet the clinical proofs of

effectiveness are numerous and carefully observed. The potentiser finds that his successive potencies have the curative drug power, that this property cannot be washed out of a vessel, and that it *can* be destroyed by prolonged heat. The only suggestion, therefore, that can be made is that homœopathic pharmacy causes at a certain stage the development of a physical force which can thereafter be transmitted to succeeding potencies. The explanation has two great difficulties to meet : First, the potencies of drugs have *specific* powers, differing for each drug, retaining the same indications for use (*i.e.*, the same tissue relations) as the tinctures from which they are made, and this implies that this force has a range of variation in quality almost unlimited. Second, clinical experiment suggests that sometimes at least the higher potencies are more powerful than the less high (*e.g.*, 200 than 30), and this is not very easy to explain. We might have expected that once the power developed it would not change much in vigour, might even (however slowly) lessen ; the opposite seems nearer the truth. For the first difficulty we can only fall back on the remembrance of the infinite possibilities of energy wavelengths for instance in light, and speculate whether, if similar variations could be postulated for our hypothetical drug force it might not be true that particular cases were best met by a particular " wave-length." For the second difficulty no explanation suggests itself. The whole subject remains obscure, and is being patiently investigated. But very few who have made the clinical experiments have been able to deny that the high potencies appear to have a real and sometimes a superlative power.

But it must not be concluded at once that high potencies are *invariably* more effective than low. It frequently happens that the high will relieve more effectively (otherwise they would never have come into use), but it also happens now and then that low potencies succeed when high have failed. Further, there are certain drugs that do not appear to " potentise " well, drugs which have apparently little or no action except in appreciable doses. If it be a fact that to potentise a drug means to develop a new energy in it, it is quite conceivable that some fact of molecular structure should prevent this energy from becoming developed in certain cases. A uniform procedure is followed in potentisation, and there may be substances to which the procedure is not fully applicable.

More probably, however, the explanation of varying success as between " high " and " low " will be found in the nature of the work which the drug is expected to perform. We can conceive of a drug as a direct tissue stimulant. This is the conception of Schulz, and probably of Schüssler (the advocate of " tissue remedies ").

Here the like remedy is chosen to ensure an effect upon the tissue principally diseased, but an appreciable quantity of it (although a small one) may be needed to stimulate it effectively and repeated doses may be required to obtain a continuous effect. Dr. Burnett (following Rademacher, as Rademacher claimed to follow Paracelsus) advocated in many cases " organ remedies," by which he meant tissue stimulants, and it is interesting to observe that these were always given in appreciable doses. Dr. Hughes, also, prescribing when possible on a basis of morbid anatomy, generally recommended the lower potencies. It is a common experience that low potencies and repeated doses are effective in acute diseases, and acute diseases have very marked tissue relationships (e.g., pneumonia, enteric, etc.). So, it will be argued, have chronic diseases (e.g., disseminated sclerosis, osteo-arthritis, etc.), but in these the tissue relationship is one of destruction and the remediable stage is before the tissue relationship becomes defined to our powers of demonstration. The inflamed lung can become functional again, but not the sclerosed nerve tissue. To give a gentle stimulus to the inflamed lung tissue by small doses of antimony or phosphorus is therefore not unreasonable, because natural forces are at work to overthrow the enemy that causes the disease ; the question of cure is a question of tiding over an emergency, and practice confirms the expectation of benefit ; but the spinal cord, threatened by some deep-acting enemy that will ultimately destroy it, may be slightly helped by gentle stimulation, but inasmuch as the natural forces will rarely suffice to defeat the enemy, cure can only be found in some remedy that will enhance this more central mechanism of defence, and that must be a general, not a local, remedy. The distinction is not to be pressed too far, because in a pneumonia or an enteric, a remedy which enhanced the production of antibodies might be preferable to one that merely stimulated the tissue chiefly attacked, and experiment shows that such remedies exist ; also without a doubt there are drugs which can affect certain tissues directly and in addition have the power to influence certain mechanisms, and sometimes one action and sometimes the other may be called into play.

But broadly it may be suggested that whenever the purpose of a drug is to improve the metabolism of a definite organ or tissue by gentle stimulation, low potencies and repeated doses are suitable, while if the aim is to influence a central mechanism of life, the higher potencies and infrequently repeated doses are of more value. By the term " life mechanism " is meant principally that system of action and interaction of internal secretions, of which in these times physicians catch a few glimpses, tantalisingly incomplete, but full of suggestion for future successes in treatment when knowledge grows and the glimpses become steady vision. Already we know that excess or defect of one or more of these secretions (e.g., thyroid, adrenal, insulin, etc.) will give rise to a symptom-picture of great complexity.

In chronic disease the resemblance of the *simillimum* to the given symptom-complex may be due to the power of the drug to affect this internal secretion mechanism in a similar way to that disturbance which is causing the illness, and the administration of the remedy may bring about a change in the amount or quality of the secretion and so tend to restore health. It may be argued that as the secretion is the result of tissue activity, the problem is still one of tissue stimulation, but it must be remembered that (apart from entire defect of secretion, as in myxœdema) the difficulty seems often to be a failure of secretion balance, of the proper adjustment of a mechanism, and a single touch, as it were, may suffice to restore this. When a secretion is tending to fail altogether, then a tissue stimulant may help, and when it has completely ceased, we can only hope to do what is so successfully done in myx- œdema, viz., supply the missing secretion from the outside. The illustrations of the action of tissue remedies and life- mechanism remedies would be rather that in the first instance we are, as it were, making the best of a somewhat damaged structure, say a mill wheel, wearing out, but capable of being patched and mended so as to serve a while longer ; in the second case we are dealing with a very delicate and finely adjusted mechanism, impeded by some grit or slight hindrance. If left to work against this impediment the mechanism will ultimately be destroyed, yet there is a time when the removal of it (even the use of a drop or two of oil, so to speak) will leave the machine once more running as smoothly as ever.*

These speculations are only profitable as indications of the need for endless experiment and observation. Probably for every case there is an *optimum* dosage just as there is an *optimum* remedy. The factors that should decide our choice will be (*a*) the constitution of the patient, some individuals being so much more sensitive than others ; (*b*) the nature of the drug, whether it lends itself well to potentisation or not ; and (*c*) the nature of the illness, whether it is mainly a gross tissue affection, or an interference with one or other of the subtler life mechanisms. It is impossible as yet to give full value to any of these factors, so that there is no way out but that of cautious experiment. One or two practical rules can, however, be laid down with some confidence.

(A) If a remedy is very well indicated by a close symptom resemblance between it and the disease, choose rather a high potency, and if possible watch the effect of each dose, treating each dose as it is usual to treat a dose of a vaccine, and not repeating until the effect of it is exhausted. (See chapter on " The Choice of the Remedy and Administration.")

An acute disease will probably demand more frequent repetition and often reacts well to lower potencies.

(B) If a remedy is well indicated, yet fails, try other potencies (both higher and lower) before changing the drug.

(C) If the resemblance of drug to disease is not very close, especially if there is any reason to think that one tissue is specially affected and that the drug has an " affinity " for

---

* Since this was written the problems of normal balance have been investigated a great deal, particularly in their relation to the central nervous system and its power of control. It is not yet possible, however, to do more than speculate on the intimate nature of drug action. The important point to emphasise is that the success of homœpathic prescribing is a matter of experience not of theory. However vain the speculations offered may ultimately prove, there will remain the fact (verifiable by any experimenter) which inspired them.

that tissue, use the tincture or low potencies and be prepared to repeat at regular intervals.

Finally, it is essential, if any progress is to be made in this difficult field, that every physician should be open-minded, swift to experiment and patient in recording his results and deducing conclusions, so long as he holds these tentatively and continually tests their validity. Probably there is a use for all potencies, from tincture to the highest ever made, and it is only by observation and experience that any trustworthy conclusions can be reached.

THE CHOICE AND MODE OF ADMINISTRATION OF THE REMEDY

The basis of homœopathy consists of a knowledge of the effects of drugs upon the healthy ; the practical application of its general conception lies in selecting out of all the remedies known, the *simillimum*, the one whose symptom-complex most closely resembles that of the case to be treated. A century and more of practical experience has given some accumulated wisdom by which the beginner (if he will) can profit, but there is no gain in hiding the fact that the discovery of the *simillimum* is seldom easy and may demand both patience and labour.

The remedies of the Pharmacopœia are now counted in hundreds, but records of exhaustive tests are available for little more than a fifth of the number and there are few indeed to whose pathogenesis future investigation may not add something of value. There may be some overlapping in the Materia Medica, certain remedies being so closely alike in their effects that one of them may finally prove unnecessary, though the infinite diversities of patients make us slow to relinquish a drug that *may* prove, if only once in a lifetime, the *simillimum* for a case. But much more significant than possible duplications are the gaps left by the unproved plants and substances, any one of which may prove to be a priceless remedy. For any given case the physician can but seek the *simillimum* from among such drugs as he knows and he has reason to rejoice that he can so often, with care, match his cases really closely with some one or other medicine.

It is not enough, however, to prepare a list of all the case symptoms and see what drug pathogenesis contains most of them. This method is both toilsome and unintelligent. True, if nine out of ten of all symptoms of a case can be matched with those of a remedy, that remedy will usually prove curative, but when (as is all too frequent) there are gaps in the compared lists (symptoms present in the case record but not in the proving), then the problem becomes one of estimation of the relative value of symptoms as guides to prescription. Resemblance, the closest possible, there must be between drug and disease, but often there are several possible claimants to the place of the *simillimum*, and their rival claims must be weighed. When no one is clearly most like, and two or three present each some symptoms of the case, it is not enough to decide on the ground of arithmetical number of resemblances. Symptoms as indications vary in value, and a close resemblance in a few more important ones may outweigh a general resemblance in many of less significance. Some criteria of relative value are therefore essential.

Guidance has been sought in more ways than one, and different physicians incline, some to one method, some to another, a fact which (rightly) indicates that each may prove on occasion trustworthy. In other words, there are cases where different physicians, though stressing different features of a case, would be led to the same remedy, and there are cases where the application of no method gives clear results, because of deficiencies in our provings which leave us in ignorance of so much of drug power : on these occasions, when there must needs be something left to speculation, now one and now another method may prove helpful.

Dr. Hughes taught that the best basis for a good homœopathic prescription was one of similarity of morbid anatomy, an obvious resemblance between tissues affected by drug and disease. Practice based on this rule has proved very successful in acute and subacute diseases : in these it is generally fairly easy to determine the tissue affected, and if the drug chosen can damage the same tissue in large doses (as revealed by proving or poisoning), it should prove a stimulant to the same tissue in a small dose : the diseased and struggling tissue may well be helped by a local stimulus (influencing blood supply and possibly cell reactions), and for the satisfactory result that often follows the physician may claim some credit. Professor Hugo Schulz worked on this principle generally and his results confirm those of many homœopathists.

But the Hughes-Schulz method has its own difficulties which lead to many failures. In the first place neither for drug nor disease is the tissue-relation always incontrovertible. Series of post-mortem examinations reveal many errors in diagnosis and clearly a diagnosis that decides wrongly as to involvement of particular tissues will lead to error in the choice of the remedy if the choice is based on tissue relationship alone : while for many drugs the morbid anatomy of over-dosing is not absolutely certain, so that error is possible on this side also.

But apart from these obvious sources of failure, the whole conception of disease in our day tends to look beyond the gross tissue lesions to a new " humoral " pathology. The pneumo-coccus may be found in a subject either apparently healthy or suffering from some lesion (a naso-pharyngeal catarrh or whatever) that is not acute pneumonia. Yet in certain circumstances the pneumococcus gives rise to acute pneumonia and clearly (granted certain conditions) lung tissue is peculiarly susceptible to its attack. An explanation of these discrepancies is gropingly sought in the mechanism of resistance and anti-bodies and it appears that a defect in this machinery may precede the illness which becomes recognisable when the lung is inflamed. But if this conception be relatively true, the patient may need treatment adapted rather to the defective mechanism of resistance than to lung tissue : yet it would not cease to be possible that once the lung were inflamed a specific local stimulant to its cells might aid them in their struggle to recover. Indeed it is not unlikely that the " specific local stimulus " to the cells of the lung would also be a stimulus to the protective mechanism of the body. If this were so not only would the remedy be doubly justified, but it would show that there is no necessary antagonism between the " tissue lesion " and the " protective mechanism " therapies.

There is yet another emergency conceivable. There may still be a danger of disaster from the breakdown of another organ which, though hardly directly attacked, may nevertheless from previous weakness be unequal to the stress of war. Thus the direct action of the pneumococcus on heart or kidney tissue may be small, but if heart or kidney be in any way defective a case of pneumonia becomes so much the more grave and clearly in such a case heart or kidney needs treating rather than the lung which (*ex hypothesi*) can take care of itself.

It is therefore tolerably clear that to consider *only* the tissue mainly involved in disease may be frequently successful as a guide to the choice of the remedy, but such a one-sided survey will surely be insufficient for many cases. But when any attempt is made to distinguish the varieties of emergency, and find an appropriate remedy for each, what guide can be found but the " totality " of the symptoms, whereof the physical signs that point to tissue involvement are a part, but only a part. If the specific anti-body resistance wants a stimulus, there will be symptoms that will not be found if it is perhaps the hydrogen ion concentration that is at fault, and in both groups of cases there will almost certainly be differences in the symptom-pictures if the cause of the defect lies in an underlying poison, such as syphilis or tubercle, gonorrhœa or alcohol. Again, in the case wherein the actual tissue upon which falls the obvious brunt of the battle is unequal to the strain, the symptom-complex should betray the need of help, or if it is a more distant organ that cannot bear the stress (as in war the civilians might fail while the soldiers retain their value and efficiency), the totality of symptoms should again show changes. If the Hahnemannian rule (that the indicated remedy is the one that most resembles in its symptomatology the given symptom-complex) be a sound one, then it matters nothing that our defective knowledge may be unequal to the precise determination of the nature of the emergency in any one case. If homœopathy be good practice we have to assume (and are justified by results in assuming) that similar symptoms in drug proving and disease, if similar not only in main outline but in colour and shading, are due to similar causes. Therefore, if symptoms due to special reactions of bodily constitution under stress of disease can be matched with similar symptoms produced in the body by drugs, it can be concluded that the drug has the power to influence the constitution in a way similar to that in which disease is influencing it, and therefore in a small dose can stimulate the mechanism which in a large dose it hinders or destroys. The essential point is that the drug should be chosen from all the symptoms and left to do its work upon the needed tissue (which may be often unknown to us), not chosen simply because of its known relation to the tissue whose involvement is most apparent to our present means of diagnosis.

The foregoing paragraphs apply mainly to problems of acute and subacute disêase. But they none the less have a bearing on the treatment of chronic disease.

Chronic disease is chronic mainly because of a failure on the part of the system involved to carry resistance to victory. If the structures involved are not immediately essential to life, or if there is enough remaining relatively normal to " carry on " with, albeit in a somewhat broken-winged way, then the curious economy of our bodies appears to tolerate the presence of disease.

Hahnemann found (as all homœopathists find) that the exacerbations of chronic disease, the periodical " flarings up " of symptoms, were relatively easy to deal with, but that it was a much more difficult matter to prevent their recurrence. He came to explain chronic disease as due fundamentally to the presence of an underlying " miasm " (or more than one), capable of being inherited, and he regarded the symptoms which bring a chronic sufferer to the physician mainly as superficial manifestations of a deep-acting cause. Consequently he sought for (and believed he found) remedies correspondingly " deep " to deal with these conditions. They were (and are) prescribed on a basis of similarity, but the endeavour in selection is to match rather the symptoms that indicate profound constitutional changes than those of the more obvious tissue involvement. These last have their value (often great and decisive value), but rank lower in importance than symptoms that express the mode of life reaction of the whole organism to the external world, and thereby indicate varieties of temperament and constitution such as make up individuality.

Hahnemann's " miasms " were three, but his actual classification is of little importance. He never used what he thought to be the nature of the poison itself as a guide to his remedy, but always the reaction of the patient as manifested in the symptoms. He placed syphilis as one great poison, for instance ; herein he was right in so far as when syphilis is present (however latent), or even when syphilis has been present, the tissue reactions of the patient will be thereby modified, and whatever his immediate complaint, his syphilis must be considered in treating him : indeed his syphilis may be the ultimate cause of many groups of symptoms not in themselves characteristically syphilitic. The same is true of gonorrhœa, of tubercle, probably, of other germ diseases (*e.g.*, pneumococcus and *M. rheumaticus*) ; Hahnemann's " sycosis " corresponds closely to gonorrhœa, and tubercle would fall probably under his heading of " psora," though many non-tuberculous disorders would figure there also, but his nomenclature to-day is of little importance. It is the underlying conception that matters.

To the extent to which we realise to-day the existence of these disease germs capable of prolonged sojourn in the body, giving rise thereby to a variety of lesions and of symptoms, we are conceiving chronic disease much as Hahnemann did when, in the days before bacteriology, he spoke of " miasms." *

But it is more fruitful for practice to think (as he always did) primarily of body reactions and only secondarily of body invaders. Not so much the germ, as the mode and power of resistance to it, matters. These resistances, it is hardly possible to doubt, come in the end back to questions of life-energy as influenced by internal secretions, their due quantities and balance and interaction with mineral salts : it is highly probable that there are infinite varieties of these adjustments, personal to individuals, counting indeed for much of bodily individuality. Some of these will be such as to render individuals immune from this or the other germ, others again will leave the possessors of them specially susceptible. These special conditions (making what the French physicians used to name a diathesis) can conceivably be inherited, and these (with all their dangers) would be the cases of inherited " miasms " of Hahnemann.

---

* Hahnemann made a shrewd guess when he suggested the poison of cholera to be a living parasite infinitesimally small : he would have welcomed bacteriology. " Lesser Writings," Dudgeon's translation, 1851, p. 851.

If, therefore, we regard chronic disease as curable at all by remedies, it will be to substances capable of modifying body reactions that we shall look. It can hardly be doubted that they exist. Outside homœopathic literature, evidence accumulates of the measurable effect on like processes of a number of substances (arsenic, yeast, etc.), and homœopathic observers have their own experimental evidence. Granted that they may exist, the homœopathist affirms that they are best chosen on a ground of resemblance, seeking always first for the closest likeness in what may be called constitutional or (as they are usually named) general symptoms. The majority of local symptoms (and this is true of acute as well as of chronic disease) are the results of tissue changes. A drug that modifies the life reactions of a tissue (as for instance arsenic and sulphur can specifically affect the skin) may be of great value as a cell stimulant, but in the endeavour to find a remedy to help the patient as a piece of life machinery, the local symptoms are less important as guides. If, for instance, some chronic sepsis has resulted in a chronic arthritis, the source of poisoning may be (with good fortune) discovered and removed, but if there were a resistance defect that first allowed the invasion to become permanent, or a metabolic defect that allowed " toxins " to accumulate, permanent recovery would require that these defects be corrected. The symptoms that serve as guides to the remedy will be the general reactions of the individual, not the aches and pains and obvious lesions in the joints, although drugs that affect tissues in and near joints may be helpers of great value. Indeed, if it is possible to correct the fundamental defects by the " similar " remedy, it is often possible to obtain recovery when efforts to discover the true initial focus of poisoning have failed, because the system thus helped can at last deal with the (unknown) invader as it should have been dealt with at first.

It remains to discuss the nature of general and local symptoms. The first in the main are the reactions of the individual to external influences, to heat (of sun or fire), to fresh air, to wind, to rain, to damp, to dryness, to thunder, to close rooms ; next the reactions to exertion and to rest, to sleep and to waking. The likings and dislikings of the patient for particular foods or drinks (fat, meat, milk, oysters, eggs, etc., etc.) may all show variations (unknown as yet but important) of constitution. A general state of hunger or anorexia, of thirst or of thirstlessness, may have value as a symptom. The mental characteristics of the patient from Hahnemann's day have been held to point strongly to the choice of the true remedy. If they are the result of disease they indicate the needed remedy, and if they are well-marked permanent characteristics, they show a certain type of individuality probably specially responsive to certain drugs, the "humours" of Ben Jonson and of so many other writers. Degrees and kinds of anger and spite, of pride and melancholy, of aversion and distrust, all are of importance to the homœopathist. Throughout we follow Hahnemann in attaching special importance to the strange, rare, and peculiar symptoms. These, however apparently fanciful, may be, if genuine, priceless indications. Here let it be premised (and it cannot be too definitely or too often said) that *no* symptom is of value except in so far as it is clear and well marked. If the patient is not sure or does not feel strongly about any of his reactions, then no stress need be laid on his answers. No leading question should ever be put to discover these reactions, but knowledge of them should be derived from observation and from the patient's own statements, supplemented by indirect questions or the evidence of friends. The "strange" symptoms to which the homœopathist will attach importance will often seem slightly ridiculous, but only because we lack the power to interpret them. Causes they must have, though we are as yet ignorant of them, and when they appear in a drug pathogenesis they are no doubt due to disturbances similar to those that give rise to them in disease. Therefore, in seeking for the *simillimum* they have claims to consideration and experience shows that they are of great importance.

Reflection on the foregoing paragraphs will leave the student in a position to appreciate practical advice as to the selection of the remedy. The homœopathist confronted with a case begins necessarily, as all physicians must begin, with the most careful investigation to determine the diagnosis, using naturally every resource to this end that modern science and modern methods have put at his disposal. Examination may reveal an illness depending on some cause for which surgical skill may be imperative, in which case clearly drug therapeutics

must (if only for a time) take a secondary place, and apart
from surgical emergencies diagnosis may reveal the need of
adjuvant measures of massage, electricity, or hydrotherapy.
The homœopathist comes to the consideration of the desirable
remedy *last*, not because of its less importance (on the contrary),
but because he must have, before he can prescribe, a clear
vision of the field of action for drugs, and a knowledge that
there is no mechanical obstacle to the drug power. Let there
be no misconception of this point : homœopathic therapeutics
are an *addition* to the physician's resources and not a substitute
for any measure of proved efficacy. They will take the place
(with rare exceptions) of other drug-giving (not highly valued
even by those who practise it, if their statements are to be
believed), and it is also true that there are cases which non-
homœopathic physicians would turn at once over to the surgeon,
which the resources of homœopathy can often deal with without surgical interference ; but here it is not that the question
of the possible value of surgery is brushed aside, it is duly
faced, and if the point is decided against the surgeon it is so
decided only on definite expectations of greater help elsewhere.

Thus, having cleared the ground and assumed that problems
of diet and nursing and air and exercise are considered and
decided by the homœopathic physician as by his colleagues,
there remains the decision as to the drug to be given.* This
is to be chosen on the grounds of similarity between the
symptom-complex of the disease and the symptom-complex
of the desired remedy. The physical signs which are all-
important in making a diagnosis are of much less value in
choosing the remedy, and the subjective symptoms and
individual reactions to outside influences (heat and cold, wet
and dry, etc.) come into the foreground. The exceptions to
this rule are the straightforward cases of acute disease (*e.g.*,
pneumonia, gastric ulcer, acute rheumatism, etc.) characterised
by few symptoms except the actual physical signs of disease,
and symptoms obviously dependent on the gross physical
changes (dyspnœa in pneumonia, joint pain in acute rheu-

* Homœopathists have always preferred a very simple and largely vegetarian dietary for their patients, and are enemies in general of tea, coffee, and
alcohol in any (even light) excess, as all these substances seem to delay metabolism, and consequently interfere with drug action. Coffee, in particular
seems to be an antidote to many drugs.

matism, vomiting in gastric ulcer). In these cases there is
clearly definite tissue involvement, and a similar tissue prescription may be the best. Even so, there will be room for
some choice. Phosphorus, bryonia, antimony will have tissue
claims in pneumonia, and the choice must be made by the
presence or absence of one or two less obvious symptoms, and
similarly, two or three drugs will compete for choice in gastritis
or rheumatic fever. But when the tissue relationship is the
most obvious ground of prescription, the choice is seldom a
very wide one, and a general similarity often seems sufficient
to ensure help from the remedy. In such cases it is best given
in tincture or low potency and repeated. Tissues appear to
respond best to stimuli thus administered, although here, too,
if the patient can be seen at short intervals (*e.g.*, in hospital),
the golden rule of the homœopathic prescriber, which can
never be too often repeated, holds good and should be followed.
This rule is, *as soon as definite improvement of symptoms sets
in, the administration of the remedy should be stopped, and no
further dose given as long as improvement continues.* When
improvement has followed a remedy and the time appears to
have come for repetition, it is often advisable to go to a higher
potency. Explain it how we may, there is much clinical
evidence to suggest that the action of the higher potencies is
often (though by no means invariably) more profound than
that of the lower.*

There remain two points to be considered in the acuter
cases, wherein the symptoms are relatively few, and chiefly
those arising from the tissue involvement. First, there are
some definite indications (and we may at any time have more
as experiment proceeds) that certain drugs enhance specific
processes of body resistance. Arsenicum appears to be almost
a general stimulant to phagocytosis, veratrum viride raises
the opsonic index to the pneumococcus, phosphorus that to
the tubercle bacillus, hepar sulph. that to *Staphylococcus
aureus*, and baptisia increases the agglutinating power to

---

* It is impossible to exaggerate the importance of the rule to let each dose
" work itself out " before any repetition is attempted. Conceiving each dose
as a stimulus the too rapid succession of stimuli can only lead to exhaustion
and a lessening of response. The rule holds even with the lowest potencies
and it is the users of these who are most in danger of neglecting it. It is very
difficult without direct experience to realise how long a response to a well-
chosen remedy can endure.

B. typhosus. Furthermore, before even vaccine therapy became general, homœopathists had begun to use potencies made from disease products, and the development of vaccination procedures has encouraged the use of potencies of " nosodes," as they are called in homœopathic pharmacy. Potencies (low and high) of tuberculin, influenza and coli germs, of pneumococcus and many others, are frequently used to obtain effects similar to those aimed at by the injection of laboratory vaccines, and there is plenty of evidence that the preparations of the homœopathist can often give good results. When, therefore, a bacteriological diagnosis can be made, should the appropriate nosode be given, or the drug which is known to affect the specific resistance mechanism ? The answer with regard to the nosode is that a dose or two at not too frequent intervals of the corresponding preparation may easily do good and is unlikely to do harm, provided the effect of each dose is watched as carefully as any injection of vaccine. Indeed, the nosodes can be used in acute conditions when most physicians would hesitate to inject the more " massive " dose of the ordinary vaccine and the use of them can be (if desired) combined with the use of a tissue remedy chosen on the grounds previously considered. But as regards the choice of baptisia in enteric or veratrum viride in pneumonia, these drugs have their characteristic symptom-complexes : when the disease presents a parallel to them they should be given at once, but not on pathological grounds alone. Homœopathic experience tends to show that if they are needed for recovery they will be indicated by the symptoms. The only reason why the nosodes are given with less exactitude is that they are relatively unproven. Those (*e.g.*, tuberculin, lueticum) for which long clinical experience has worked out a kind of proving, can be treated even as baptisia and its congeners, and given on symptomatic grounds rather than bacteriological.

The second practical consideration concerns the use of remedies in alternation. The giving of an intercurrent dose of a nosode has already been alluded to, but in general homœopathic practice occasionally two remedies are given in alternation for cases wherein no single remedy seems to cover the symptom-complex satisfactorily. It must at once be admitted that practice of this kind often gives good results, but it is open to grave objections which should make it a practice " more honoured in the breach than in the observance." In the first place, in the event of success it is impossible to allocate the praise to either drug with confidence, or in the event of failure to be sure that it may not have been due to drug antagonism rather than disease stubbornness. Thus, knowledge becomes less definite and the practice of medicine loses.* Secondly, to give two drugs in alternation is generally a confession of the lack of knowledge to determine which is the better indicated, and it should be the aim of the physician to correct this deficiency. Closer examination will generally indicate which remedy has the greater claims. Let it have the first chance to cure. If it fails, re-examine the symptoms and try again. It must often happen that when two drugs are given, cure is really due to one only. To determine this is to make a contribution to clinical experience.

To sum up then : in cases of acute disease, examine the entire symptom-complex, noting especially any strange or peculiar symptoms, any general reactions to outside influences (heat, cold, etc.), any mental and temperamental symptoms, and lastly all the local symptoms, whether obviously dependent on the tissue involvement (e.g., character of pain, cough and fever, etc., in pneumonia) or accompanying it (e.g., skin eruptions, etc.). If the totality indicates any drug clearly, give it preferably first in a medium potency (12–30), and as far as possible watch the effect of each dose, repeating at first perhaps every two or three hours.† If improvement sets in, well and good, stop the remedy, or at least lengthen the interval between doses while improvement lasts. If improvement ceases, reconsider the case, to determine if perhaps the indications now point to a change of remedy. If they do not, repeat the first

* The objection of the homœopathist to mixtures of drugs is an objection to the combination as *unproved* and therefore incapable of exact choice. Doubtless satisfactory mixtures could be made, but before they can be used with exactitude they must be proved. Drug alternation is not drug mixture, but it is not far removed from it, and there is little knowledge as to the possible interactions of remedies which have exact enough indications when given singly.
† Unless the physician has deeply studied in the Materia Medica, a dictionary of symptoms, a so-called Repertory will be necessary to determine the *simillimum ;* nothing but prolonged experience will enable the physician to dispense with this, and there should be no hesitation in using it.

chosen drug and preferably in a higher potency. If, however, a drug, apparently well indicated, fails to relieve in the first selected medium potency, and also on a higher one, give it a trial in a much lower potency before deciding that it has been wrongly chosen. As the case proceeds, however satisfactorily, fresh indications must be constantly sought, especially any that may point to some fundamental condition of constitution in need of correction. When a remedy of relatively swift and temporary action (*e.g.*, aconite, belladonna, gelsemium) has brought the immediate condition well towards recovery, a corresponding remedy of more profound action will nearly always be of benefit, but there should never be any haste to give any drug so long as progress is steady.

In chronic disease the search for the best remedy is more difficult. It is of the utmost importance to take enough time in considering the choice. To put a chronic disease (not showing any symptoms of pain or discomfort that call for speedy relief) on a placebo for a while is often very desirable. It gives time for suitable study of the case, and it also gives opportunity for the effects of suggestion and so-called mental influence to become apparent. Every physician knows that wonderful results are thus obtained now and then, and it is as well, scientifically, to give such influences fair play, uncomplicated by drug therapeutics. If, however, the *simillimum* is apparent readily, it should never be withheld, for although the attempt to explain all therapeutic successes in terms of " suggestion " has often been made, the explanation has never been conclusively established.

In choosing the remedy for a case of chronic disease, the essential is a complete symptomatology. The question of diagnosis and adjuvant treatment is, of course, to be considered with the same thoroughness as for acute disease, but for the selection of the remedy let it be said once more, subjective symptoms, and especially any reactions to external influences (heat, cold, damp, thunder, etc.), are of great importance. Here a necessary proviso must be made, necessary for that matter in all attempts to choose a remedy for any case of disease. A symptom is of value precisely in proportion to its " weight," to the degree in which it is marked, and in selecting the remedy, if a symptom is prominent in the case, it should be equally prominent in the drug pathogenesis. Remembering this, then, every " curious," unusual symptom becomes of great importance as a guide to the remedy. A symptom that is ordinary in one kind of disease may be unusual in another : thus, it is not at all wonderful that a febrile case should be thirsty (though even so the character of the thirst may have a distinctive value), but for a febrile case to be without a thirst *is* unusual and such a symptom should have prominence. It is common enough for sensations to be described as " burning," but when burning seems to accompany every kind of sensation in a case, then the symptom gains in importance. Symptoms are often conveniently classed as general and local, but the distinction need not be forcibly maintained ; it is generally easier to realise which symptoms are consequences of gross physical tissue changes (these are of *relatively* less importance) and those which have a functional basis. These in many cases indicate quality of life resistance and adaptability and, representing thus the resources of the patient, are better taken as guides to his remedy.

Cases fall into two great classes :

(A) Those with many symptoms both objective and subjective, both general and local.

(B) Those with objective symptoms of tissue change and others clearly dependent on the changes, but with few subjective symptoms.

In choosing a remedy for a case in class A the course is now tolerably clear. If the patient presents very well-marked reactions of a general kind, say an intense aggravation of suffering from heat or cold, or a marked aggravation at a definite time of day, these symptoms can confidently be used to narrow the field of selection, eliminating drugs which do not present them. Then choose another group of well-marked symptoms (general ones if possible) to narrow the choice further. Presently (the aid of the repertory—symptom index— being all but essential, as a rule) the *simillimum* will be found to lie between some three or four drugs, even if one does not at once stand out above all the rest. To make the final selection it may be necessary to compare in detail the pathogenesis of the drugs with the case symptomatology, but often this labour can be spared by the use of the minor local symptoms, which may at once give the clue required. Having finally decided, give a single dose (or two at a short interval of hours) and give it a reasonable time to produce an effect.* The results may be entirely negative, or positive in a variety of ways to be presently discussed. If no result *at all* follows after ten or fourteen days, the drug is probably wrongly selected † ; there is nothing for it but to restudy the case. In so repeating the investigation, even more attention than at first should be given to possible inherited tendencies, to possible latent disease, such as syphilis, gonorrhœa and tubercle, to possible drug or diet habits, which may be antidoting the remedy. If considerations of these kinds bear any fruits, treatment by a nosode (virtually a potentised vaccine) may be necessary, or previous drugging may need to be combated. Especially may this be necessary when purgatives and analgesics have been much taken, and remedies like sulphur, nux vomica, or pulsatilla are often of great value for this purpose, even in the absence of any very close indications for them. However, often the physician fails to produce an effect, yet if the case has a well-marked symptomatology and the tissue change has not progressed far in the direction of destruction (*e.g.*, sclerosis), it is salutary for him rather to conclude that the fault lies *in his inadequate application of the homœopathic principle*, and to devote yet more study and patience to his task.

So much for a negative result to the first prescription. A positive result may be perhaps (a thrice fortunate one but often obtained by the good prescriber) an immediate improvement. In this case the choice of the drug is justified and all that remains now is not to spoil the case by injudicious handling. A chronic case that is of months' or years' duration must be allowed time to recover. Never repeat the remedy as long as

---

* Even in very chronic diseases potencies below 30c. can be very effective and produce permanent results. Unit doses of tinctures have at times scored heavily. Even in such desperate cases as those of malignant disease potencies like 3c., 6c. or 12c. have also a claim. But the essential point in practice is that whatever potency is chosen should be given at intervals as long as possible. Dilution, as it were, in time is even more important than dilution in space.

† The chance that the case is incurable, having no power to react, has to be considered, but such cases, as will be seen later, are very seldom those now being considered, which present a good variety of symptoms.

improvement continues ; when improvement ceases give the remedy in the potency first chosen ;· but if improvement does not follow this time give a higher potency and so proceed, remembering that practice suggests (inexplicable as the results are at present) that as a rule the higher potencies maintain their effects for a longer time.* If the general course of a case is towards recovery, the minor incidental aches and pains should not be separately prescribed for ; it is a great mistake to multiply remedies. At the same time, there is evidence that if an intercurrent symptom (e.g., sleeplessness or neuralgia) is very troublesome, and apparently unaffected by the main remedy which is improving the general condition, then there is no harm, but only good, in the use of an intercurrent remedy to relieve it. This should be chosen from similarity to the particular symptoms in question, and will often be found to be related to the main remedy (as aconite is to sulphur) in curative power. It should be given, however, in a *low* potency, and never *lightly* given at all. From time to time the symptom-complex should be reviewed as a whole, for changes may occur in it which will call for a new remedy. It is a curious but frequent experience that in the course of a recovery there may be a return of symptoms of old, and often forgotten, previous troubles. These are not to be regarded as indications for a new remedy if they can be so identified. It is a general rule that symptoms disappear curatively in the reverse order to their appearance, the last observed being the first to go.

Instead of immediate improvement there is sometimes seen a marked aggravation of symptoms. If the aggravation is mainly of local symptoms (e.g., pain, or intensification of a skin affection or joint swelling), and if simultaneously the patient has (as often he does have) a sense of improvement, then the aggravation is to be regarded as favourable rather than the reverse. A parallel phenomenon is the negative phase of Sir Almroth Wright, after a vaccine injection, and though it calls for caution, it is not, unless very severe, an untoward incident. It will almost certainly pass over into an improvement (positive phase), which improvement is then to be treated exactly as described in the foregoing paragraph for an initial favourable response. Only, since the patient has shown a tendency to

* Occasionally a lower potency works better than a higher one.

become temporarily worsened, even more care is needed in repeating drugs and in using higher potencies.

If, however, the aggravation does not pass over into ameli- oration, and particularly if the symptoms that become worse are the more deep-seated ones, the outlook is more grave. There are undoubtedly certain cases (e.g., advanced phthisis) wherein there is not vital energy enough left to eradicate the disease, but where a careful husbanding of the strength will carry the patient along, albeit in a somewhat inefficient way. To give a deep-acting remedy, like silica or sulphur, to such cases, is occasionally to induce a violent reaction, which uses up a great deal of the patient's strength, yet, not being enough to produce cessation of the disease, leaves him ultimately worse than before he was thus treated. Tuberculin treatment in other hands than those of homœopathists has led to similar failures. The true wisdom lies in exercising great caution at first in testing the ability to recover of any patient concerning whose powers of reaction there is any doubt. If a deep-acting remedy is indicated, do not use it at first in potency higher than the 12th, and only proceed higher with much care. If there is reason to believe that recovery is impossible, there is still much to be done by attacking the problem from the tissue side (the local symptoms). Many a chronic tuberculosis of the lungs, incapable of true arrest, can be carried along in comfort with remedies like arsenic and stannum, iodine and sanguinaria in low potencies and repeated doses. Symptom similarity remains the guide to the choice of the remedy.

If the danger has been incurred and the aggravation persists, it is sometimes possible to antidote the effects of the remedy with another drug. Occasionally even when the aggravation is not regarded as dangerous, it involves so much suffering that it has to be combated temporarily. Many drugs have more or less specific antidotes in homœopathic therapeutics, and nux vomica, pulsatilla, coffea, camphor, etc., are general drug antidotes.

Finally, there are cases (e.g., advanced cancer) wherein sub- jective symptoms are few and unimportant, and local symptoms and gross physical signs hold the field. In these the disease has reached what is often called the " ultimate " stage. 'Broadly speaking, a symptom-complex that has many subjective symptoms in it may be regarded as evidence of the body reaction to disease ; when this reaction is poor or absent, the chances of successful cure are not good and palliation may be the only resource. In any case, the attention will now be directed rather to low potencies and tissue remedies and frequent repetitions. Dr. Cooper, indeed, records some very striking cancer cases recovering under rare doses of strong tinctures of certain drugs, and though the grounds of choice appear to some extent empirical, the aim is to employ similarity as the clue to them (notably the use of ruta for rectal carcinoma). If all else fails, and pain has to be relieved, the employment of morphia is naturally a resource, but homœopathists find that by studying the character of the pain they can often find a similar remedy more effective than morphia with none of its attendant evils. It is fair to say that, so long as any symptom similarity whatever can be found between the disease and any drug pathogenesis, that similarity affords the best guide to the most suitable remedy.

In all arts old men speak of laws, using the laws of harmony to browbeat the young composer, the laws of prosody to check the budding poet. In these concerns (and also in others) the word law is a dangerous one. Even in science it can mostly stand for little more than a brief way of recording general experience, not hitherto subject to exceptions that cannot be accounted for. *Thus we should do better to call the law of similars a generalisation from experience, valid within the bounds of our knowledge*, and, in regard to the practical application of it, even more caution is required in laying down instructions and rules. The " laws " of the arts are actually the accepted practices of the masters. Each new genius has a way of breaking the laws of his predecessors, or ar least widening their bounds, till his rebellion succeeds and his practice, which at first roused intense opposition from the pedants, becomes a new weapon for the armoury of the pedant's never-failing progeny. Thus Mozart and Beethoven are denounced as blasphemous innovators until presently their practice is used to confute Wagner. History, therefore, gives little encouragement to those who wish to stereotype the practice of an art, even the art of therapeutics, and it would be an ill service to the student to leave this chapter of practical instruction without a reminder that it represents the results of experience, but no more. The rules indicated above are those that the most careful and practised prescribers have found most generally valid. But greater knowledge and wider experience may lead to more effective practical rules, and it is for the physician not to fall back supinely upon the judgments of others, but to make his own rules, and, if he may, add a stone or two to the temple of therapeutics. Hasty dogmatising has long been the curse of medicine. Our ignorance is still vast, and we still grope in a darkness that is not made more penetrable by hailing every will-o'-the-wisp as the dawn of day. Humility, patience, and freedom from prejudice, which will lead to endless experiment and courageous record of experience, can alone be counted on to forward the time when the medical profession shall live in the full sunlight of assured knowledge.

MATERIA MEDICA

ACONITE

Aconitum Napellus—Monkshood : Tincture of whole plant (including root), when beginning to flower.

ACONITE has an old-time reputation for causing sweating and relieving certain cases of rheumatism and sciatica, but precision in its use is due to the provings of it on the healthy which were made by Hahnemann. It is most closely associated with the early progress of homœopathy (and early antagonisms thereto), because largely by its use Hahnemann and his followers were able to dispense with the blood-letting fashionable till after the middle of last century for almost every disorder. Modern research has isolated an alkaloid, aconitine napellus, and allied species yield similar substances. Delphinine, the alkaloid of staphisagria, is similar in effect to aconitine but less poisonous. Aconitine is a very deadly poison : many of the symptoms of the aconite pathogenesis are due to this alkaloid ; but there is little doubt that other constituents of tincture of aconite count for a good deal. Specially to be noted is the presence of phosphate of iron (ferrum phosphoricum) ; the provings are of the tincture, and when they are suitably matched with cases, it is the tincture or a potency of it that should be preferred as the remedy.

Aconite first stimulates and later depresses sensory nerve endings, more especially those of common sensation. As a result, reflex sneezing, coughing, salivary secretion and vomiting occur ; but some stimulation of medullary centres also is not unlikely.

It seems to act upon the circulation by first (in relatively small doses) stimulating the medullary inhibitory heart centre and so producing a slow pulse ; possibly also it acts on the vaso-constrictor centre ; at any rate, as will be seen, the provings bring out a marked condition of relatively high tension. Aconitine experiments have been mostly made on animals and with increasing doses, so that the finer effects of the more gradual provings cannot be expected. Large doses of aconitine appear to act directly on the heart, producing a quick, irregular pulse, with lessened conduction of impulses and finally fibrillation and death. In these circumstances the blood pressure tends to fall, with occasional temporary rises to a fair though not great height. The respiratory centre is affected early and directly and its depression causes dyspnœa and sometimes death before the heart fails.

Since the publication of Dr. Ringer's " Handbook of Therapeutics " (a volume of perennial interest to the homœopathist as a " conveyor " of certain instances of homœopathic practice), aconite has been praised by orthodox physicians for febrile conditions, but its use seems if anything to be less frequent among them to-day. The explanation of its disuse has a certain significance. From Hahnemann onwards, the homœopathist has known that aconite is of great value in febrile disorders whenever the rise in temperature is associated with definite symptoms, whenever, in fact, the case as a whole is " similar " to the aconite provings. Its value is as great to-day as ever ; but if other aconite symptoms are not present, the mere presence of fever is not sufficient indication for the remedy and its use will be followed by disappointment. It cannot be too often reiterated that homœopathy seeks remedies for individuals, not for the names of diseases, and to use aconite as a " febrifuge " irrespective of any other symptoms is neither homœopathy nor good practice. Dr. Ringer gave quite precise indications for its employment, but the haphazard routine use of the drug has led to its being discredited by many, and high authorities to-day have no recommendation for it ; yet for the homœopathist it reigns as supreme as ever, an invaluable remedy for suitable cases of disease. Its true spheres of action must now be made clear. Aconite is a remedy of powerful but short-lived action and correspondingly is most suitable to diseases that set in suddenly and violently, but run a brief course. The violent storm which quickly passes is the type of disease to which it corresponds most closely. It will be found of value in a few more chronic cases (neuralgia, etc.), when detailed symptoms of drug and disorder can be matched, but most often it is called for in acute and sub-acute diseases and among them those of sudden onset and immediate violence.

An acute disease is one wherein the body resistance is swiftly mobilised, wherein the tissue is not long in doubt and victory for one side or the other a matter of days. Such a disorder is, as we say, a self-limited disease and the possibilities of natural recovery considerable. Nothing is more difficult in therapeutics than to estimate the real effect of drugs in such a case, but the very power of resistance that causes the difficulty of judgment is an enormous enhancement of the physician's ability to help. Since recovery in any case can only take place through a prearranged bodily machinery, and since the effect of any remedy can only be exerted along this pre-existing channel, it is clear that the more powerful the machinery the better it may be influenced by a drug stimulus. The body generally possesses reserves of resistance to disease, and, broadly speaking, the drug therapeutics are attempts to use these reserves ; in acute diseases they are usually being mobilised fairly effectively without the help of remedies, but clearly there is room for efficient action if it is rightly directed. In some cases it is conceivable that the extra stimulus of a well-chosen remedy may make the difference between victory and defeat ; in many more cases it affects the speed and ease of recovery than on the bare result of life or death. If there is no adequate machinery of resistance to respond, no drug will avail, since no drug brings in any new force, but only influences pre-existing forces. Yet a drug stimulus may bring the forces to bear more swiftly and may even sometimes bring into action reserves, which without its aid would be unused or used too late. For with such knowledge as we possess of bacterial diseases it is readily conceivable that if the (necessarily limited) power of resistance could be used at once in great volume, it might overwhelm the enemy, but used in driblets against an increasing foe may prove ineffective. Yet the total power used might well be less in the first instance than in the last. Vaccine therapy works with some such conceptions behind it and drug therapy (at least in homœopathic hands) is influenced by similar considerations.

Aconite, then, is pre-eminently a remedy for acute conditions. Fever will nearly always be present, of a kind to be presently described. Now modern research has brought us to consider fever largely as a reaction to disease by no means always (or even usually) unfavourable. The practice (still too common) of attempting to reduce fever without regard to any other symptoms is seen to be faulty when it is known that anti-body production is frequently more effective with a raised temperature. Fever is of many types and wisdom seeks to adjust the appropriate remedy to each type.

The mechanism that regulates body temperature is complicated and a high thermometric reading may be due (no doubt is due) now to one cause, now to another. But when it is a response to a call for increased anti-body production it is likely that the result is obtained through the action of the cerebral heat-regulation centres and there are grounds for thinking that aconite influences these centres. Homœopathic experience finds the drug to correspond to acute affections in apparently strong, healthy, often full-blooded subjects, where the attack of disease meets with a violent response. The young need it more often than the old and respond to it swiftly. After its successful administration the temperature often falls at once and the storm subsides. Two explanations are possible : if the rise of temperature was to enhance anti-body production, its rapid fall after aconite (with return of the patient to health) might mean that the aconite had so encouraged this process that the raised temperature was no longer needed. But since the drug appears to act mainly on the cerebral centres this is unlikely : it is more probable that the initial rise was, strictly speaking, unnecessary, that the body was equal to the emergency without it and that the disturbance was of the nature of a false alarm. The effect of aconite may then be to quiet this needless disturbance thereby leaving the field clear to the forces of recovery. The nearest analogy would be that of a beleaguered city with a frightened civil population whose disturbance hampers the garrison. Aconite would correspond to the forces of persuasion and confidence that should quiet the civilian anxieties and leave the soldiers to do their own work more effectively.

Whatever the final explanation, the homœopathist is seldom in doubt as to the true indications for aconite. There are few drugs so related to a definite causation as is aconite. Acute intense conditions brought on by chill, especially the chill of cold, dry, bitter winds or in hot, dry weather and especially the heat of the sun, shock, fright or surgical operations are exciting conditions producing the aconite symptomology.

The essential nature of aconite was accurately summed up
by the late Dr. Hughes in the one word " tension." There is
emotional and mental tension shown in great anxiety, restlessness and fear. The fear is usually unreasoning and intangible,
though the fear of death is characteristic ; tension in the
arteries with the pulse full, strong and rapid, sometimes finding
relief in hæmoptysis or arterial hæmorrhage from the nose ;
tension in the muscles ; in the involuntary muscles as is seen in
the violent action of the heart ; in the special sense where
sensation is heightened. It is often the first remedy in acute
inflammatory conditions, but the invasion is sudden and violent
and accompanied by anxiety, restlessness and fear. Such a
state is especially seen in the acute condition in strong robust
individuals, frequently full-blooded, even plethoric.

The symptoms indicating aconite are apt to present themselves in patients of a quick, lively, sanguine temperament,
who enjoy as a rule good health. The vigorous individual
succumbs rapidly to a violent invasion, when the characteristic
mentality appears. Every ailment, however trivial, is
accompanied by forebodings, anxiety, restlessness and fear.
The face assumes an anxious expression, the mental tension of
the sufferer is expressed by fear, often indefinite, and, being overwhelmed by the violence of his condition, his forebodings take
definite shape, as fear of death, and he may predict the hour of
death. There is often a quite unwarranted fear out of all
proportion to the gravity of the case. The anxiety causes much
tossing about and restlessness, with considerable mental
exaltation or even violent delirium. There is heightened
sensibility ; the pains are severe, sometimes intolerable (numbness and tingling may replace pain) and the special senses
respond to stimuli more violently than is normal. These cardinal symptoms therefore, restlessness, anxiety, fear and
exalted sensitiveness, with rigor and a sharp rise of temperature
and a full hard pulse, are the main features of the aconite case,
and these features are impressed on the character of the
symptoms whatever part of the body is affected. The head is
heavy, hot and burning, the pain is violent and intense and
accompanied by fear. Such headaches occur in plethoric
individuals from exposure to cold, dry winds. On rising from
the recumbent position, the red face may become deathly pale,

or the patient becomes giddy. The vertigo met by aconite is always aggravated by rising from the recumbent position.

The first stage of catarrhal inflammation of the eyes prior to exudation, with aversion from light and the lids swollen and red following exposure to dry, cold winds, reflection from snow or after extraction of foreign bodies are promptly relieved by this drug. With similar causes, a sudden inflammation in the ear is produced accompanied by cutting pain. Together with this earache, the external ear is red, hot, painful and swollen.

The heightened sensibility of the special sense is shown in this organ by the sensitivity to noise; music is unbearable. Aggravation of symptoms from music is a not uncommon recorded symptom and appears under the heading of several drugs. To one who is sensitive to music the statement may require qualification; for any discriminating lover of the art could at any time be disturbed, even annoyed, by some kinds of music. When the symptom is recorded it is to be read as a heightening of the musical sense so that the music which is never liked becomes intolerable and even that which is generally appreciated is avoided, either because the auditory apparatus is at fault and the sounds come to the hearer jangled (this is the rarer condition, and there will be other auditory symptoms) or because the physical response is so overwhelming as to be undesirable. Coryza, with much sneezing, comes on suddenly, possibly accompanied by nose-bleed, headache, fever, thirst, anxiety and fear. The sense of smell is often acutely sensitive. The aconite face has an anxious frightened expression. Severe neuralgia, especially of the left side of the face, accompanied with restlessness, tingling and numbness may be present. The mouth is dry, hot and tingling, the tongue swollen and coated white with tingling at the tip. It is a great reliever of tooth-ache which may occur even in sound teeth following exposure to cold, dry winds. The teeth are sensitive to cold. The throat is red, dry and constricted, accompanied with the typical aconite symptoms. Gastric catarrh, especially from drinking iced water, will often require it. There is bilious vomiting with profuse sweats, some hæmatemesis, increased urination, with anxiety, restlessness and fever. The thirst is intense for cold water. The patient craves pungent things, brandy or beer or bitter things ; everything tastes bitter except water.

The abdomen is tense, tympanitic and sensitive to touch, and is accompanied by fear and anguish. The colic of aconite _nay be so severe as to cause the sufferer to double up, but actually no position relieves the pain. Acute hepatitis and jaundice with violent fever and anxiety resulting from exposure to cold may occur. There is an urgency to stool with tenesmus ; the stool may be of a choleraic nature while the patient is collapsed, restless and anxious. Affections of the urinary system show the usual aconite violence and intensity. Inflammation of the bladder is acute with constant urging to urinate, though the urine is scanty and may be admixed with blood. Retention of urine, especially in children, resulting from exposure or shock is accompanied by restlessness and crying (cf. Rhus Tox.).

Acute conditions in plethoric, vigorous, excitable women call for aconite, especially such as are brought on by emotional excitement, fear or exposure to cold. So, the menses may be suppressed ; during pregnancy, abortion may be threatened ; after delivery the milk fever is accompanied by delirium ; the breasts are hot and hard and tense with scanty milk.

Many acute conditions of the respiratory tract require aconite in the early stages. Laryngitis is spasmodic, the cough is hoarse and dry, breathing is oppressed and laboured. This condition is found in children after exposure to cold. The child wakes from his first sleep or after midnight with fever and intense excitement, dyspnœa, laboured breathing and feeling of suffocation ; the cough is dry, short and hacking and aggravated by drinking and lying down. The child must sit up.

Acute pneumonia or pleuritis may set in with general symptoms that indicate aconite. It is rare for aconite to suffice for the whole course of such an illness, though occasionally a lobar pneumonia will seem to respond marvellously. The early stage of a pneumonia suggesting aconite presents the suddenness of onset and intensity always associated with the drug. The patient is one who apparently in robust health previously, succumbs to a sudden high fever accompanied by rigor. He feels intensely ill. The face is hot, dry and flushed ;

the conjunctivæ injected. Generally, the patient is very distressed, anxious, restless and in a state of fear. The cough is short and continuous, the sputum scanty and, within a short time, may be streaked with bright red blood (not rusty coloured as in bryonia). There are violent pains in the chest ; the tongue is dry and there is intense thirst for cold water or something bitter. The fever is high and the pulse full and bounding. The patient has difficulty in lying and finds the greatest ease in being propped up. The course of a pneumonia with this violent onset may be aborted by the administration of aconite. Though such may be the case, it is usually advantageous to follow up such treatment by giving a few doses of SULPHUR. The latter drug is a deep-acting remedy which has the closest relation to aconite, and whenever a case has indicated aconite and done well on it up to a point, sulphur will generally complete the cure. Similarly, rheumatic fever with sudden onset as resulting from exposure to cold, dry winds may be aborted by aconite. The attack usually begins at night with high fever accompanied by restlessness and anxiety. The joints are red and swollen, sensitive to touch, aggravated by heat, motion and shift from one joint to another.

In all such acute conditions, the sleep is apt to be disturbed. There is sleeplessness with restlessness ; there may be anxious dreams or nightmares. The restless insomnia of the aged, even without pain, is often much helped by aconite.

Good subjects for aconite are frequently full-blooded, even plethoric, and in later life when arterial tension arises and apoplexy becomes a possibility, the drug is often called for to meet emergencies. Its effect is too transient to deal with actual arterial changes for which remedies like BARIUM are better adapted, but it is invaluable for times of special stress. After cerebral hæmorrhage, if tension remains high, it will deal with it at least as well as blood-letting.

There is some evidence that after prolonged and gradual poisoning, aconite affects finally the spinal motor centres and it has been, therefore, recommended for acute anterior poliomyelitis. Broadly speaking, homœopathic experience does not find it very frequently indicated in this disease, but if the general symptoms called for it, its possible pathological tissue-relation would add weight to the decision. Failing the general symptoms, it is doubtful if the pathology alone should be allowed to determine the choice of it.

Dr. Hughes valued aconite for acute (ulcerative) endocarditis on the ground of its (undoubted) direct action on the heart. But here again most homœopathic observers agree that it is seldom symptomatically indicated and its use is disappointing. Such endocarditis is a bacterial disease and the main hope lies in combating the cause through the body resistance mechanism. There is no evidence that aconite affects these ; any effect it could have would be as a possible direct stimulant to the heart, that is to say, palliative, not curative.

Sudden disturbances of special senses (especially that of vision), dependent probably on vascular temporary defects (high tension), can be swiftly relieved by aconite and sudden inflammation of the eye structures after exposure to strong light or other stress will be benefited.

It is a great reliever of pain, rivalling CHAMOMILLA and COFFEA, especially when recent, aggravated by exposure or emotion and accompanied by the characteristic restless tension. The pains that call for it are very severe : tearing, cutting, accompanied often by numbness or tingling. They may follow the course of nerves, or centre round joints.

Generally speaking, the patient who needs aconite does not feel chilly or desire heat. He is worse in a warm room. Fresh air relieves and with fever the warmth of the bed is intolerable, the bed clothes will be thrown off. He feels better when uncovered. Rest frequently ameliorates the symptoms, but during the night in bed, the pain becomes unbearable. Unquenchable thirst is a prominent symptom : everything but water tastes bitter. Conditions requiring aconite are brought on by exposure to cold, dry winds, cold bathing, overheating or exposure to the heat of the sun. Emotional disturbances such as fear, fright or shock are important causative circumstances. The aggravation of complaints is intensified at midnight.

Aconite being a remedy of swift action and limited range requires as a rule somewhat frequent repetition.

ANACARDIUM ORIENTALE

Marking nut.   Preparation :   layer of nut between shell and kernel triturated.

The cashew nut is anacardium occidentale, growing in the West Indies, and anacardium orientale is the marking nut and grows in the East Indies.   The latter is the more fully proved, but such symptoms as are known of the former resemble closely those of anacardium orientale, so that it is possible that they may be regarded as virtually interchangeable although naturally the one would be preferred whose symptoms were known.   The cashew nut skin symptoms are very prominent in poisoning cases.   Those of anacardium orientale are similar in character but perhaps less severe.   If, therefore, in a case that suggested anacardium the skin was very notably affected, it might be preferable to use the occidentale.   But the point probably need not be stressed.

Gross Effects on the Body

Anacardium is virtually unused in therapeutics except by homœopathists.   Cushney speaks of the anacardium occidentale as containing Cardol which is a powerful skin vesicant applied locally.   Lewin records œdema, erysipelas and persistent eczema following the external use of it, and violent colic as a symptom when it is taken internally.   The provings, as will presently be seen, develop many skin symptoms.   Clarke speaks of erysipelas and œdema under anacardium occidentale as Lewin does, but records them as the result of cashew nut poisoning in a way that seems to imply that the conditions followed the taking the drug internally.   Certainly similar, though less severe, skin symptoms have followed the use of anacardium orientale so that Clarke's statements are probably well founded, though he may have recorded together symptoms that ensued from both external and internal use.   It is a constant homœopathic experience that a drug (e.g. rhus) that produces violent effects through contact, displays its power over the skin also after internal use.   The irritant remains an irritant after absorption into the blood stream sufficiently to affect the cells of the skin after repeated (even small) doses.   In susceptible persons (and a good prover is necessarily one susceptible to the drug proved) minimal quantities may elicit symptoms. The conclusion is that skin symtoms that follow external applications may be indications for the internal use of the drug and if internal administration confirms them at all, then the physician can speak more positively.* The tincture of anacardium is made from the layer that encloses the kernel below the outer shell. The similar layer in the occidentale nut is black and semi-fluid. It is the part used in pharmacy., Botanically, anacardium is related to the rhus species, and its action on the skin resembles that of this group. It can antidote the effects of rhus poisoning as far as these concern the epidermis. Further resemblances are in the general characteristics of chilliness, sensitiveness to draughts, relief from warmth.

Comparison with Rhus Tox

There appears a marked aggravation of pain on the first movement of the affected part which is like that of rhus. But whereas in the latter case continued movement progressively relieves and rest aggravates pain, with anacardium rest often relieves and the increase of pain on first movement is not eased by continuation of it. Nor does anacardium show the affinity of rhus for joints, fasciæ and fibrous tissues generally, nor are the abdominal symptoms of the two drugs comparable. The cases that do well on this remedy sometimes show an intermittence in their symptoms. There is no definite periodicity, but after a few days of suffering there will be freedom from it for a space independently of treatment.

Mental and Emotional Symptoms

The great interest and importance of the remedy lie in the mental sphere. It is one of the most noteworthy instances of drug effects on consciousness. It appears as though symbols emanating from the unconscious continue to reach the conscious mind until a sense of dual personality is established, a

* It is, of course, possible that skin symptoms following external use may be caused in some instances more mechanically than chemically. Thus *Dolichos Pruriens* causes intense irritation from the microscopic hairs on the plant and it is not clear that the symptom is an indication for the drug to be given internally. On the other hand, provers of it showed general increased sensitivity (and other symptoms). Internally therefore in potency it might lessen hypersensitiveness and so relieve skin symptoms. The help there would be indirect.

feeling as of two wills, usually contending. Sometimes the
division goes farther and there are delusions that mind and
body are separate, or that the other will is that of an evil spirit
tempting him.   He may feel as though he were living in a
dream, often hears voices, usually ones that he knows, but of
persons dead or distant.   Irritability is usual and there is a
marked tendency to swear or blaspheme, going beyond even
the modern freedom of speech and, of course, more noticeable if
the patient is normally not addicted to bad language. This is
due to the removal of an inhibition and accentuates sometimes
the sense of duality, the patient feeling as though he were
urged or compelled thus to express himself.   Further evidence
that it is not just an explosion of bad temper and annoyance is
found in the fact that although the patient blusters and asserts
himself, actually his courage is not great.   He is readily cowed.
The oaths are of the nature of a camouflage for a deep sense of
inferiority.   Indeed, anacardium in potency is used to restore
courage which is failing in anticipation of some ordeal. The
power of anacardium in this respect has earned it a reputation
as a remedy where there is fear of an ordeal like an examination,
particularly viva voce.   Memory in anacardium subjects is
poor, and this adds to the fear of failure very naturally and
increases dread of the examination. Many a student has found
anacardium a present help in such time of trouble and it will be
effective even if few other symptoms of any kind are present.
In potency it reverses its poisoning effect, shutting off disturbing thoughts, concentrating power in the present.   Sense
illusions are not uncommon, blunting of the special senses, of
hearing, or of smell, more often than of vision.

Commentary on the Influence of Homœopathic Remedies on Psychopathic Symptoms

This curious mental state has parallels in the symptomatology of other drugs, but it may be suitable here to discuss
the general question of the relation of drugs to consciousness,
apart from the gross power of some of them to abolish it temporarily. It is on the emotional side particularly that there is
likely to be scepticism, e.g. as to the claims of homœopathy
that fear, jealously, suspicion, hatred and desire to harm and
such emotions are both characteristic of certain remedies and

can be modified by the use of them. The pioneer work of Freud, Jung, Adler and their followers has undoubtedly increased and clarified our (still scanty) knowledge of the modes and mechanisms of our minds. It is accepted that consciousness is a very complex thing, but probably the idea that a material agent like a drug can modify conditions attributable to complexes, vary the interplay between consciousness and the unconscious and assist in an harmonious balance between the two, might be one unacceptable to the psychoanalyst. It is, however, common knowledge that drugs can produce marked mental phenomena, hallucinations, maniacal disturbances and moral perversions. Furthermore, post-encephalitic conditions are only too often accompanied by deplorable changes in character. Therefore there is a starting point at least for the homœopathist, and, as always, he turns to clinical experiment. No one who will patiently test the matter can doubt that the rightly chosen *simillimum* is as potent in the mental sphere as the physical, and further, Hahnemann's claim that mental symptoms are of all guides to true similarity the most certain is a well-founded one. But it is none the less strange for the beginner to think that a particular fear or dream in a patient may be a good guide to a remedy. The final test is, of course, experiment. Experiment can be trusted to confirm the claims, but some discussion of the difficulties may make the road of experiment easier to take. Psychoanalysis finds the explanation of phobias in the repression of certain (often infantile) experiences. Such past experiences may enter consciousness again in a distorted form and express themselves characteristically in daily life by fears of a definite kind. If this be so, how can a drug have a general association with any one of them ? Dreams, again, may sometimes be veiled expressions of experiences whose memories are troublesome. Where does a drug come in here ? The first comment to make is that it is obvious that certain drugs can diminish power of inhibition. More or less lack of usual control is frequently recorded in drug pathogenesis and the disturbing mental effects (*e.g.*) of hyoscyamus are familiar enough, and every " dope " taken tends to loosen moral control, whether be taken morphine, heroin, hashish or cocaine. But besides the power to lower the standard in inhibition, different drugs have varying actions on the body generally ; cannabis or hyoscyamus, for instance, stimulate the sexual organs and centres. It is, therefore, not strange that with these the lowering of inhibition should show marked evidence of the sexual stimulation in erotic ideas, dreams, visions, etc. Should a similar condition arise in the course of disease, the drug (cannabis or whatever) would so far match the symptoms and be a candidate homœopathically for choice as a remedy.

Fear in general again appears to be associated with sympathetic overstimulation and overactivity of such hormones as the adrenal secretion. A drug or disease that disorganises the sympathetic—parasympathetic nervous system, or over-stimulates the suprarenal glands, would be associated with fear and similarity could be found between drug and disease symptoms.*

Argentum nitricum is one of the greatest remedies for fears of many kinds, and there is other evidence suggesting that it can effect the suprarenal gland. Exactly what kind of fear pre-dominates will depend on the character and life experiences of the individual, but a drug that can control favourably the supply of a hormone will lessen any kind. Homœopathy, however, claims to find good indications in specific fears, e.g. of insanity, of thunder, of knives, of disease or death, of the dark, etc. For some of these again a reasonable explanation can be found. Any sensitive person who feels mind control slipping away whether from drug or disease, will have a fear that his reason may be in danger ; so that a drug need not do more than produce an inability to think as clearly as before, to remember accurately, to realise external relations precisely, in order to cause mental anxiety. There are many drugs that produce brain confusion in varying degrees. Nevertheless, there are others in which the specific fear of insanity is more definitely associated than with others. This may mean no more than that the prover of it was sensitive on that particular point by reason of some personal experience. So that a fear that might remain vague (though concerned with mind control) in others, became very definite in him. That precision would still make the drug

---

* Certain physiologists consider that diarrhœa brought on by fright is probably due to sympathetic exhaustion following overstimulation, thus allowing the vagus to act unopposed.

indicated for a patient who showed the same definite character in his fear, for it would indicate particularly some similar life experience causing a similar " trauma." Fear of death often indicates a vague realisation that the bodily state is grave. But a patient's condition may be serious and yet the fear is not present, or as, *e.g.* with aconite, the fear may be out of proportion to the danger. These variations will depend on constitutional differences and in so far as they indicate these conditions become good reasons for choosing a " similar " remedy. Thus the best patients for aconite are often the robust who have not had much illness. Such patients, suddenly struck down, will be more alarmed than more weakly subjects familar enough with minor ailments. The serious cases which yet have no fear may have the sense of illness inhibited through a profound toxæmia, or with a possibly better hormone balance can control their anxiety. Again, there will be different types needing different remedies. Fear of thunder implies a sensitiveness to electrical changes which will infallibly have led to some startling experiences in thunder storms, but this sensitiveness again is constitutional and a hint for the homœopathist.

But there still remain the special fears, of knives, of fire, of enclosed or open spaces, of falling and so forth. There is good reason to trace such fears to definite repressions, and they can be relieved, sometimes, at any rate, by the analysis that recalls the root of them. But experiences that appear to cause them are nearly always found to be of so usual and general a character that not one in a hundred of the population can have escaped them in the course of growth from infancy onwards. What child is there that has not had experiences of fire and cutting edges that were at the moment disturbing, but how seldom do these childish experiences leave any mark ? The comparative rarity of serious trouble suggests that these experiences ought to be forgotten : " sunk without trace " ; and that if they are not, there is probably some physical defect in the bodily nerve mechanism. The most probable defect would be an increased permeability of the threshold of consciousness to messages from the unconscious. If this be so, then, as something of the kind is clearly produced by some drugs, the administration of them should homœopathically strengthen the barrier and lessen the fear. Clinically, this suggestion has been tested and proved

effective in many cases. No experienced homœopathist doubts
that much can be done remedially for phobias, persistent
dreams, abnormal haunting wishes which are so opposed to the
normal desires that they are resisted but return in sleep and
during unguarded moments. Such are, for instance, the
temporary revulsions from loved ones which may even be
accompanied by thoughts of killing or injuring them. If, then,
we class the drugs which are remedial in such cases as all
possessing the power to make the threshold of consciousness
more permeable, it might be argued, as already suggested, that
in provings, the phobias and whatever that appear are dependent on the prover's experience and that strict correspondence
as to their nature need not be demanded in prescribing in order
to achieve success. This is so far true that, whenever there is a
general resemblance between drug and disease symptoms (and
the phobias will be but one, albeit an important one), the
similar drug can be confidently given, even if the character of
the phobia or dream or abnormal desire be not identical for
patient and prover. For instance, the fear of robbers appears
strongly under ARSENICUM, but a different kind of fear would be
no bar to the prescription of it did the rest of the picture fit
the drug.

The point can be illustrated by two provers' experiences with
JABORANDI (q.v.). One prover recorded a haunting nervous
experience with a fixed idea that she would kill her family with a
hatchet. A single record such as that, though appearing while
testing a drug, can at first be only tentatively attributed to it.
The cause might be something in life apart from the proving, so
that further confirmation is desirable. But a second prover,
unaware of the experience of the first and therefore not open to
any suggestion, found himself similarly haunted ; not with a
desire to kill his wife, but a terror that he would be impelled to
do so against his will. A cutting instrument was the one
continually in his mind. In both instances the thought of
killing loved ones arose with the drug proving and disappeared
on ceasing to take it. It is difficult to resist the conclusion that
the drug was causal. The differences in the details of the
obsessions illustrate the conception put forward above : that
the drug affects the permeability of the threshold of consciousness to urges proceeding from the unconscious mind, but what

reaches consciousness, or the way in which it reaches it, will depend on the nature and life experience of the patient.

It is, however, necessary to add that certain drugs are associated with definite phobias and other psychopathic disturbances, and that patients not only on occasion record experiences exactly like those of the provers, but find the mental symptoms cured by the use of the similar remedy. We can only tentatively conclude that certain temperaments and constitutions, due very likely to varying hormonic balances, incline some of life's common experiences to stimulate the activity of the unconscious to produce in the conscious mind processes from the forgotten experiences of life and establish complexes, so that a tendency to have mental symptoms of a special kind becomes a sign of such a constitution and therefore a good guide to a remedy. Thus anacardium possesses a general power to lower the barrier between the conscious mind and the unconscious, and thus comes about that sense of duality that has been stressed above. There is also the removal of inhibition and lessening of moral restraint. But specific fears are relatively rare and so are fixed ideas and morbid desires.

It has been convenient to discuss the general question of the effects of drugs on mental phenomena at this place, but other remedies offer more striking instances of precise and detailed mental symptoms, e.g. cannabis, opium, stramonium, etc.

Skin Symptoms

There remains for consideration anacardium symptoms affecting the alimentary and respiratory tracts and the skin. The last have already been mentioned, but here can be described in detail as burning, itching, increased by scratching, the formation of vesicles sometimes as large as a pea, with burning sensations and tendency to develop warty excrescences.

Gastro-intestinal Symptoms

The alimentary canal shows many important symptoms and the drug is useful in a number of cases of chronic dyspepsia. The tongue is coated and food tastes offensive, indeed unpleasant taste and smell are often present apart from food.

Thirst is usually present but the gastro-intestinal symptoms are aggravated by cold drinks and often worsened by taking soups. Gastric pains are relieved by eating, freedom from pain and distress continuing for two hours after the meal when pain recurs and lasts until food is again taken. Generally the pain is relieved by warm food and aggravated by cold food. The bowels may be constipated but there is often an urgent call to stool which is, however, expelled with difficulty. A very common abdominal pain is described as a pressive sensation as though by something blunt which also causes a sense of stoppage or plugging. This may be felt in the epigastrium or rectum. Gastro-intestinal symptoms brought on by emotional excitement and strain is a valuable indication and in addition to the local modalities, the typical anacardium mentality, intense irritability and bad temper usually presents itself.

Respiratory Symptoms

Violent convulsive paroxysms of coughing appear not infrequently and the dull pressive sensation may be felt in the chest. The cough is related to eating, as though the pneumogastric nerve connections were a factor in producing the condition. Sometimes eating starts the cough ; sometimes notably relieves it, but a relation between the gastric and respiratory symptoms is generally noteworthy.

Patients in general are easily fatigued and weary, and in spite of the fact that excitement or anxiety may induce the appearance of symptoms, the anacardium patient, in other ways, is not liable to be disturbed by his immediate environment. (It can be observed that acuteness, or blunting of the special senses produced by a drug is usually associated with a corresponding awareness or insensitivity to surroundings.) Patients feel the cold and dislike particularly draughts of cold air. Sleep is often heavy and unrefreshing and accompanied by dreams of fire, of danger, of disease, of death ; thus the normal recuperation from sleep is not obtained.

ANTIMONIUM TARTARICUM
(K.Sb.O.)(C4H4O6)
Tartar Emetic.   Trituration of Solutions and Potencies from both.

Antimonium crudum (the sulphide of antimony) and antimonium arsenicosum, the arseniate, are used as well as antimonium tartaricum, but the last is the most important member of the antimony group of compounds. It is well known to the dominant school of medicine and some of its uses therein have a distinct flavour of homœopathy. But on the whole the non-homœopathist tends to use it less in these days, while the followers of Hahnemann, holding to their guiding principle, find its precise application relatively easy and the results of it as satisfactory as ever.

Locally, tartar emetic irritates the skin, causing a papular eruption and later the development of vesicles and pustules not very unlike those of small-pox. The openings of the skin glands and hair follicles are the points where the pustules begin. Injected hypodermically it causes great pain and often local suppuration and sloughing, so that this mode of administration is undesirable ; the intravenous route is preferred when the drug is administered in orthodox practice. The skin effects are most easily brought out by local application, but appear from homœopathic and other experience (see both Schulz and Lewin) to follow occasionally the internal use of the remedy. Also the eruption sometimes appears not only where the application has been made, but on areas far removed, suggesting a more than local influence. Regarding these skin effects, therefore, as a specific skin reaction and noting the characters of the eruption, homœopathists use ant. tart. for cases of small-pox, when other symptoms correspond and apparently with much success. As will be seen below, the characteristic early backache of variola finds a parallel in the pathogenesis of ant. tart.

As its name suggests, the effects of tartar emetic show readily in the gastro-intestinal tract. Small doses cause little but slight perspiration to healthy individuals, but larger ones cause great nausea and violent vomiting, with profound depression, salivation and sweating. The pulse is quickened. The later vomitings contain much slimy mucus and even blood. With the vomiting appears a profuse watery diarrhœa and great muscular weakness sets in, and often symptoms of general collapse. The skin becomes cold and covered with sweat, the face cyanosed, the voice weak, the respiration and temperature depressed and in fatal cases life ends in coma. Albuminuria is a fairly frequent symptom of poisoning. The vomiting and diarrhœa appear to be largely due to the local irritant action, for though they will follow hypodermic injection, the drug is largely excreted into stomach and bowel and produces its local effects in this way. The symptoms of chronic antimonial poisoning are depression, headache, giddiness, confusion and drowsiness. There is loss of appetite and discomfort or pain in the region of the stomach. The patient gradually becomes weak and exhausted. Profuse diarrhœa may occur. Later there is a loss of flesh, albuminuria and finally collapse. Pustular eruptions have been reported from the prolonged internal use of antimony tartrate. Ulceration of the small intestine is said to appear and Payer's patches to be specially affected. Blood pressure falls after poisonous doses ; œdema of the lungs and congestion are common, and, in animal experiments, catarrhal inflammation of the bronchi and pneumonia have been observed. Certain secretions such as sweat, saliva and that of the respiratory mucous glands are stimulated. After chronic poisoning there is evidence of fatty degeneration of certain organs (*e.g.*, liver), as with arsenic. Small doses stimulate the kidneys, large doses cause nephritis. The drug appears to have specific power of destroying trypanosomes in the blood even in dilutions of 1 in 500,000. It has therefore been employed in sleeping sickness and in syphilis and has proved remarkably successful in kala azar and has become the remedy for bilharziasis.

The effects of these poisonings and results of these direct experiments on animals make clear that antimony acts profoundly upon the body and has special points of attack in the gastro-intestinal tract, the respiratory system, the skin and the kidneys. But for effective use by homœopathists these broad outlines need to be made more precise in detail. When drugs are " proved," they are taken in relatively small doses over a period of time. The " shock " effects of the large quantity of a poison are less evident, but the finer shades of response become more manifest. It is by means of these that the decision is made for the choice of not only a similar drug, but the most-similar possible. In all that follows, therefore, while the information derived from poisoning effects is by no means neglected, the physician is depending very largely on the provings of the drug on healthy human beings. Clinical experience also over more than a century has added a good deal to our knowledge. Thus homœopathic experiment and experience make clear the detailed indications for its successful use.

The association of nausea and vomiting with symptoms showing irritated inflammation of the smaller bronchioles and lung have led to the use of antim. tart. in the sequelæ to ether anæsthesia. The practice of the Glasgow Homœopathic Hospital for some years has been to give the drug beforehand (one or two doses), and it is claimed that patients so treated have a much pleasanter experience and give far less anxiety than the average etherised subject. If chloroform is to be the anæsthetic, phosphorus (q.v.) is the drug of election. There is not as yet enough experience of the more recent anæsthetics for dogmatic pronouncement though here too phosphorus has been advocated.

The outstanding feature in the study of the homœopathic use of this drug is that it is especially applicable to acute conditions superimposed upon debilitated and weakly constitutions. Thus it becomes indicated in complaints at both ends of life ; in feeble children and in affections occurring in old people ; it further applies to the complaints of individuals with broken down constitutions. From both orthodox records of poisoning and homœopathic provings, antimony tartrate is shown to have a marked action on the respiratory system, but it is seldom that the drug is required during early stages of acute conditions affecting the lung. But in the later stages of lung trouble, where reaction is failing or when weakness has been present from the beginning, the typical state of affairs requiring antim. tart. is to be found. The patient is prostrate ; there is little fever, he is cold and covered with a cold sweat.

Two other characteristics of the drug may be mentioned. In nearly all complaints the symptoms produce drowsiness ; often there is an irresistible inclination to sleep. The second characteristic relates to the state of the skin ; there is coldness and the patient is bathed in a cold clammy sweat. Eructations ameliorate symptoms. Children resent being touched or even looked at.

The mental and temperamental symptoms which characterise the drug are distinct and well marked. The mentality of the patient may be summarised by Hering's rubric " bad humour." If a child, he is cross and peevish and will whine and complain continually. Though he may cling to those around and want to be carried, he resents being touched, refuses to move, refuses to obey any command ; will show, in fine, " a fractiousness " which is a torment to nurse and relations, but a clear guide to the physician. Both chamomilla and pulsatilla are frequently needed in gastric complaints of children : of these pulsatilla suits a tearful state, desiring consolation and company, but usually without any ill-temper—a mood of " softness " in fact ; while although chamomilla is fitted for very ill-tempered children, there is with these an underlying wish for sympathy and help, however ungraciously overtures may be received. When antimony (in any preparation) is to be thought of, the ill-humour is without any desire for consolation and attempts to give it worsen the temper : the child's chief desire is " to be left alone." Older patients will have more control, but the peevish ill-temper will be noticeable enough. He is ill-humoured and prefers to be let alone ; he is irritable when disturbed and does not want to be bothered. Great dejection accompanies this persistent bad humour and such despondency may increase till the patient passes into a state of the greatest anxiety, so much so that such a patient, anxious, prostrate and with surface of the body covered with a cold sweat, may resemble somewhat the picture of the arsenic patient. A somewhat contradictory state may supervene, but one illustrating a general modality of the drug. If the patient be allowed to be quiet he may become drowsy and fall into a sleep.

The face of the antim. tart. patient is pale and sickly, and covered with a cold sweat, the lips pale and parched. The alimentary canal is the seat of many definite symptoms. The tongue is heavily coated white with red edges. In the mouth there is a copious flow of saliva. Nausea is a marked symptom in this patient. With all stomach and abdominal symptoms there is a constant nausea which tends to intensify the anxious state of mind and is frequently followed by vomiting if food is taken. Nausea, retching and vomiting with faintness and prostration are symptoms marked associated with all complaints requiring tartar emetic. Vomiting temporarily relieves nausea.* The general characteristic is again seen in this con-

* This is not the case with ipecacuanha patients.

nection. Vomiting is apt to be followed by a feeling of langour and drowsiness. Generally there is a disgust for food with an especial aversion from milk which produces nausea and vomiting. In some cases the patient may crave acids or acid fruit, which, if taken, have a similar result. In most complaints the patient is thirstless (but thirst for cold water little and often is not unknown).

Pain in the abdomen appears, but more discomfort and uneasiness, and the motions are loose, frequent, slimy, generally yellow or brown and occasionally contain blood. Summer diarrhœa, when vomiting is a marked symptom, with collapse and cold sweating, yields to this remedy. The presence of gastro-enteric symptoms in pneumonia or small-pox is a strong indication for antim. tart.

Its sphere of action on the respiratory organs is great. Antim. tart. is one of the most valued remedies in homœopathic prac- tice for pneumonia. It is especially to the broncho-pneumonia of weakly children and of the aged that it corresponds. But whatever the affection of the chest, be it broncho-pneumonia, whooping cough or asthma, there is a characteristic rattling of mucus, though very little is expectorated as might be expected, because the sufferer is too prostrate to have the power to raise it. Such expectoration as may be brought up is white. All the respiratory complaints are accompanied by the general state of this drug : prostration, irritability, tendency to drowsiness, pallor, and cold sweat. Respiration is rapid, short and diffi- cult ; the patient desires to sit up and, if a child, is better when carried in the upright position. Such oppressed breathing tends to be at its height about 3 a.m. An interesting extension of the antim. tart. generalities is seen in weakly, chilly, pale children suffering from whooping cough. The paroxysm of coughing is preceded by angry temper or a fit of crying—after eating or drinking or getting warm in bed. After the attack has sub- sided, another antim. tart. symptom supervenes : the child becomes drowsy and falls asleep.

It is interesting to note that Trousseau, who valued the drug in some acute chest affections, observed that it acted when there were gastro-enteric symptoms, *i.e.*, when from a homœo- pathic point of view it was better indicated by the whole symptom-picture.

The picture of the symptomology in pneumonia can be made more detailed and precise. The pneumonia which would suggest aconite has already been described, the case that requires antimony is different in many respects. A physical diagnosis can legitimately turn a physician's thought toward a certain group of remedies, but he will do best if he is constantly on his guard against routine prescribing. In every case the decision must be made on the symptoms present in the actual individual case. No human being exactly resembles another and each case needs its own remedy.

As was mentioned above, the use of tartar emetic is found in the later stages of pneumonia, especially in individuals of feeble constitution. It applies to the type of pneumonia that has not responded, the patient being severely ill. He is prostrate, with the face pale and drawn, the lips pale or cyanosed, he is cold to the touch and there is a profuse cold clammy sweat. The mental condition is that always associated with this drug. He is depressed, irritable and peevish. He wants to be let alone and if left undisturbed will lie quietly enough, making few demands on those attending him. There is marked respiratory distress, the chest is full of mucus, rattling can be heard as the patient breathes, but expectoration is very scanty ; such sputum as is brought up is white and the effort to expectorate causes retching or even vomiting. The respiratory distress is aggravated by the warmth of the room ; his most comfortable position is sitting upright. The patient is usually thirstless ; there is an aversion to all food, especially milk, though there may be a desire for acids or acid fruits. The stomach and abdomen are distended with flatulence and with this there is constant and intense nausea.

In the genito-urinary system, homœopathy does not make much use of the power of the drug to produce nephritis. Unless kidney symptoms are accompanied by others elsewhere that suggest antim. tart. they seldom by themselves lead to the choice of it. Nor does it much influence the sexual organs. It seems to have some power over papillomata and has had clinical success in gonorrhœal warts.

The skin suffers from obstinate itching and a pustular generalised eruption is characteristic and gives a local indication for the use of the drug in small-pox. Hering mentions the value of the drug in several skin conditions where pustular eruptions occur. Dr. Tyler emphasises its efficacy in impetigo contagiosa.

Another indication is found in the very severe backache affecting the lower part of the spine and corresponding to the well-known early symptom of variola. But similar aching from other causes can be relieved by antim. tart. if the peculiar symptoms of the drug be present, e.g., in lumbago. Movement aggravates the pain, the slightest effort may cause retching and the patient breaks out into a cold clammy sweat. Joint pains appear in the provings ; in these rheumatic conditions there is a passive swelling of the joints which is especially troublesome during cold damp weather.

The complaints requiring antimonium tartrate generally are aggravated by warm weather, warm clothing and a warm room, though cold damp weather is liable also to aggravate the symptoms. Symptoms are usually increased by lying down, sitting up relieves ; they are aggravated by anger or vexation. With the nausea there is an aversion from food, especially milk. Many symptoms are aggravated at night, especially about 3 a.m.

APIS

Apis mellifica—the poison of the honey bee : tinctures made with alcohol.

The effects of bee stings on sensitive persons are often general as well as local. These symptoms, supplemented by deliberate provings of the tincture and checked and extended by clinical experience, make up a characteristic drug-picture of a remedy valuable in a variety of diseases, principally, though not exclusively, acute and subacute affections. In many places there is a popular belief that bee stings relieve or cure rheumatism, and instances of the apparent remedial effect of them even in chronic long-standing cases have been recorded by physicians. Homœopathic experience confirms the remedial relationship of apis to certain joint disorders and justifies the popular belief, while defining the cases likely to respond to the drug.

Locally bee stings usually give rise to considerable œdema

and the general effects of the poison include probably some lowering of blood coagulability, for a tendency to urticaria and to serous effusions develops.

Apis acts especially on the outer parts of the body ; the skin and cellular tissues, also upon the coverings of organs and serous membranes generally. Consequently recent serous effusions, acute inflammation of the kidneys and other parenchymatous tissues, are conditions that suggest apis to the homœopathist. Particularly it is valuable in a number of local inflammations of the skin and mucous membrane, e.g., erysipelas, pharyngitis or tonsillitis may respond to it. Recent pleural effusions (non-purulent), pericarditis and synovial effusions come into its sphere of action. In every case, however, the guiding symptoms are present which lead to the choice of the drug. Like the other great poisons of the animal kingdom—the serpent poisons—it is a remedy suited to those who bear heat badly. The patient is generally aggravated by warmth in every form ; a warm room, warm clothing, a warm fire, warm drinks. The local condition is similarly aggravated by heat and relieved by cold.

Most complaints requiring apis are associated with a degree of œdema, and this is accompanied with stinging, burning pains and extreme hyperæsthesia of the affected parts ; there is great sensitivity of the surface to touch and general soreness is marked. The aversion from touch or pressure has one exception, the head pains are definitely relieved by external pressure. There is also an aversion to tight clothing. Such symptoms recall similar ones produced by lachesis. But while the sensitiveness of lachesis is almost entirely a nervous irritability, that of apis is accompanied by a general sensation of soreness and a weary bruised feeling that often produces an effect as of great bodily fatigue. The final result of these sensations is a condition of debility that may go on to actual paresis, more functional, however, than organic, although, as will be seen later, the poison can cause muscle spasm and the end-result of that undue stimulation would be depression. With all this discomfort, however, there is a marked restlessness, even fidgetiness.

Restlessness again recalls the effect of arsenic, but with this drug it is rather a mental symptom ; with apis, more the result of bodily suffering and the attempt to find ease by change of position. So that as a symptom it is really more closely allied to the relief from movement of rhus, to which drug apis has points of resemblance. However, the apis pains are not markedly aided by the movement : the involuntary search for relief in restlessness is not successful.*

There is evidence of effect of the bee poison on the nerve centres, for trembling, twitching and jerking of muscle groups are prominent symptoms in the complex. These spasms may be followed by stiffness (e.g., of the jaw or the tongue). These motor nerve symptoms (as well as the pains) show a preference for the right side of the body (opposite to that of lachesis).

The conditions leading to the apis state are frequently associated with such emotions as grief, fright, anger and jealousy and especially are apt to ensue from suppressed eruptions.† The complaints have a violent onset and develop rapidly so that in certain cases the patient becomes stuporous or unconscious. The severity of the patient's suffering is usually at its height in the late afternoon.

Mentally there is generally an anxious, tearful restlessness of demeanour. In the less severe condition the patient is depressed, inclined to weeping without cause, fidgety and exacting : there is a general whining tearfulness.

In more severe infections, such as erysipelas or diphtheria, the mental state tends more to indifference, listlessness and inability to think clearly. In the most severe grades of infection, this apathy may increase even to stupor or unconsciousness ; consequently apis has been used with considerable success in meningitis and hydrocephalus. The patient gradually passes into a state of unconsciousness. This condition is characterised by the accompaniment of sudden shrill, sharp cries or screaming as if he were experiencing severe pains in the head. A muttering delirium may supervene, again accom-

---

* " quella inferma
Che non puo trovar posa in sulle piume
Ma con dar Volta suo dolore scherma."

† It has been often observed that in exanthemata such as measles and scarlet fever a poor development or a retrocession of the rash is accompanied by severe and often dangerous symptoms, in fact a more profound toxæmia. Such occurrences turn the thoughts of the homœopathist to certain drugs which clinical experience has found to be very useful. In many more chronic skin diseases there is a firm belief also that stimulating local treatment may bring about the disappearance of the eruption without removing its cause and that this is undesirable and may be followed by symptoms in other organs.

panied by that peculiar sudden piercing cry. It must be noted that the general aggravation from heat is extended to the mental state. All the mental symptoms are markedly aggravated by heat in any form : a hot room, warm clothing, a hot bath ; thus, for example, such a patient, in a stuporous condition when put into a hot bath, is liable to be thrown into a state of twitching and convulsion. Heat in any form aggravates every symptom, mental and local, in the apis patient.

In conditions requiring apis, the head is usually hot and congested, accompanied by sudden stabbing pains, which are aggravated by movement and definitely ameliorated by external pressure (a contradictory modality, as generally the pains of apis are aggravated by touch and pressure). In meningitis, acute or chronic, this modality of amelioration from pressure is especially demonstrated. The child bores its head into the pillow. Here the general mentality is one of stupor, accompanied by occasional piercing screams.

Many inflammatory conditions affecting the eyes such as ophthalmia, staphyloma of the cornea, serous iritis, keratitis, find their remedy in apis. All such conditions are characterised by a serous exudation : considerable œdema, sudden stinging pains and a marked aggravation from heat and therefore desire, usually with temporary relief, from the local application of cold.

The face of the apis patient varies according to the manifestation of the disease presenting itself. In acute infective fevers it is usually red and burning ; in kidney disease the face is waxy, pale and œdematous. Apis is of value in the treatment of erysipelas affecting the face ; generally the infection extends from the right side to the left. The pain is described as stinging, the face is red and swollen, the œdema is out of proportion to the intensity of the pain.

In acute fevers, the tongue is fiery, hot and red, even hot and dry ; in low fevers it may be hot, dry and trembling, resembling the tongue of lachesis.

Regarding the alimentary canal, the pharynx is very sensitive to the action of apis, and tonsillitis with œdema calls for it. With all throat conditions there is œdema accompanied by burning, stinging pains. The condition is relieved by cold drinks or sucking ice and aggravated by heat in any form. The tonsils and uvula are swollen and red in appearance. In the early stages of scarlet fever which requires apis, the throat is bright red and œdematous, and is painful on swallowing. Generally, the patient is hot, wants to uncover, craves air and open windows, and suffocates in a warm room. Furthermore, he is usually thirstless. It is similarly valuable in the treatment of diphtheria, in cases where the throat is painful and œdematous (the membrane is often not extensive), with aggravation from heat. Mentally the patient may be inert and listless, even stuporous.

The stomach presents few characteristic symptoms. In most conditions the patient is thirstless, though the opposite modality may occasionally present itself when there is insatiable thirst. The apis patient has a craving for milk and oysters.

When the abdomen is affected, the general superficial sensitivity peculiar to apis is found. Here there is a sore, bruised feeling of the abdominal wall; and the whole abdomen is extremely tender. Peritonitis with great tenderness and stinging pains with the apis generalities may occur.

In the genito-urinary sphere, the drug is indicated for some inflammatory conditions of the kidney, especially during or subsequent to eruptive fevers. Acute nephritis with albuminuria and casts may be met by apis (e.g., scarlatinal nephritis). In such cases there is aching in the lumbar region with soreness over the kidneys, and this associated with tenderness of the abdominal wall. The nephritis is accompanied by much œdema, especially in the face and upper part of the body. The skin is dry, and the patient himself may be restless and thirstless or, if more acutely ill, he passes into a state of stupor.

In the male there is usually an increase of sexual desire; but apart from local inflammation with marked œdema, when apis is a valuable, if temporary, remedy, there is little call for it in diseases of the male genital organs.

In the female its effect is more marked, apart from local inflammations. Dysmenorrhœa and recent affections of ovaries and tubes (especially right-sided), when pains are severe and tingling, are often helped by apis. Neuralgia of ovaries, especially of the right ovary, are accompanied by stinging pains and a bruised feeling over the abdominal walls. As always in the apis case, there is an aggravation from the application of heat. Apis has prevented threatened abortion where the patient experiences stinging pains in the ovarian region, she feels hot, wants to be uncovered and is thirstless. Suppression of the menses, especially in young females, accompanied by a hot, flushed face and followed by cerebral symptoms, such as intense excitement or even mania, alternating with stupor, have found a remedy in apis.

The affinity of apis to serous membranes is seen in its effect on the pericardium, where there is soreness over the region of the heart, scanty urine, swollen limbs and the general apis modalities. Thus, pericarditis may find effective remedy in this drug.

In the respiratory sphere, besides being indicated in pleurisy with non-purulent effusion, the pathogenesis contains the symptoms of a violent, dry spasmodic cough, with great soreness and sensitiveness of the larynx. Dyspnœa of an asthmatic character is also a symptom. There is a feeling of suffocation, the patient feeling as if he could not draw another breath and an inability to lie down.

The power over the joints is a general one on synovial membranes. Homœopathists find it most useful when the joints are swollen and shiny, when the pains are sharp and stinging, sensitiveness marked, effusion considerable, and where there is marked restlessness and an aggravation from applied heat.

Urticaria is a prominent affection of the skin that suggests apis. Itching is intolerable and swelling considerable. The condition is accompanied by stinging, burning pains, and the skin is sensitive to the touch.

The patients who need apis are often drowsy, but sleep badly, being wakened by pain or anxious dreams. Children often awake screaming when suffering from acute affections that otherwise suggest the use of this drug. There is also in the apis symptom-complex some measure of that aggravation from sleep that characterises so strongly lachesis and its allies.

The general features of the apis patient are therefore, firstly, that heat in any form causes an aggravation of all symptoms. Patients are worse in closed and heated rooms ; stinging pains are associated with most conditions which are made worse by touch and pressure. The exception is that head pains are ameliorated by external pressure. There is generally an aggravation of all symptoms in the late afternoon about five o'clock, and some aggravation after sleep. The right side of the body is more affected and the trouble tends to extend to the left side. There is always an amelioration of symptoms from open air, uncovering, cold bathing and the application of cold water. The action of the drug develops much more slowly than does that of aconite or belladonna, so that care must be taken, if it seems well indicated, not to abandon its use too early. The effect of aconite in acute conditions will often be seen in a few minutes, but apis often requires an hour or more. All potencies are praised.

ARGENTUM METALLICUM

A trituration of pure metallic silver.

General Remarks

Before the advent of colloidal solutions, pure metals were little used by orthodox medicine, with the important exception of mercury, during the last century. In the middle ages, silver and gold were prized on (mainly) astrological grounds. With the " collosols " various uses have been found for the metals and silver has now a place in therapeutics. It is given in strengths of 1 in 2,000 and less (between 3x and 4x in homœopathic pharmacy), and is thought of mainly as an antiseptic for local use in such affections as ophthalmia and gonorrhœa. It is given internally for stomach and bowel conditions, locally in a spray for asthma, and claims are made for it in septicæmia.

In this drug study it will be found that homœopathy has a significant word to say on all these points except that of septicæmia, where for us, the drug is seldom suggested.

But while the study of colloids was in its infancy (and before), Hahnemann had found that his method of potentisation by trituration could convert substances virtually inactive into powerful remedies and was using the metals among other agents in this way. Further he discovered that when triturated to the third centesimal potency the material became soluble and could be treated as a solution therapeutically and for further potentisation. In fact, as Boyd and Judd Lewis have shown, the procedure had resulted in a colloidal preparation. Thus once again Hahnemann is justified in a claim long derided as charlatanry. As so often he was right and his arrogant critics wrong, since they, as usually when considering homœopathy, preferred assertion to experiment.

Among other metals, silver has been potentised and proved, and argentum metallicum as a remedy is the result.

It is a constant observation among homœopathists that the therapeutic properties and uses of an element vary when it enters into combination with others. Naturally resemblances can be traced as easily, e.g., all sodium salts have much in common, but the added element or elements make a different entity and in the exact prescribing, which is the aim of homœopathy, there is need now for one compound : now for another.

Although the cyanide and the iodide of silver have been used, our real knowledge of the silver salts rests on the provings of the metal and the nitrate. There are important differences in symptomatology ; the two are by no means interchangeable. Their principal points of attack correspond up to a point but the nature and the intensity of the effect varies. It is impossible with our present knowledge to say how this variation comes to be but the facts are clear and can be verified clinically.

It is likely, and it is true at any rate of the provings, that ingestion of small quantities with any persistence induces more profound and far reaching effects than will follow the larger amounts which the body neutralises in " argyria." But it still remains a problem why, since both drugs affect the nervous system profoundly, they should present different results there, and why the metal shows an " affinity " for cartilage which cannot be deduced from the action of the nitrate. But the business of the homœopathist is to fit symptoms of disease to those of drug, and he will use metal or compound as these indications command.*

---

* It has to be remembered that hardly any provings reach an ideal standard. All tend to be fragmentary and incomplete, the real marvel is that so often they are ample and adequate. If both of these remedies were more exhaustively tested on human beings, more resemblances might appear. Personal idiosyncrasy must play a large part in determining the response of any prover. No one is 100 per cent. perfect in every cell and if the body is exposed as a whole to any poison there must be a tendency for the less perfect tissues to give rise to symptoms first unless, for any reason, they are shielded from the attack.

Action on the Nervous System

Metallic silver (like gold or lead) affects the body slowly but profoundly. It bites deep. Always the nervous system shows important symptoms. It can affect peripheral nerves but it seems largely to begin its effects from the outside : the nerve sheaths. The brain cells can ultimately soften and degenerate under its power. It is the rational, intellectual side of mental processes that suffers most. Emotions and affections are little influenced and this is of especial significance in that arg. nit. disturbs the psyche profoundly on the emotional side, particularly in producing phobias and unexplained anxieties.

Arg. met. appears to disturb the intellectual faculties of the individual, there is inability to think and general mental weariness, so that he becomes increasingly nervous and sensitive to his surroundings. In such patients the memory fails and he becomes forgetful. Thus it is pre-eminently valuable for those whose life centres largely in thought ; for brain workers of any kind. As pain of one kind or another is generally a predominant symptom this naturally disturbs and distracts the thinker even more and the palliatives to which he is likely to resort, being all more or less inhibitors of brain activity, do not improve matters but the reverse. The patient is fatigued but sleep helps not at all. He is apt to feel worse after sleep and the morning for him is a terrible time of strain, only by an effort of will can he attack his day's work.

When the intellect is thus hampered the patient naturally becomes confused and may at first sight resemble one in whom emotion, such as anger or fear has upset the balance. But the origin of the confusion is intellectual, not emotional. True he may be irritable, easily angered, even full of wild sayings of rage. But this is the result of control slipping because of increasing awareness that his reason (on which he prides himself) cannot be trusted. Similarly in society he is not inclined to talk. He has lost confidence ; fears to talk foolishly and on occasion if pressed may both say and do foolish things.

Jerking of the limbs is a noteworthy symptom. It comes on especially when lying down to sleep.

The end of the mental picture is a nervous breakdown which may be profound. Nutrition suffers, bodily weight goes down and the patient becomes increasingly sensitive and more and more nervous, and physically, increasingly thin and sickly.

At this stage particularly odd things will be said and done, unbalanced behaviour that lead to charges of " hysteria " from acquaintances, even friendly ones from whom they are averse to any sympathy.

When a profound state of nervous prostration is present the skin may show symptoms. The patient likes heat and sun baths may be tried. Their effects need careful watching for the skin may begin to itch and burn unduly and that leads to scratching and so to sore places whch are slow to heal. The areas affected, look not unlike those suffering from frost bite. Homœopathists are frequently reminded of the embryological fact that both skin and nervous system are ectodermal in origin. But the relationship between skin symptoms and nerve symptoms are difficult to trace with confidence.

The relation of the metal to both gonads and the intellectual faculties and the nitrate to the adrenals and the emotion of fear is sufficiently interesting for speculation as to the correlation of drug action on the cortex and the endocrine glands.

There is hardly a drug in homœopathic experience which does not to some extent develop symptoms in the nervous system. The more deeply they are proved, the more likely are such symptoms to acquire significance and the more valuable such indications become as guides to the prescriber, as Hahnemann maintained long ago. Nor is it difficult to understand that the nervous system, the director of the body, should be susceptible to influences which, if noxious, have to be met and dealt with. The psyche is so closely related to the brain that modifications of its activity in such circumstances are almost inevitable.

It follows, therefore, that in considering (and cautiously speculating about) these relationships and their possible explanations, now one drug and now another, will seem to illustrate an aspect of the whole question. It is probably best in the present state of our knowledge (and our ignorance) to discuss these matters piecemeal as the effects of a particular remedy offer suggestions, but there will of necessity be a little repetition of ideas under different headings. With coca and cocaine, for instance, will be found some paragraphs which have a bearing on these that follow. It is an interesting problem to consider as to how far creative mental work is related to the sexual pattern of the individual. If we regard (and in this matter we should) chiefly the greatest artist creators it becomes increasingly clear that they nearly always have a background of more or less thwarted sexual desire.

Whereas Freud derives the creative power from personal experience and regards great personal achievements as the result of sublimation of intense passions hindered in their normal satisfaction, Jung considers that the creative faculty is not a compensation and an escape but that it emerges as an autonomous symbol from the unconscious. As creation appears to demand a certain femininity of approach (in the sense of surrender of the ego to subliminal impulses), then periods of sexual inhibition should encourage artistic creation. It matters not at all that the great artists may have had at times numerous, even promiscuous, sexual experiences. These have been attempts, which have failed, to find satisfaction for deeper desires that have persisted. The probability is that physical sexual activity and creation are incompatible and that it was during periods of sexual inhibition in their authors that the masterpieces of the world have resulted.

Of course, we have to realise that apart from their sexual pattern and the surrendering of it to creative work, there lies behind special gifts and that ability to use subliminal messages which are probably the nearest we can get to a name for the inspiration of genius. Life's experiences and the power to transmute aggressive sexual activity into a channel for what emerges from the unconscious only releases such springs of creative life as are latent : the amount and quality of it must depend on other factors. It remains, we think, that those readily satisfied sexually (e.g. Casanova) and also those of little or no strong sexual desire have never produced creative work of the first rank. They can be entertaining, witty, intelligent, excellent critics of other's work, benefactors to the race in many ways, they make often admirable scientific workers (though not scientific creators, for repetitive work is the antithesis of creative work). They can be valuable citizens but the highest flights in any direction are not for them. It is fascinating, by way to follow, to suggest that the general failure of women to rival men in the highest artistic achievements is due to the fact that motherhood, physical creation, takes for them the place of it. This is not to underrate the creative part played by the male physically but the labour of building up the single cell of male plus female into a human being falls on one partner only. Those women who have achieved most in artistic work have seldom had the physical side of their natures completed. Women, themselves, naturally stress rather the disabilities imposed upon their minds through centuries by the dominant male. The powers, they claim, are there, but they have not had chance to develop. Whether they are right or whether the suggestion thrown out above, namely, that artistic creation diminishes when sexual functions are normally fulfilled, will have a chance to be settled by experience in the next century or two, unless indeed the folly of mankind destroys civilisation as it now exists.*

Returning now to argentum metallicum, its action on the gonads would incline us to think of it when patients have been brain workers, even creative ones, for we should say that their potency as to the sex hormones would be an important factor in their health. We should expect their sex glands to be sensitive but a little below the average in power so that disease, attacking the less well-defined parts, would weaken them further, and the drug helping the resistance locally, would make more available the brain stimulus which was lessened by illness.

Of course there is plenty of evidence that silver affects nerve cells but, on the whole, it seems to attack those that influence the psyche. The mental symptoms of silver may very largely be caused indirectly but mainly through the effect of the drug on the gonads.

In women the effects might show more on the physical side, their particular creative sphere, in men on the mental and emotional. It must be remembered always that while for the human race only the greatest achievements are important, there is plenty of secondary temporary work to be done which has in

* The reversibility of bodily functions and psychical activities are especially to be observed on the plane of creative work.

it creative elements. It may very well be that it is among these lesser folk that silver finds its most frequent uses. The great artists are in any case few and far between and, as a matter of fact, recalling what we know of them there are not many, at the moment we recall none, who would be considered a good subject homœopathically for arg. met.

The relation of sex hormones to personality is another point of great interest. Under platinum we suggest that the over-weening conceit that characterises the drug should be associated with its undoubted power over the gonads leading to a disturbance in hormone balance.*

Since silver, not to mention gold and other agents, acts on these glands, it is interesting to follow up possible effects on character and disposition now that we have discussed the possible effects on creative energy. We must promise that our working hypothesis in this field is that of belief in free will and the power of education to modify and control tendencies due to such factors as hormone balance and its variations. Naturally we realise that individuals vary without limit in the tendencies with which heredity and circumstance and disease endow them. That is why personal moral judgments are so futile though mercifully they are *not* among the physician's duties. To " compound for sins we are inclined to, by damning those we have no mind to," is as easy as it is foolish. Those who aware of the possibilities of disease in these directions will find it easier to refrain from that habit.

We have good evidence that certain drugs are associated with certain defects of disposition. When similar defects arise in obvious disease or exist in subjects as a result, presumably of this physical make-up, the appropriate remedy will influence them for the better. The suggestion that the mechanism involved may be one of hormone balance is an attempt to relate the clinical facts to current physiological opinions. But the facts and the practical application of them remain even if the explanations prove faulty.

The ground thus cleared, we can return to Arg. Met. Unlike platinum which suggests disordered excess, arg. met. suggests

---

* It is not impossible that hormones themselves may at times be slightly modified in structure. This would add another factor to the disturbance, but failing direct evidence we can work on the hypothesis of disturbed general balance through excess or defect of one or more internal secretion.

defect of sex hormone. Its subjects lack confidence and are not conceited. Self consciousness often goes with a sense of inferiority and this may be present. The camouflage for this state is sometimes a forced assertiveness, but it does not amount to vanity unless the whole complex remains deep in the unconscious. If there is any (however slight) conscious realisation of failure and defeat, vanity does not appear. Indeed the mechanism behind vanity is not an easy one to examine. A distinction must be drawn between conceit and vanity. Rarely they may co-exist but either can be present alone.

Conceit is a fixed conviction of superiority (arising from an inferiority feeling) that does not depend on evidence but manufactures it from every incident of life. Every personal act becomes important. Every achievement magnificent in the opinion of others is of no importance. Opposition and criticism excite anger but no shaking of the ingrained belief. This is the platinum state and is almost certainly associated with perversion of the sex hormone. Benvenuto Cellini is a typical example in history of the type. But *vanity* is a desire to be noticed and appreciated, a longing for the limelight, and although the vain person delights to have himself and his work praised and can absorb unlimited flattery, he is often reasonably critical himself of his achievements and not overweeningly proud of them. Adverse criticism even he can endure for it is, at least, notice of him. Now this type when well marked very seldom has strong sexual power. He is often affectionate and kindly and his vanity has a certain quality of childishness which supports the idea that sexually he is a minus and not a plus subject. These people are seldom, if ever, among the greatest creators, though they often produce admirable secondary work ; ingenious, witty, charming. Probably with the lessened sex hormone goes rather an excess (small) of thyroid and pituitary. They usually have good health and are energetic.

Finally, it should be added that the very greatest creators in virtue probably of their will power and control are neither vain nor conceited. Dante, Leonardo and Beethoven were well enough aware of their powers but had neither the uneasy desire for praise of the vain nor the self-centred contempt for others of the conceited. Dante confesses to his pride but true

pride values the realisation of power with control in its manifestations and the deep sense of responsibility for it which may
mean humility before God. It is the lesser men and women who
fall to conceit and vanity, and this conception helps to place
those whom we feel to have some of the equipment of genius who
yet fail to achieve the work that we think was possible for them.
They are often weak in moral control also, and it is probably in
this failure of will that the trouble lies. The great are either
gifted with or painfully acquire the power to control their
physical equipment. So that with them subliminal impulses
can be shaped and used by all the conscious faculties without
let or hindrance from temporary emotional influences. Silver
might help the vain rather than the conceited, but as already
suggested is seldom the remedy for the greatest spirits among
men.

Arg. met. meets certain types of mental exhaustion found in
business men and brain workers. The memory fails and the
power to think and concentrate is impaired. The sufferer
wakes up unrefreshed in the morning ; it is with difficulty that
he can set about the mental activities and physical effort
required of him during the coming day.

He is sensitive to his surroundings and so becomes readily
annoyed or even angered with his family. Anger aggravates
his symptoms.

Some of the anxiety and anticipation found in the arg. nit.
subject, present itself in this drug also. The expectation of a
coming engagement arouses fear and anxiety, perhaps resulting
in an attack of diarrhœa.

Headache may be frontal or occipital, more commonly
frontal. Hemicrania is a frequent feature, especially right-
sided headaches. The pains gradually increase but cease suddenly. Heat relieves them, though close rooms aggravate the
patient and may produce vertigo. The headaches often show
periodicity and the hour of noon is a favourite time for the
onset of head and other pains. Pressure and bandaging also
relieve. The arg. nit. headache has similar features, but oddly
enough the arg. met. patient is chilly and likes warmth while the
arg. nit. patient in general likes coolness. This different
reaction to temperature shown by closely related drugs is not
common but occurs, e.g., with pulsatilla (desiring coolness) and

silica (desiring warmth).   Yet silica follows puls. as well or better than any remedy.*

As has been mentioned, symptoms suggest an action on the gonads of both sexes, though oddly enough they appear in the female mainly on the left and in the male the right testis is more often affected. With arg. nit. appears a marked aggravation of symptoms at the menstrual period. With arg. met., however, the glands appear to be affected in all respects and tissue damage in them has cleared up under this remedy. It is also likely that the internal secretion of the gonads is modified and increases the nervous symptom-complex in the direction of lack of control. The tissue changes that suggest arg. met. in the glands are those of chronic infiltration. Chronic orchitis, for instance, is often helped by it and if it has a gonorrhœal origin the metal has a special value, for its power over mucous membranes brings it into the picture for urethritis. The especial indication for arg. met. in gonorrhœal urethritis is that the discharge continues as a thick yellow or greenish yellow condition ; an unusual manifestation of gleet which is usually noted to be a thin colourless discharge. There is absence of pain. Thus, it is for the chronic case (with these modalities) that persists after much treatment that this drug is likely to be of value. On the other hand, given the susceptibility of the locality to the metal in provers it may be that now and then in a sensitive it might do more harm than good. Strong local " antiseptics " are not much favoured by homœopathists who prefer to work from within outwards. The general asthenia which silver causes naturally affects the pelvic supporting tissues and sagging and prolapse are common in women. Cervical ulceration again is likely to be chronic and the drug has a place in uterine carcinoma, especially when associated with a purulent offensive discharge.

Arg. nit. has a marked power to produce conjunctivitis. The metal attacks the eye region, but the eyelids rather than the eye. Blepharitis with infiltration and thickening and free discharge of mucus which may contain pus but often is simply

* Dr. Gibson Miller, as fine a prescriber as homœopathy has ever seen, stressed this reaction to heat and cold and attached much importance to it. It has great value when strongly marked though the paradoxical relations noted above have to be remembered. There are, however, many " Laodiceans " neither hot nor cold and they should not be forced into either category.

grey and tenacious. Thick grey mucus like this comes from other mucous membranes also, and arg. met. ranks as a " catarrhal remedy." Although the outer eye structures are less obviously affected (cornea, lens and iris) there is often dimness of sight but its relation to a tissue is not determined.

In the alimentary canal the symptoms are less marked than with arg. nit. but there is a catarrh of stomach and bowel to be noted and muscular enfeeblement inclines to constipation, which may be very obstinate unless the catarrh is enough to cause an irritable diarrhœa.

Polyuria is often noted and both albuminuria and diabetic conditions indicating silver (in broken down constitutions especially) have cleared up under its use.

A very prominent action of arg. met. which does not appear strikingly under arg. nit. is its power to affect cartilage. Thickening and infiltration of connective tissues has already been noted, but this action on cartilage goes deeper still. Joints, ears, nose, any of these regions may show cartilaginous hypertrophy and infiltration with thickening and hardening. Whenever, therefore, cartilage is attacked by disease, arg. met. should be thought of, and other symptoms pointing to it will usually be found. This power of infiltration and thickening has led to its use in cancer and with a good deal of success, at least in relieving cases and some actual disappearances of new growths are recorded. Schirrus is particularly likely to be helped by it.

The marked effect on the larynx is to be associated with its action on cartilage. Laryngitis develops and possibly aphonia, especially after excessive use of the voice as in singers and speakers. There may be more or less paralysis of the vocal cords. Add the deep inflammatory power of arg. met. to the picture and it comes to be thought of for tubercular or even malignant ulceration.

There is constant rawness and soreness and a sore spot at the bottom of the trachea is not infrequent. Talking and laughing aggravate the cough which is repeated till a little grey tough mucus is expectorated. The fits of coughing are not as violently spasmodic as with bryonia or drosera, but persistent and hacking. The chest feels " weak " as though the muscular power were insufficient for effective respiration and this makes coughing more difficult. With this often goes palpitation, fluttering, and, as with many other symptoms of arg. met., rest does not relieve but worsens the trouble.

Nerve pains are common and can be severe particularly in the lower extremities. Such pains are much aggravated when at rest ; the patient, though possibly exhausted, is compelled to walk about.

The pains are sometimes described as "like an electric shock." They come on suddenly, especially when he is about to fall asleep.

Among the joints, the wrist joints are favourite sites of chronic thickening and a history of gonorrhœa is an additional hint to the prescriber.

General Modalities

Pains in general are aggravated during rest ; often the patient cannot keep still however he tries.

Cold and damp bring on pains and heat tends to relieve, indeed the patient is generally chilly and prefers heat though he likes the open air.

Many of the complaints are aggravated during rest and are better from motion : all symptoms are worse after sleep.

Noon is also a time for the appearance or aggravation of symptoms.

Arg. met. should be studied with arg. nit. : now one, now the other is to be preferred, and their differences are sufficiently distinct to make the choice easier than might be imagined from their structural similarity.

ARSENICUM ALBUM

The White Oxide of Arsenic, As_2O_3.   Solution and Trituration.

The sinister and deserved reputation of arsenic as a deadly poison changes into a fame correspondingly great as a beneficent agent in many cases of disease, when the generalisation of homœopathy is accepted and made the basis of practice. Beginning with the criminal cases of it in the sixteenth and seventeenth centuries, it passed into therapeutics (though arsenical compounds in medicine were not known very much earlier), and to-day orthodox medicine regards it as a valuable "alternative," while it is an essential ingredient of compounds like atoxyl and salvarsan and more recent inventions designed specifically to exterminate certain parasites. The homœopathist notes with interest how frequently its " alternative " action (*e.g.*, in certain skin diseases) corresponds more or less closely to Hahnemann's doctrine, and finds much to discuss in the problem of the " great sterilisation " of salvarsan, though the early hopes of achieving that end have had to be much modified.

Knowledge of the effects of large doses of arsenic is considerable, derived not only from cases of criminal poisoning, but also from many accidental poisonings. Arsenical dyes, arsenical preservative solutions and contaminations from impure sulphuric acid (such as led to the poisoning epidemic of 1900, when the glucose used for cheap beer carried arsenic with it from the sulphuric acid employed in its manufacture) have been responsible for chronic body effects that are often difficult to diagnose, but once realised, are invaluable for the homœopathist. There are few drugs whose " morbid anatomy " is better known, and those who prefer to find a ground for their prescriptions in definitely damaged tissues naturally turn often to arsenic. The presence of the poison is easily recognised even long after death, and this fact has led to a great diminution of the criminal use of it.

Acute Poisoning by arsenic speedily produces constriction of the throat, gastric pain rapidly becoming violent and accompanied by vomiting and watery diarrhœa, the latter soon taking on the character of the typical " rice-water " stools of cholera, shreds of mucous membrane, disintegrating in a watery fluid. Stools and (more often) vomit may contain blood. The urine is diminished or even suppressed : muscular cramps, giddiness and headache accompany the other symptoms and collapse ensues, passing into coma and death, preceded sometimes by convulsions. These are the symptoms of a large dose, and already the homœopathist would be led to think of arsenic for Asiatic cholera and certain severe cases of enteric or other bowel affections. The remedy has often justified the homœopathist doctrine in such cases. Sometimes there are few symptoms but collapse and coma, and this again is a phenomenon not unknown in cholera.

Chronic Poisoning may follow a single large but not fatal dose, but more often is seen when arsenic is gradually absorbed, *e.g.*, from wall-paper (dust inhalation) or beer or wine. *The symptoms of chronic arsenic poisoning may be divided into three phases.*

At first the patient complains of general weakness, loss of appetite, nausea, vomiting and gastric discomfort ; at this stage constipation is more common than diarrhœa.

Presently the respiratory mucous membranes become affected : the conjunctiva inflames the surface of the nose, pharynx and larynx, so that coryza, sneezing, hoarseness and cough appear. Jaundice is occasionally seen. The skin is notably influenced ; the eruptions may be vesicular, papular or erythematous, but nearly always there is considerable formation of the epidermal scales ; pigmentation is usual, but is due neither to normal pigment nor to an arsenical compound, but to some other organic substance. The hair and nails fall off. Herpes is not uncommon and is to be associated with the other nerve phenomena characteristic of prolonged poisoning. There are persistent headaches and neuralgic pains.

" In the third stage, there are sensory and motor disturbances in various areas of the body."

First the nerves are irritated and formication, pain and variations in sensitiveness to heat and cold appear, while later, sensation is dulled or lost, and the gait may become ataxic therefrom. The motor nerves being irritated cause cramps and spasms, and later there is paralysis. If the spinal centres are affected they are only influenced secondarily ; the primary and important lesions are those of the peripheral nerves. The affected muscles degenerate so that recovery is very slow and sometimes partial. An apathetic, almost demented, mental condition has been observed from severe poisoning and also epileptic attacks have supervened.

The effects of increasing quantities of arsenic on mucous membranes are not corrosive, but resemble those of phosphorus. The cells show cloudy swelling and fatty degeneration, and the tissue is generally congested. Peyer's patches are special sites of arsenical action (*cf.* use of the drug in enteric). These signs are present in gastric and intestinal mucous membranes, however the poison is absorbed ; they are specific, not only

local, and the power of the drug to cause irritation and ultimately fatty degeneration of mucous membranes is clear.
The increased fluid (" rice-water " fluid) in the intestine appears
to be a result of vascular action. Small doses of arsenic given
to dogs increases the gastric secretion, and it is, to say the
least, noteworthy when the power of large doses thus to damage
and destroy these tissues is so certain, that small doses should
rightly have the reputation of encouraging digestion, for
although Arndt's generalisation as to stimuli is generally
admitted, only homœopathists (and Professor Schulz) consciously use it as a ground for prescription.

The heart is not obviously affected by arsenic, except that
in fatal poisoning the muscle degenerates. The blood pressure
falls (as arterioles dilate from effects of the drug on the muscle
coat) and more blood accumulates in the splanchnic area :
this is the ultimate cause of the increased fluid in the bowel.
The provings, where the arsenical absorption is very slow,
as will be seen, show a good many subjective cardiac symptoms
and the iodide of arsenic has a deserved reputation in some
chronic heart cases, but the iodide element without a doubt
counts for much in this action.

*In chronic arsenic poisoning eruptions on the skin are common
and appear to be due to the direct action of the drug on the skin.*
The tendency to proliferation of the epidermis with formation
of scales has been already noted. The growth in thickness
and cell multiplication may go on to epithelioma. Arsenic
has certainly the power to influence the body towards the
appearance of malignant disease.

There is some evidence that arsenic diminishes the number
of red blood cells, but it is not conclusive. *It appears to have
a direct action on the bone marrow. When arsenic is administered
to normal animals the bone marrow is found to be in a state of
increased vascularity, with a greater number of red blood corpuscles. It has been stated that in pernicious anœmia the
administration of arsenic increases the number of newly formed
red cells, though the number of mature cells is diminished. After
hœmorrhage, the blood appears to regenerate more quickly if
arsenic be given.* Persons chronically poisoned by arsenic are
usually anæmic, however, and seem to be more susceptible to
microbic diseases, especially if under-nourished.

It has been asserted that the leucocytes will absorb minute quantities of the red sulphide from the blood stream : this would suggest that arsenic might prove in small doses a stimulant to leucocytic action and it has been stated that phagocytosis is encouraged by the presence of minute quantities. It would follow that large doses would impede leucocytic action, and thus chronic arsenical poisoning cases might be less resistant to infections, having in mind the part played in resistance by the white corpuscles. Conversely, therapeutic doses should stimulate resistance, and since it is very doubtful if the action of arsenical preparations in malaria, sleeping sickness, or syphilis is that of a pure parasiticide (see below), the leucocytic stimulation may count for something when favourable results follow its use.* In fermentation of sugar by yeast, the presence of small quantities of arsenic definitely accelerates the process, while that of large quantities retards it. The drug does not encourage the multiplication of the yeast cells ; it is a stimulant to a function rather than to tissue building.

As regards general metabolism, small quantities of arsenic (like small quantities of phosphorus, but less intensely) accelerate autolysis : large doses arrest it by destroying the ferment. Fatty degeneration occurs in poisoning, not only in mucous membranes, but in liver and kidney, heart and other muscles, blood vessels and lung alveolar epithelium. If the fatty degeneration of the liver is considerable, pressure on the bile ducts may cause jaundice. Arsenic is excreted largely in the urine and may irritate and inflame kidney tissue in the process. Homœopathy finds it often useful in nephritis. It is said that under the influence of arsenic quantities of sugar can be assimilated, such as would normally cause glycosuria—but the mechanism by which this effect is produced is obscure.

A tolerance to arsenic can be acquired and the Styrian arsenic eaters are famous. They believe it improves their powers of respiration. The effect of it on complexion and hair (it is given to horses to improve their coats) is readily explained on Arndt's generalisation (homœopathically), for since large doses of the drug inflame the skin and damage it

* Enlargement of lymphatic glands has been found in arsenical poisoning cases and also enlargement of the spleen.

and cause hair to degenerate and fall, relatively small doses should stimulate skin and hair nutrition. The orthodox therapeutic use of arsenic for skin diseases is particularly noteworthy by the homœopathist, since it is for psoriasis, chronic eczema and lichen rubra that it is chiefly recommended, and on the whole these are the diseases it can most readily counterfeit. Homœopathic provings, as will be seen, endorse its use for asthma (when other arsenical symptoms are present) and its presumed effect on leucocytes is recalled by the use of it in lymphoma and leucæmia. Neuralgia and cachexia are among its effects and it is praised as a remedy for both. In chorea some physicians prize it highly : the lesser degrees of poisoning induce spasm of muscles but when large doses are given with cessation of symptoms the effect is more probably on the conduction of nerve impulses. When the case is one that in its whole complex suggests arsenic to the homœopathist, potencies (much too minute in quantity to produce any gross tissue effect) will cure chorea and their action can only be interpreted as a reversal (homœopathically) of the spasmodic effects of the disease poison by an agent itself capable of producing spasm.

Acute arsenical poisoning should be treated with prompt, copious and repeated washing out of the stomach. Chronic poisoning will tax the patience and resource of the physician, but sulphur and pulsatilla are often called for by the symptoms.

The general effects of arsenic are made by Professor Schulz the basis for its use in many conditions on his well-known view of drug action which so closely resembles a (somewhat) crude homœopathy. His own provings bring out many of the finer points of arsenic symptomatology similar to the homœopathist, and he treats with it not only neuralgias, chorea, malaria, asthma and chronic skin diseases, but also choleraic diarrhœas and cholera (using the arsenite of copper) and a variety of chronic conditions wherein he finds drug symptoms and disease symptoms to correspond.

Before, however, proceeding to homœopathic provings of arsenic and the therapeutics founded on them, the question of arsenic (especially of salvarsan and allied compounds) as a parasiticide must be briefly referred to. The use of this compound has unquestionably been of great service to sufferers from syphilis, but it is no great surprise to the homœopathist that many cases (and especially the severe cases from which salvarsan won its first laurels) should respond to arsenic, for on a purely symptomatological basis arsenic is often called for in this disease. Broadly speaking, arsenic corresponds more frequently for the homœopathist to primary syphilis and such tertiary symptoms as ulceration, while mercury is more likely to be indicated for the secondary stage (although arsenic may also be needed then) and although most followers of Hahnemann use low potencies of both drugs and continue the administration of them, yet in no case are large enough amounts given to make any parasiticidal action credible. In other words, here as virtually always, the homœopathist endeavours to stimulate a body reaction rather than directly to attack a body invader. In this connection it is of interest to recall that the older physicians were well aware of the value of arsenic in syphilis and Donovan's solution remains in use as evidence of their knowledge to this day.   Therefore, to Ehrlich and his followers the homœopathist is inclined to say : " Arsenic as a remedy for syphilis I value, and your preparation may have a special virtue, but before conceding your claims that it acts as a direct parasiticide I require much more evidence. If you can establish the fact, I shall gratefully employ the agent : indeed if I am convinced that its effect is à good one (better than I can otherwise obtain), I will use it thankfully, suspending final judgment as to its mode of operation.   But I note that you confess to certain risks in its use, from which at least my smaller doses are free and your claims for speedy and complete cures are not now made with that confidence that at first filled newspapers with rejoicing optimism.   Gone is the belief in the ' great sterilisation ' and instead we have statements as to parasites becoming resistant to arsenic to the point of invulnerability. Meantime one expert at least maintains that the drug effect is principally indirect and that commends itself to me on the grounds of much experience with drugs and their actions.   If the virtue of arsenic in syphilis is to stimulate a body resistance, as I more than suspect, I doubt if ÿour large dosage (with attendant risks) is needful : at least I add the comment that I frequently find arsenic called for on homœo-pathic grounds and suspend my judgment as to its value when not so indicated." Such in brief is the general attitude of homœopathy to the parasiticidal action of arsenic, in sleeping sickness and malaria, as well as in syphilis. When indicated by the symptom-complex as a whole, the homœopathist expects it to prove its value without any excessive dosage and attributes success to the body reactions aroused and encouraged by it. If not indicated homœopathically, he would doubt if mere increase in quantity of it would achieve a cure. Similar doubts attend the parasiticidal action of quinine in malaria and emetine in amœbic dysentery, and it is noteworthy that opinion thoroughly orthodox begins to question, as does homœopathy, whether the effect of either drug on its appropriate parasite be the sole or even principal cause of the undoubted success that often attends the use of each.*

The Homœopathic uses of Arsenic

The way is now clear to the consideration of the indications for the use of arsenic (arsenicum album unless otherwise noted) as a homœopathic remedy.

There are some grounds for thinking that arsenic acts more powerfully on vegetable-eating animals than on flesh-eaters : it is often useful correspondingly for ill-effects of excessive eating of melons, strawberries, etc., and for various disorders when affecting vegetarians. In this respect it is the opposite of nux vomica. The Styrian arsenic eaters are mainly vegetarians and they are said to believe that the arsenic which they swallow is the more needed by them because of the absence of meat from their dietary.

Arsenic is a profoundly acting remedy with a wide range of action : it meets both the most severe and also mild and trivial conditions. Where it is applicable there is to be found to a greater or less degree a restless anxiety and fearfulness which may even induce prostration. The patient is easily

---

* Since this was written arsenical preparations have multiplied and their multiplicity at least suggests that the ideal treatment has not yet been found. The general view of the homœopathist remains as stated above. Meantime bismuth is being largely used for syphilis in its later stages. It is not possible to claim much similarity for this metal as it is for both mercury and arsenic, although our provings of it are less extensive and there may be similarities of which we are as yet unaware. But our minds turn much more to gold and to silver for the late effects of syphilis, for similarities between drug and disease are there much more readily found.

exhausted even in trivial complaints and this gives rise to the characteristic irritability and weakness out of all proportion to the nature of the illness. It corresponds to constitutions that are very susceptible to cold and damp, especially to cold. Heat and sun or fire or clothes relieves symptoms of pain and discomfort, except for headache. The headaches of arsenic are relieved by cool air and cold applications, but apart from headache, the patient is shivering from the least exposure and desires heat.

The pains that indicate arsenic, whether definitely neuralgia or the result of gastritis, enteritis or whatever, are severe and unbearable and notably burning. This burning quality appears in the pains of sulphur and phosphorus also to a high degree, but there is no drug of which " burning " is more characteristic than arsenic. And the " burning " is relieved by heat, while sulphur patients are notably averse from heat and though phosphorus subjects are in general " chilly " folk, the stomach pains characteristic of this drug crave for cold food and drink and violently resent hot things. The troubles of arsenic, on the other hand, are relieved by heat throughout, with the one exception noted, of the headache. Thus, a dyspepsia that is caused or aggravated by ice water or ices will often find its remedy in arsenicum.

Hyperæsthesia of all senses is a feature of arsenicum, the patient is over-sensitive to everything : smell, touch, noise, excitement and external surroundings. This over-sensitiveness is projected on to the mentality of the patient who is characteristically precise, punctilious and fastidious.

Periodicity and a definite time aggravation of complaints is marked. Symptoms may recur every day, every third day, every week, and so on. There is weekly headache well known to brain workers, that recurs regularly at the end of the week when the tension of routine is relaxed, as though the bill for fatigue were deferred till the time of stress is temporarily over. Such a headache often yields to arsenic. The time of symptom aggravation in the twenty-four hours is at midnight and after, a little later than that characteristic of aconite. Pains, fevers and delirium are apt to worsen notably then ; asthma paroxysms habitually coming on between 12 p.m. and 3 a.m. often respond to arsenic. The time of onset of an asthma paroxysm or of any recurrent complaint is of great value as a symptom for the choice of the remedy.

The secretions and excretions of arsenic are not profuse but acrid, excoriating and unpleasant, so the discharge, be it from the eyes, uterus or lungs, tends to be irritating and offensive.

It is especially suitable to complaints of profound prostration, often out of proportion to the obvious tissue lesions and whenever patients are manifestly overwhelmed and exhausted in the struggle with disease, arsenic is a remedy to be considered. This is accompanied by intense fears, excessive anxiety, even anguish, great restlessness going on to prostration.

It must be remembered in considering the study of drug symptomatology that the intensity of a symptom is apt to vary in direct proportion to the severity of the illness, so that in a mild case, provided a symptom is clearly marked, it would be a good indication even if it were not present in a very high degree. Thus a chronic skin disease that in no way threatened life might have a sense of burning in the affected areas relieved by heat and this might be specially observable about midnight. There would be two indications for arsenicum and might determine the choice of it if other symptoms were also in agreement.

Again, in the more acute conditions there are anguish and intense fears. The greater the suffering, the greater the restlessness which is shown by continued tossing about, every movement being followed by exhaustion. In less severe conditions the patient is restless and, though not continually prostrate, easily and suddenly becomes exhausted. Hahnemann says in this connection : "That symptom of a not very important character and otherwise trivial affection induces a sudden and complete sinking of the strength." Thus, in very acute conditions the most intense anguish and fear is found, but even in illnesses of less severity the patient is still fearful. He fears the dark, fears being alone or going out alone ; there is a fear of anything unusual, and with these fears the patient finds comfort—if a child in the presence of his nurse or parents, if an adult by the presence of his friends. At the same time the candidate for arsenic is often of a suspicious nature and does not make friends readily.

The drug in its general picture corresponds to states so

frequently found in the more profound bacterial poisonings and produces on the healthy a definite state of fever with a daily rhythm or one of longer range. Thus it is a great remedy for enteric (varieties of paratyphoid, too), especially when the usual loose stools are present. Poisonings show its affinity for Peyer's patches. The constipated type of typhoid more often requires bryonia. Influenza ordinarily is too short-lived a disease to need arsenicum and seldom requires more than gelsemium or baptisia, but if a case drags on, arsenic symptoms may appear. Early tuberculosis often calls for it, when acute or sub-acute. Pneumococcal affections less often : here phosphorus, the congener of arsenic, is more likely to be indicated. In general it can be briefly stated that any quality of " malignancy " in any acute or sub-acute disease (measles, scarlet fever, diphtheria, enteric, etc.) should always suggest the use of this drug. The drug causes a rise of temperature comparable to that of all these conditions, as well as so many other symptoms apt to go with the fever. Hectic temperatures, if occurring without much formation of pus, often benefit from it. Considerable suppuration (e.g., empyemas) seldom show arsenic symptoms : as a rule, when arsenic is wanted, leucocytosis is not marked, even though in general it would be looked for in the disease in question. There may even be leucopenia. In more chronic cases, however (Hodgkin's disease, leukæmias, etc.), arsenic has a value, but these show not reaction leucocytosis, but pathological increases in white cells and the indications for arsenic are here more general, as also in pernicious anæmia. It is unfortunately true, however, that in these serious disorders, though arsenic palliates (considerably when well indicated), it seldom cures.*

Prolonged irritation from arsenic undoubtedly can cause epithelioma, and for the homœopathist it is an important cancer remedy. Whatever shall prove to be the mechanism of body resistance to cancer, unquestionably that mechanism is sometimes effective, since " spontaneous " recoveries from undoubted cancer multiply on investigation, however rare they are. If, therefore, the body can ever defeat this deadly disease,

---

* Since the introduction of liver therapy the greatly increased power to deal with pernicious anæmia also improves the " adjuvant " value of the similar remedy.

conceivably it can be helped to do so if the defensive mechanism can be encouraged, and since massive doses of arsenic tend to impede the mechanism, the homœopathist would expect small doses to support and stimulate it. Here, as always in medicine, there can be no routine treatment and the remedy indicated by the whole symptom-complex should be given, but cancer cases usually lack even a fair number of distinguishing symptoms, leaving the drug choice to be made on less assured and more empirical grounds. For the present it is very doubtful (in spite of many results of promise for the future) if the physician considers the chances of interference good. But the field of the physician, though thereby restricted, remains important. There are, unfortunately, inoperable cases, recurrences and others : these should be attacked, and though clearly they will be more difficult to deal with than the early cases entrusted to the surgeon, yet helpful results, if obtained, will be more significant. Secondly, surgical removal of a growth is not in itself a cure for the cause (problematical at present) of the growth : that cause, persisting, makes a tendency to recurrence which surgery can minimise perhaps but never eradicate. The physican, from the moment of operation, or before, should attempt to deal with this cause on the basis of the homœopathic generalisation. Such considerations have led the late Dr. George Burford to advocate the routine administration of arsenic for long periods after operation and his results as to nonrecurrence are encouraging. Probably indications should be sought for a closer adaptation of drug to patient. High as are the claims of arsenic, there are others to be considered, notably thuja and carbon and a group of vegetable remedies such as symphytum, ruta, ornitholgalum, lobelia erinus, etc. These last are mainly prescribed in occasional " unit " doses of tincture by the method of the late Dr. Cooper, who did most to find and fix their places in the Materia Medica and have apparently tissue relations of some significance. Dr. Burford advises the cacodylate of soda and gives appreciable doses persistently. If arsenic symptoms (general or local) were clear, potencies would almost certainly be preferable.

In the mental sphere, the patient who needs arsenic is both irritable and despairing : he shows anger, even fury, with hopelessness and misery. Many cachexias of serious disease produce

a combination of sadness and irritability and arsenic reproduces this (as well as the physical symptoms of cachexia) and
will aid it whether the cause be syphilis or tubercle, cancer or
malaria, or overdosing with such drugs as quinine or mercury.
No reader of the symptoms of chronic arsenical poisoning, outlined earlier in this article, can fail to see that arsenic produces
cachexia. The homœopathist concludes, therefore, that it can
relieve disease cachexias which show its characteristic symptoms and is justified by the results of such treatment.

Returning to the mental sphere, the angry melancholy that
belongs to arsenic has one pervading characteristic of restlessness. Even if delirium sinks into stupor, fits of restlessness will
occur and generally the patients constantly toss about shifting
their position and are anxious and filled with fear of death or of
worsening of their symptoms. These features recall aconite,
where is also restlessness and fear of death, but arsenic shows
none of the tension that goes with aconite. The patient's
power of reaction seems poor, his tension lowered rather than
raised, and it is seldom that the prescriber hesitates between
aconite and arsenic. The restlessness is often accompanied by
jerking spasms of groups of muscles, especially when the patient
is on the point of falling asleep. When, for instance, such symptoms appear in chorea, arsenic might be given with confidence
and other nervous diseases of an acute or sub-acute type often
need it, notably, of course, neuritis and neuralgia. It is less
often indicated in chronic nervous diseases of spinal cord and
cerebral tissues. Thus the mentality of the arsenic patient is
one of anxiety and restless fear. The sufferer cannot rest in any
place and changes his position continually. If strong enough,
he moves about from chair to chair or gets out of bed and sits in
a chair. If confined to bed, he tosses about, unable to find ease
or comfort. The restlessness is always followed by sudden
exhaustion which may go on to prostration. In very acute
conditions there is a sudden sinking of strength accompanied by
intense fears, as fear of death : the patient being bathed in a
cold sweat and soon becoming exhausted. In less acute states
calling for arsenic the patient is restless, always doing something and easily and suddenly tired out by his exertions. He is
" nervy " and frightened. He fears the dark, is timid of being
alone or going out alone.

The general hyperæsthesia is manifest in the mental sphere by a sensitivity to disorder in his external surroundings, so that any untidiness distresses him. The arsenic child is almost morbidly tidy, particular about the care of his toys or the soiling of his clothes ; the adult is equally fastidious and precise. The type of headache yielding to arsenic is frequently periodic in its occurrence and shows the general symptomatology just described. The pains are throbbing and burning, accompanied by anxiety and restlessness, though the pain is aggravated by motion and the head sensitive to touch. There is a definite time aggravation after midnight or about 3 p.m. Unlike the pains generally, the headache is ameliorated by cold air and cold applications. It should be noted, however, that neuralgia of the scalp has amelioration from heat.

Turning now to the more local symptoms of arsenicum, it must be noted that mucous membranes, peripheral nerves and skin are principally attacked. The effects on mucous membranes are similar, whether they are respiratory, gastro-intestinal, or genito-urinary. The tissue is violently irritated and ultimately inflamed and ulcerated : swelling and free secretion of pus are generally lacking : the surface is dry, sore and burning, the discharge watery and irritating. Thus, all inflammation of the eye is characterised by hot burning pains, excoriating lacrymation, frequently accompanied by photophobia and swelling of the lids. When these symptoms are present, it has been found useful in ophthalmia and inflammation of the cornea.

In the inflammatory conditions of the ear, similar burning pains occur. Otorrhœa is accompanied by a thin excoriating offensive discharge causing the skin of the ear to become raw and burning.

Again, acute coryza and hay fever requiring arsenic present a watery excoriating discharge. Violent attacks of sneezing occur which fail to give relief to the patient. Such colds frequently spread to the throat and chest. An acute coryza may be followed by a sudden attack of asthma. The coryza of arsenic is aggravated in the open air and relieved indoors. The arsenic patient takes cold easily ; he is chilly and always aggravated by cold damp weather which gives rise to the coryza as described.

As is clear from the accounts of arsenic poisoning and from the provings, the drug is especially applicable to cachectic conditions and thus the face presents a typical appearance. It is pale and puffy, even in fever, and definitely so in all conditions of the gastro-intestinal tract demanding this remedy. In the more acute conditions the face is pale, sunken, pinched and covered with cold sweat. The anxiety and fear, so characteristic of the drug, is depicted on the face which reflects the sufferings of the patient. In the acute conditions of children the same pinched and drawn expression is to be seen. The face looks worn and haggard : the child can be described as having the face as of an old man. Facial neuralgia, with burning tearing pains, accompanied by the general indications, relief from heat, a midnight aggravation, restlessness followed by exhaustion, is met by arsenic.

The alimentary tract is perhaps the most important of all the many sites of action of arsenicum, and meets many cases of acute gastritis, gastric ulcer and gastric carcinoma. The patient presents the general symptoms of the drug. He feels very ill ; he is restless, fearful and chilly.

The tongue is dry and cracked, seldom heavily coated, often red and angry looking. He usually craves cold drinks which aggravate his trouble, as does milk to a marked degree. The arsenic subject frequently craves fat.

Inflammation of the throat occurs, with the typical burning pain aggravated by cold and relieved by warm drinks. Arsenic is valuable as a remedy for the later stages of diphtheria when a typical condition applicable to the drug is to be found. The membrane looks dry and shrivelled. There is a burning thirst in such diphtheritic conditions, the breath is fœtid, there is restlessness, the patient may try to get out of bed, eventually profound prostration supervenes.

In conditions of the stomach requiring arsenic, this organ is irritable, often so much so that the least food causes distress, nausea and vomiting and may be accompanied by diarrhœa. Such digestive disturbances are brought on from exposure to cold, following drinking of ice-cold water, eating ice cream, or indulgence in watery fruits such as melon or strawberries. Very characteristic is a constant thirst for small quantities, preferably of hot fluids. " Little and often " is the thirst which calls for arsenic, cold drinks aggravate the pain. There is general relief from heat : external application of heat and warm drinks produce temporary amelioration. Thus, the most violent attacks of gastro-enteritis are met by arsenic when the characteristic symptoms are present : extreme irritability of the stomach which will retain but little ; burning pains : intense thirst, together with the anxiety, fears and restlessness going on to prostration. Arsenic meets many disturbances of the lower intestinal tract. Colic and burning pains prevail over the abdomen, accompanied by great anguish, inability to find rest or ease in any position, but with some amelioration of the pain from hot application and warm drinks. The stools are nearly always frequent and loose, seldom profuse, passed with violent pain and tenesmus : they are at first yellow or greenish, but become more and more watery. Blood may be evident and mucus and shreds of tissue. The attacks of diarrhœa are brought on by eating and drinking, especially cold drinks, the attacks occurring usually after midnight. The diarrhœa is preceded by the most violent burning pains and followed by extreme exhaustion.

Cholera, enteric, dysentery, colitis, all of these are conditions that may need arsenicum. Cramps are a feature of the drug and confirm the choice in many cases. In cholera and choleraic disorders when they are very severe indeed the arsenite of copper (*cf.* Professor Schulz) is particularly valuable. Finally, as regards the alimentary canal, the subjective sensations of provers suggest that the appendix region is a favourable site for the action of the remedy ; but the drug should not be chosen without some definite general symptoms of arsenic and these seldom appear at the beginning of this disease, while now that early operation is the rule (rightly) the grave conditions that might suggest it seldom obtain. Belladonna at the earliest signs and one of the serpent poisons (lachesis or crotalus) up to operation, and if necessary afterwards, are usually the most appropriate drugs.

The arsenic symptom-complex may apply to both acute and chronic nephritis though more usually the latter. In kidney conditions requiring the drug, the urine is usually scanty ; generally there is œdema accompanied by great thirst, an irritable stomach and the general symptoms of the drug.

The drug corresponds to many serious affections of the heart. Arsenic produces on the heart subjective symptoms of intolerable palpitation and irritability and has a real value in the last condition. But inasmuch as prolonged use of it tends to fatty degeneration of heart muscle, it is as a general remedy to encourage and make stable compensation that it is deservedly prized. To this end the iodide is frequently used. The drug appears to help compensation, and in young children with hearts crippled early by rheumatic fever such treatment persisted in with judgment over months and years seems of real and abiding benefit. The iodide element is here of considerable importance. Where the heart has been so affected by a rheumatic infection, the pulse is small, rapid and feeble : there is the usual prostration and anxious fear. It is useful in the irritable heart of excessive smokers and tea drinkers. In angina pectoris the agonising præcordial pain is attended by anxiety, difficult breathing, the attack occurring after midnight and aggravated by the least motion.

Many conditions of the respiratory tract find a remedy in arsenic. For example, it meets attacks of asthma brought on by exposure to cold changes of temperature, the attack occurring after midnight frequently presents arsenic symptomatology. The patient is pallid and has a sense of suffocation and burning in the chest. There is a dry wheezing cough, dyspnœa which compels him to sit up in bed, there is an anxious restlessness and the subsequent exhaustion always associated with the drug.

Arsenic is a drug of the utmost value in the later stages of pneumonia where the patient is seriously ill. The face is sunken, drawn and grey, the surface of the body is cold and covered with sweat : he is intensely chilly and wants to be covered, though the head may be unpleasantly hot for which he wants cold application. He is restless and consumed with fear. As the condition increases in intensity, the restlessness subsides and the patient becomes prostrate. He is then collapsed ; with pallid face, the lips blue and cold, the mouth and tongue dry and offensive. There is incessant thirst for sips of cold water. The cough, with offensive sputum, produces great exhaustion. Such a serious condition is liable to occur after midnight or in the early hours of the morning. It is then that the administration of arsenic produces a definite reaction in the patient who becomes less prostrate, less terrified and experiences a general improvement of all his symptoms.

In the locomotor system the prominent symptoms of arsenic are those due first to the irritation and then to the paralysis of the peripheral nerves, motor and sensory. Thus neuralgias (sharp, cutting and especially burning), twitches, cramps and spasms are prominent, also loss of sensation and paralysis. Whenever neuritis can be diagnosed, arsenic becomes of prime importance as a remedy : but here, as always, it acts in a very definite proportion to the degree in which the whole symptom-complex calls for it. The red sulphide seems a particularly useful preparation in this disorder. It may be remembered in epilepsy also.

Those who require arsenic are generally poor sleepers at night, because of the usual aggravation of symptoms from midnight onwards. But on the whole, drowsiness is a marked symptom of the drug and shows when the pain remits by day or by night. Sleep is unrefreshing and dreams terrifying ; but it is interesting, since sleeping sickness finds a remedy of some power in arsenic, that the drug should show in its pathogenesis a definite drowsiness, although probably the homœopathist would find it even better indicated in many cases by the general symptoms that underlie the grave nature of that severe affection.

Finally, the skin is a site where the action of arsenic is marked and persistent. Most often the eruptions are scaly (psoriasis, etc.), but urticaria, herpes, ulcerations (characteristically sluggish, with burning pain and scanty acrid secretion), papules and pustules, all of these have appeared under the use of it, and for all it may be indicated. All skin conditions requiring arsenic show, as a rule, intense itching and burning. Falling of the hair occurs in the pathogenesis and can be helped by the drug. Sweating (worse at midnight and after) is heavy as a rule when arsenic is required.

In all the numerous conditions to which arsenic is applicable, it is essential always to follow the general indications of the drug. The patient is chilly, worse in wet weather, from cold of every kind, cold food, cold drinks. He frequently experiences an aggravation of symptoms when near the sea. In all conditions (except headache) there is a general amelioration from heat. Lastly, arsenic is predominantly a right-sided remedy.

In the course of this discussion allusion has been made to various preparations of arsenic. Arsenious acid, arsenicum album, transcends by far in importance of every other compound. Of the remainder, the iodide has great value in chronic heart and lung conditions. All potencies of arsenic, high and low, are prized. Material doses of the cacodylate have been given for cancer.

Though an extensively used remedy, with a wide range of action, the patient must present the symptoms of the drug if success is to follow its use.

BAPTISIA
Baptisia Tinctoria.   Tincture of fresh root and its bark.

Baptisia is one of the important remedies introduced into the Homœopathic Materia Medica after the death of Hahnemann. It came very rapidly into use, because the indications for it are clear and because as they generally occur in acute or sub-acute diseases its value can be speedily tested and thereby established.

Baptisia corresponds to febrile complaints of a definite type, the fever that indicates either a slower or less effective reaction to infection or a more poisonous invasion than is the case, for instance, with the fever that calls for aconite. Its analogies are rather with bryonia, arsenicum or gelsemium, and indeed, either of the first two may be needed to complete the favourable reaction which baptisia may initiate.

When baptisia is indicated the patient from the first is obviously more or less overwhelmed by the invader. The onset of the disease is sudden, the patient rapidly becomes very seriously ill. Very shortly he becomes drowsy. His countenance is dark red with a besotted appearance, his eyes are bleary and his head aches severely. He is very restless and constantly tries to find a more comfortable position. He experiences great muscular soreness : the bed feels hard (cf. arnica, which does not, however, present the drowsiness, redness and besotted condition of baptisia).

The sweat is profuse and offensive, as are the discharges. The throat is dusky and may ulcerate and discharge an offensive mucus.

The patient is usually intensely thirsty, which may produce nausea.

Baptisia is therefore applicable to the treatment of serious acute fevers such as scarlet fever, diphtheria, influenza, typhoid fever and septic conditions of the blood.

There is great mental confusion and an inability to think. It may amount to stupor or suggest intoxication. The patient is drowsy and will fall asleep when being spoken to or when speaking. When aroused he attempts to speak only to fall asleep again in the midst of his answer. Concentration is very difficult, the mind wanders.

A curious mental symptom is very characteristic of the drug and in some degree is quite frequently encountered in practice if the physician is alert to notice it. It is a sense of a divided personality, expressed in a variety of ways : sometimes the patient thinks in delirium that his body is double or scattered in some way with the pieces retaining separate consciousness : or there will be a feeling of two contending wills. Naturally these illusions and sensations are heightened by the rising temperature and may go on into actual delirium. This is usually rather stuporous : the patient can be roused and will answer questions often vaguely or in such a way as to indicate the characteristic " divided personality," and then sink again into sleep. Yet there are indications through the heavy drowsy condition of considerable mental restlessness. It happens that R. L. Stevenson has left on record an account of a personal experience which gives a masterly description of phenomena, analogies of which are not seldom met with, though the sufferers from them have not the power either of analysis or of description to relate them clearly. The experience was during a bout of fever the result of an exacerbation of Stevenson's old enemy, tuberculosis. This fact makes the symptom more significant for such emergencies. Stevenson relates that every day as his temperature rose he became aware of a conception arising in his mind that his sufferings were caused by the failure to join the ends of a certain piece of string. If the ends were joined (so his self of fever averred), the whole of his troubles would end. Simultaneously, his normal " non-febrile " self knew that this was an absurd delusion and struggled to hold back the expression of absurdity. But not finally with success, for on at least one occasion he puzzled and distressed his wife by angrily asking in the person of his " febrile self " why she did not join the ends of the string and terminate the suffering. This is an admirable instance of a condition suggesting baptisia. Recent studies of personality have rendered familar (even to the popular Press) the conception of it as no longer one and indivisible, but as a compound of subliminal and supraliminal selves with the liability of the invasion of the supraliminal " normal " consciousness by " uprushes " (in Meyer's phrase) from the subliminal.* These " uprushes " are coherent and beneficent in the inspirations of genius, incoherent if not harmful, in delirium and madness. If, then, this conception, well fortified by many facts, corresponds to reality in the mental sphere, the brain as the organ of mind has presumably a condition or a structure which represents the " threshold " dividing subliminal from supraliminal, and now permitting, now inhibiting, uprushes. It is upon this structure or as influencing this condition that baptisia may be held to act, but only in the way in which the general circumstances of fever act upon it. The delusions and illusions of insanity are not often helped by baptisia, it is when the delirium of fever takes this particular form that the drug is so well indicated. When the " threshold " wears thin, as it sometimes does, as a result of overwork or mental stress, with any approach to actual insanity, the drug whose indications oftenest come to the surface is anacardium orientale. It also seems to act on this region or condition that constitutes the " threshold," but not in the " febrile " way of baptisia.

Side by side with the mental state of baptisia there are to be noted a variety of subjective and objective symptoms. Objectively the eyes are " bleared," the eyelids heavy, the countenance vacant with a dusky flush, almost besotted.

Subjectively, the head feels large and numb : there is a

* Modern psychology makes little or no use of Meyer's terms, but he was one of the very first to put forward an illuminating conception of personality and although the " subliminal " field has been much elaborated since his time the general idea of a threshold of consciousness is convenient for the discussion of the therapeutics of a number of remedies, notably baptisia and anacardium.

bruised, aching soreness of head, especially in the occiput, with drawing sensations in the muscles at the nape of the neck. The light tries the eyes, the lids may be even partly paralysed, the eyeballs are sore. The limbs ache, the back aches : numbness and soreness appear here also. The feet feel heavy and difficult to move, but it is a functional not an organic paresis. The pharynx is often inflamed and ulcerated. Baptisia meets certain serious diphtheritic conditions. The patient is stuporous, semi-comatose or delirious. The face is dusky ; there is a most offensive odour from the mouth ; there is great difficulty in swallowing solid food, only liquids can be taken ; but the throat is as a rule less painful than its physical appearance would suggest.

The tongue is swollen, dry, parched, cracked or ulcerated, with a yellowish-brown centre coat and a good deal of thirst, but no appetite. The tongue feels burned.

Nausea, retching and vomiting occur early with gastric and general abdominal pain, distension and soreness of the abdominal muscles. The right side of the abdomen is markedly affected. Empty sinking sensations are frequent. The stools are frequent, loose and very offensive. In abdominal affections requiring baptisia there is a foetid exhausting diarrhœa which causes excoriation.

Symptoms are worse on waking (as with the serpent poisons, which suit the profounder septic cases), worse on movement, worse from open air and cold. Numbness, soreness and drowsiness recur over and over again in patients that need baptisia.

When this well-defined symptom-complex is reviewed it will be no matter for surprise that baptisia has won such laurels in influenza and in enteric. It may be indicated also now and then in dysentery or colitis or ill-defined intestinal conditions, and it has been highly praised in some epidemics of small-pox when patients presented symptoms resembling the type of fever described. Its value in acute tuberculosis is considerable and from time to time other febrile disorders may present a case that calls for it, but influenza and the varieties of typhoid are the conditions wherein it leaps to the mind of the homœopathic physician. Not that it is to be used as a routine remedy ; its indications are clear, and unless they are present it is not likely to avail, but they are shown in these diseases with great frequency. If influenza exhibits much coryza or acute pain, gelsemium has claims, but the ordinary attack, with its weary aching and prostration, especially if gastric symptoms supervene, yields to baptisia with great rapidity and leaves much less weariness behind than when the drug has not been used.

The case for the use of baptisia in typhoid is founded, for any homœopathic observer, on the symptoms as detailed above. It is particularly valuable at the beginning of the disease ; even before the diagnosis is certain the indications often appear. Baptisia given then aborts a certain number of threatening cases, such as our predecessors used to call " gastric fever " or " low fever." It cannot confidently be claimed that all or even some of these would, if untreated, have proved to be typhoid, but a fact of great significance has recently been reported from America. Dr. R. Mellon,* working with young students, has shown that baptisia possesses the power of producing in the blood of healthy individuals as agglutinin which will agglutinate typhoid (Eberth) bacilli. Considerable doses are required to produce the phenomenon, but Dr. Mellon's experiments were conclusive as to its reality and definiteness. It was no mere shadow of a reaction that was produced, but one as clear and well marked as would more than suffice for a confident Widal reaction and diagnosis. From this experiment emerges the significant result that a drug which on grounds of general symptomatology is indicated homœopathically for many cases of enteric, is found to possess the power of producing an anti-body which can act as a specific resistance to the bacillus of enteric. The laboratory finding endorses the claim of the prescription from general likeness of symptoms between drug and disease.

One or two points suggest themselves for comment. First, although the agglutination reaction begins when regular doses of the $2x$ or even of the $3x$ are taken, it does not become unmistakable until the $1x$ and tincture are used and in large quantities. Yet cases of disease seem to respond favourably to drop doses of tincture or of potencies such as $3x$ or much higher. But it must be remembered that the production of

* Medical Century, 1914.

typhoid agglutinin is not normally part of the body's work and it may well be that in health a massive stimulus may be needed to encourage it suitably. In the provers, persistent dosing with the drug ended in a cessation of agglutinin production, that is to say, the power to make it was exhausted by over-stimulation. This is a result only to be expected, a simple illustration of Arndt's generalisation as to stimuli. In practice, baptisia produces favourable results in potencies, in other words, when the disease itself is making for agglutinin production, a very slight drug stimulus can encourage the process.

It might be deduced from this apparently specific reaction that all enteric cases should have baptisia as a routine treatment. But the homoeopathist, while agreeing that such a procedure would probably be generally useful, should seek for a symptomatological resemblance between the drug and the given case of disease before giving baptisia with full confidence. For the problem of recovery from an infective disease is not always simply and solely a matter of resistance to a given germ. The resistance may be effective enough and yet life, or at least health, be threatened through existing organic weakness and the temporary effect on it of disease. The point has been discussed in the introductory chapters : it is enough here to repeat that if the case requires baptisia symptoms will appear that call for it and if such symptoms are absent it is doubtful wisdom to give the drug on its laboratory virtue alone.

The cases of enteric fever requiring baptisia show the stuporous condition of the patient associated with the drug. There is restlessness and possibly a muttering delirium. The face is dusky, there is foetor of the breath and body, the stools are characteristically thin and offensive. In such conditions there is frequently to be found great sensitiveness of the right iliac region.

If given when not indicated it may conceivably check resistance process, which was going forward without it, and meantime, for lack of another remedy indicated by the symptoms, some serious damage elsewhere may occur.

The baptisia patient is notably aggravated by humid heat and when indoors, though there is an aversion to the open air. All symptoms are apt to be aggravated on awakening.

Rhus toxicodendron presents a good many symptoms similar to those that call for baptisia in enteric. It is desirable to test this drug also as to its agglutinating power. Other remedies that resemble it in much of its symptomatology are arnica, gelsemium, bryonia, echinacea, lachesis and nitric acid.

BELLADONNA

Atropa Belladonna—Deadly Nightshade. Tincture of whole plant when beginning to flower.

From belladonna are derived the closely allied alkaloids, atropine, hyoscyamine and hyoscine or scopolamine. These are also found in the drugs hyoscyamus and stramonium. It is consequently not wonderful that the three possess many points of resemblance, but the tinctures none the less give rise to symptom-pictures in provers which are by no means identical and the three drugs have been effectively proved but not the alkaloids (though some data exist for the use of atropine), wherefore the homœopathic physician relies on the well-tested tincture of belladonna, valuing, as usual, precision of indication beyond possible concentration of power. As, however, the alkaloids are largely preferred by non-homœopathic prescribers and are held responsible for the main actions of belladonna, it is important briefly to give an outline of their effects, which are at any rate important features of the drug symptom-picture.

Atropine is a stimulant to the central nervous system : that is the cardinal feature of its action. A dose of $\frac{1}{25}$ grain (which is a large dose) will cause in man the following symptoms : Marked dryness of skin and throat, thirst, difficulty in swallowing, hoarseness, nausea (sometimes vomiting), headache, flushed face (except during vomiting), and giddiness, the pupils dilate, the respiration quickens and the pulse rises to 100 or over. Redness of the skin is common and inflammation of the conjunctiva. If the drug is pushed still further, the pulse rate runs up exceedingly, restlessness and garrulity lead to confusion of speech and finally to maniacal delirium. In milder degrees, the delirium consists of pleasing illusions and delusions and of mimetic acting. The patient may carry out in dumb show simple actions like dusting, knitting, playing the piano, etc., accompanied by muttering and smiling. Marked muscular tremor and convulsions appear and gradually the stage of excitement passes over into a coma : "respiration and pulse become slow and irregular, the face pallid and death from asphyxia ends the story. Some such symptom-complex is seen as the result of accidental deadly nightshade poisoning, which is not so very uncommon. Oliver Madox Brown in the Dwale Bluth gives a very excellent description of it as seen by a layman with great power both of observation and description.

The cause of these symptoms is briefly a stimulation followed by a depression of the central nervous system. Unlike strychnine, which affects principally the spinal and medullary centres, atropine stimulates most the brain centres. Not reflex, but co-ordinated movements are made more active (speaking, etc.) ; reflex sensibility is also heightened, but this is much less marked a feature of the drug action. Yet the part of the brain affected is not so much that which rules the highest psychical function, but chiefly the motor centres. These being stimulated become less and less controllable and increased action follows until at last depression ensues as the result of over-stimulation.

Most secretions are diminished by atropine, saliva, gastric and pancreatic juice, mucus, sweat. This is the result of failure of the nerve impulses to these glands, not to an action on the gland cells. It is interesting to note that as far as salivary gland is concerned the action of atropine is on one set only of nerve ends (chorda tympani nerve ends, not sympathetic), a specialised action which is a good instance of the fact so well known to the homœopathist that drugs seem to pick and choose among bodily structures, sometimes with extraordinary precision. The secretion of bile is checked also and the conversion of glycogen into sugar. Milk is not affected : it is well known that this secretion is little controlled by the central nervous system.

Unstriped muscle (except in arteries) is affected by atropine. The pupil dilates as the result of unopposed sympathetic nerve action, the ciliary nerve ends being poisoned by the drug : at the same time power of accommodation is paralysed. In the bronchial muscle fibres atropine seems to paralyse the vagus nerve ends which cause contraction. In stomach and bowel, however, vagus and splanchnic nerves are unimpeded by atropine, but abnormal peristalsis (of non-vagal causation) is controlled by it. Large doses seem to increase peristalsis and may account for the vomiting and occasional purging of poisoned cases. Spleen, uterus and bladder also continue to respond to normal nerve stimulation after atropine, but are then immune from the poisons which otherwise induce violent contractions. Poisonous doses often produce a desire to micturate without ability to perform the act after preliminary emptying of the bladder as an early effect of the drug.

In the heart atropine inhibits the action of the vagus. There seems to be some direct action on the heart muscle which causes a preliminary slowing of the pulse. This is followed by acceleration, the vagus control being removed.

Sensory nerve terminations are depressed by atropine causing numbness, but the unbroken skin prevents local absorption.

Atropine causes a definite rise of temperature, perhaps from an action on the heat centres in the brain.

The gross effects detailed above will be recognised in the provings, but these also add the finer shades which clinical experience has elaborated into trustworthy indications for the use of the drug as a remedy. It must be noted again that tincture of BELLADONNA is the subject of the provings and contains more than atropine. For instance, among its mineral constituents phosphate of magnesium is prominent. Homœo-pathists know this as an agent to relieve pain when the general symptoms of the case correspond, and it is possible, seeing that atropine shows little power to cause pain even in large doses, that the undoubted efficacy of belladonna in certain painful affections is due to mag. phos. which it contains. This, of course, would not be the explanation of relief from it in, say (biliary) colic : there its successful action would have to be explained as a relaxation of spasm.

Primarily, belladonna acts on the brain ; unless symptoms of cerebral origin are prominent, it is not likely to prove the desired remedy for any complex case.* Herbivora (especially

* This does not apply to simple cases, e.g., ordinary sore throat.

the rabbit) are all but immune from its poisonous action, and it has been suggested that the explanation of this is to be found in the relatively poor brain development. It seems, however, more probable that in rabbits and other herbivora atropine is broken up in the blood by a mechanism that does not exist in carnivora or in man. It is, nevertheless, a good observation that the more mentally developed respond on the whole better to belladonna than do the less developed. Hufeland, Hahnemann's famous contemporary, even said that on idiots it hardly acted at all. It would, however, be a mistake to push this idea too far. The deep acting drug that corresponds most closely to belladonna is CALCAREA CARBONICA, which is notoriously often of extreme value in rather stupid children, though even here a qualification may be made, in so far as it is not so much congenitally stupid children that respond as those who suffer from mental deficiency as the result of disease. For instance, slight degrees of defect in thyroid secretion often become normal under calcarea and the slow backward child becomes intelligent (see calc. carb.).

Belladonna is on the whole a remedy of swift but not very prolonged action, suitable for acute and sub-acute disorders, especially applicable to the complaints coming on in vigorous and intellectual persons and bright precocious children. Such individuals are usually in an apparently good state of health and are attacked by an infection whose onset is sudden, the illness runs a regular course and subsides equally suddenly. Suddenness is the essential feature of all belladonna symptoms.

The most marked characteristic in its pathogenesis is hypersensitivity—both general and of the special senses. Every stimulus becomes almost unbearable ; light, noise and motion or jar will aggravate suffering. Response is very quick and the heightened sensation causes great alertness and irritability. Its general reaction to heat is one of relief : subjects that need it are chilly, made worse by cold air or applications, the head is notably sensitive to cold so that complaints requiring the drug are induced by exposure of the head to cold, even by washing the head or having the hair cut. There is general and local relief of symptoms from warmth. The pains developed in its provers are severe and of great variety, throbbing, burning, cutting, but all relieved by heat. It is characteristic of them to come and go suddenly and that they are paroxysmal. Paroxysmal pains relieved by heat resemble the pains produced by mag. phos. and it has already been suggested that possibly the presence of this mineral in belladonna is responsible for the causation of belladonna pain and the power of the drug to relieve it. It is also noteworthy that both mag. phos. and belladonna affect predominantly the right side of the body.

The pains that call for belladonna are often those accompanied and caused by acute local inflammation, and the classic signs, heat, redness and burning, appear notably in the belladonna pathogenesis. When the symptomatology of the drug is present it will modify or abort acute local inflammations. Over inflammations of the serous membranes, especially of the peritoneum, its remedial power is very marked. Acute appendicitis, salpingitis, or other pelvic peritoneal inflammation, whether operation be needed or not, will certainly benefit from its administration. When applicable to such acute inflammatory conditions, the characteristic picture, of course, must present itself. The attack is violent, the onset sudden with severe paroxysmal pain, high temperature, rapid full (not tense) pulse, bright red flushed face, dilated pupils and throbbing carotids. The exposed skin feels burning hot, though the covered parts are bathed in sweat. The pains (apart from joint pains) are often aggravated by lying down, which leads to attempts to move about unless the illness is very severe. The pains are aggravated by touch, movement and cold and thus in pleurisy the candidate for belladonna lies for choice on the sound side. There is little thirst, anxiety or fear as is found in aconite. The patient may pass into a semi-stuporous state frequently broken by sudden starts, cries and an outbreak of delirium.

Such a symptom picture as that detailed above may appear in many acute conditions and whenever characteristic will call for belladonna. The facts that with belladonna the pharynx is dry and inflamed and the skin shows a smooth red rash have naturally led to the use of the drug in scarlet fever, but it is an error to suppose that it is always indicated in that disease. It is necessary for the kind of symptom-complex to be present which has been described ; and the characteristic rash is the smooth, even, scarlet rash which does not appear in all scarlatina epidemics or cases. From the time of Hahnemann, physicians have believed that belladonna has a prophylactic value in epidemics of this disease : if the prevailing type is really similar to the belladonna pathogenesis, a prophylactic use of the drug is possible enough to make it worth while to give likely sufferers the benefit of the doubt. But it is neither proven nor even likely that it will ward off any and every infection of scarlet fever. To establish its value in this respect is far from easy. Experiments made at a big fever hospital in America were entirely negative as far as concerned the existence of any protective value as a result of the repeated administration of low potencies. But before the point can be regarded as finally determined further experiments are desirable. Whatever the protective body mechanism may be that wards off scarlet fever infection or modifies its virulence, it can only be by a stimulation of this (if at all) that belladonna possesses a prophylactic value. Presuming that it can stimulate this resistance, analogy to vaccines would suggest that the healthy should receive rather one (or two) large doses than repeated small ones. Conceivably also high potencies (in single doses) might develop resistance. Baptisia only causes the appearance of specific agglutinins in the healthy after large doses, and until belladonna has been tried as a prophylactic in full doses of tincture (one or two) or in high potencies, its claims cannot be finally dismissed.

In the mental sphere belladonna is characterised by symptoms of violence and excitement which may precede delirium. The excitement and agitation comes on during the fever : in the early part of the fever the delirium is very violent, but as the condition progresses the patient passes into a semi-comatose state, lying with a hot dry skin, red face, dilated pupils and throbbing carotids. The interesting symptom is recorded that the excitement and delirium is often ameliorated by eating a little light food. In his delirium the patient may jump out of bed, or is disposed to bite and strike those around him. Fantastic illusions occur, terrors and fear of imaginary things from which he endeavours to run away. There is starting in his sleep (especially at night ; the marked dread of darkness is characteristic of stramonium which has some resemblance to belladonna).* Acute mania sometimes calls for belladonna. The mania is furious, the patient attempts to bite or strike those around him, but is not obscene : the latter state is more often met by hyoscyamus.

Acute headaches are often much helped by this drug. Hyper-æmia of the head, with flushed cheeks, dilated pupils and a throbbing pain that comes on suddenly, lasts indefinitely and ceases suddenly : these are the characteristic features. The hypersensitivity of belladonna is manifest in the head pains which are aggravated by every movement, by light, by the slightest noise. The headaches are worse when lying down, sensitive to cold (cf. glonoin aggravated by heat), ameliorated by holding the head back and by gradually applied pressure. The pains of belladonna generally are aggravated by pressure, and so the scalp is sensitive to the least touch, but an amelioration of the head pains is experienced if gradually increasing pressure is employed, such as the application of a bandage.

The headache in the early stage of meningitis is met by the drug. The intense pain is accompanied by the hot head, flushed face, throbbing carotids, bright eyes, frequent full pulse, nausea and thirst. Spasms and twitchings are frequent symptoms of convulsions. If exanthemata in children begins with violent convulsions, belladonna is often the remedy to give the case a good start. Paroxysmal spasm and convulsion of cerebral origin are so characteristic of belladonna that it is naturally thought of in epilepsy and to the prominent symptoms of an attack it can show a close parallel in its pathogenesis. The attacks are preceded by a hot heat, flushed face and throbbing carotids and followed by nausea and vomiting. It is not, however, a deep acting remedy in such cases so that its undoubted value is mainly in quite recent cases or as a temporary aid to diminish the frequency of attacks. It is usually desirable to follow up the treatment of the condition with remedies of deeper action.

With the special senses, the dilating effect on the pupil is well known. Acute conjunctivitis with little secretion may be

* The delirium of belladonna is violent and is accompanied by intense burning heat, redness of the face, the fever is remittent. The delirium of stramonium is similarly violent, accompanied by some heat and redness, but is found in continuous fevers ; in that of hyoscyamus there is little or no fever, little violence, the face of the patient is pale and sunken.

helped by it ; the inflammatory conditions of the eye are accompanied by heat, redness, burning and intense photophobia. The sudden onset of strabismus in acute affections of the brain with flushed face, dilated pupils, throbbing carotids may be met by this drug.

The mucous membrane of the nose, mouth and throat is made dry and burning by belladonna, though coryza with much sneezing occasionally occurs. It is especially applicable when the sudden stoppage of a coryza is followed by a general sense of burning, marked headache, hot head and cold extremities.

Inflammatory conditions of the ear which proceed to suppuration rarely indicate belladonna, but sudden attacks of acute otitis media with the general symptoms of the drug are controlled by the remedy. Reactions to sense stimuli are generally heightened. Two cases of poisoning resulted in complete deafness. This was almost certainly due to a central cause and Dr. Cooper reported some success in chronic nervy deafness with belladonna in " unit " doses.

The mouth is dry and parched with thick viscid saliva. The tongue is red, dry, hot and cracked with the papillæ erect, sometimes coated, especially in brain affections. Toothache from inflammation, with redness and swelling of the gums, often obtains relief from belladonna when pain is violent, paroxysmal and relieved by heat.

The throat is bright red, dry (even glazed), burning and painful : swallowing and talking are alike painful, as is swallowing, especially the swallowing of fluids. The early stages of acute tonsillitis where the tonsils are bright red, swollen and intensely painful, the pain relieved by heat, may be checked by belladonna. Follicular tonsillitis generally needs phytolacca or mercury, diphtheritic cases cyanide of mercury, lachesis or lycopodium. There is a craving for lemons and lemonade which frequently proves beneficial. With the thirst there is sometimes considerable hunger. Acute gastritis occurs often, brought on by exposure and accompanied by general distress, burning pain aggravated by the slightest movement or pressure and relieved by bending forwards. With this is often associated nausea and vomiting ; these latter symptoms being amongst the most persistent effects of the drug.

The abdominal pain is severe, burning and cutting and the

distended abdomen is very sensitive to touch or even to jarring of the bed. It may be accompanied by vomiting. Sudden attacks of infantile colic which appear and leave suddenly are relieved by belladonna. There is fever, the face of the child is hot and red and the pains are relieved by bending forwards or firm pressure.

The patient who requires belladonna is more often than not constipated. Spasm of the anus and tenesmus are common symptoms ; sometimes there are attacks of diarrhœa with frequent small loose stools, marked straining, with heat, redness and burning in the face ; hot head and cold extremities. Hæmorrhoids are intensely painful, red, swollen and inflamed and very sensitive to touch.

In the genito-urinary sphere belladonna is useful for incontinence of urine (though in enuresis of children calcarea is usually of more permanent value for the cases whose type suggest belladonna). Spasmodic retention will benefit from it when other symptoms agree. The inflammatory conditions of the bladder are accompanied by tenesmus and burning scanty urine.

It has value for spasmodic dysmenorrhœa where the pains come and go suddenly. There is general sensitivity ; the pains are aggravated by excitement, movement and jarring. The menses are likely to be premature and profuse, the flow bright red and hot as it passes. Whether this is due to the actual heat of the blood, or (more likely) to sensitiveness of the parts, it is in conformity with the hyperæmic condition induced by and curable by belladonna. Sharp pain appearing to start in the vagina and shooting upwards, internally, is a well-known and trustworthy confirmation in the pains of pelvic hyperæmia, whether menstrual or other. It is helpful in the spasmodic ineffectual labour pains if other symptoms confirm the choice. It controls uterine hæmorrhage whether from congestion or other causes when the usual symptoms of sensitiveness are present. The patient herself is generally sensitive and excitable, sensitive to touch, to jarring, the whole condition often accompanied by fever. The " bearing down " pains present in conditions of prolapse are often aggravated by lying down and relieved by standing.

Soreness of the vulva and vagina associated with free secretion calls for other remedies, but where acute, dry and sensitive belladonna may be very useful for a few hours to control inflammation of these parts as in the early stages of vulvitis, vaginitis and urethritis, specific or simple.

The power of belladonna to cause local congestion leads to hæmorrhage with some frequency in its pathogenesis : various bleedings (uterine, hæmorrhoidal, nasal, etc.) appear.

It is valuable in acute inflammatory conditions of the breasts. The patient is restless, sensitive, the face flushed and fever is present. The breasts are acutely painful, sensitive to touch, all movement aggravates the pain.

In the respiratory tissues the effect of belladonna on the nose in drying up secretion and causing irritations is continued into the larynx and trachea. Consequently it becomes a remedy for laryngitis with a dry, tickling, spasmodic cough and with a sense of constriction and painful stitches in the chest : the cough is excited by any touch on the larynx, by the slightest attempt to talk, by every movement. The onset of the condition is sudden, the cough is worse at night ; some relief is experienced after a paroxysm of coughing which may end in an attack of sneezing (cf. Sulphur). The orthodox prescription of the drug in whooping cough could often be justified on grounds of homœopathicity.

Pleurisy cases may suggest belladonna as do certain definitely developed pneumonias in the early stage. The typical condition requiring the remedy usually occurs in robust people following exposure. This history is very similar to aconite, but the intense anxiety and fear of the latter is not usually found in belladonna. The patient, on the contrary, is excited, hypersensitive to light and touch and violent delirium may supervene. The skin is dry and intensely hot, the puplis dilated, the patient feels hot and may complain of a burning heat ; the tongue red and very dry. The cough is dry and the sputum stained with bright red blood. The hyperæsthesia of belladonna is notably found over the affected chest and the patient cannot lie on the affected side. Some of the dyspnœa of belladonna is due to its action on the heart : symptoms that call for it here are tachycardia and violent palpitation. Asthma cases are not often of the general belladonna type, but the drug should not be forgotten when the spasmodic element is predominant and there is little or no bronchitis. The tachy-cardia suggests also its use in Graves' disease and it can show tremor in its pathogenesis and some indication of its effect on the thyroid gland. It has been used in the 1*x* potency for extreme degrees of thyrotoxicosis. Nevertheless, the use of it is seldom efficacious in this disease, for such resemblance as there seems to be is really superficial and the disease has, as a rule, too profound a causation to be much influenced by a drug of (relatively) brief and shallow action.

In the nerve-muscular sphere the neuralgias characteristic of belladonna have been mentioned already. The patho-genesis shows many pains in joints and limbs, with cramps and tremors : the pains are severe and show the sensitiveness to external stimuli characteristic of the remedy. Its use may now and then be suggested in rheumatic fever from sudden exposure to cold in plethoric individuals, or in sub-acute rheumatism or gout. Many or all of the joints are swollen, hot, red and burn-ing. The joints are sensitive to cold, uncovering and to draught, and are relieved by warmth. Although the general reaction of belladonna is that symptoms are made worse by rest, this does not apply to joint pains which are aggravated by movement, the patient must lie perfectly still. In these rheumatic condi-tions there is considerable fever and copious sweat on the covered parts of the body.

The effect on the skin is to cause an erythema which may assume an erysipelatous appearance. Local redness, swelling, heat and pain are all belladonna symptoms and it has a real value in acute skin inflammations (erysipelas, etc.). As stated previously, it is also applicable to the scarlet fever where the eruption is perfectly smooth and scarlet.

Laboratory evidence of its power is lacking as yet, but from the pathogenesis and clinical evidence it is quite probable that it would be found to have a specific influence on at least some varieties of streptococcus.

In general, belladonna is indicated in acute illnesses with marked excitement and violent reaction. There is a great tendency to hyperæmia of parts and general sensitiveness to external stimuli. The time of greatest suffering is usually at night rather than by day, although from three to four in the afternoon (earlier than with lycopodium) there is frequently a secondary time of exacerbation of symptoms. The excitement passes into a semi-stupor for a time, and on the whole there is a good deal of somnolence in cases that call for the drug : the patients start from sleep or have terrifying dreams and the stupor is broken by paroxysms of violence and excitement, but in the course of twenty-four hours a considerable amount of sleep is usually obtained.

The fevers are not continuous but remittent, so the drug is often required in inflammatory, catarrhal, rheumatic and puerperal fevers. The violent delirium of typhoid is not fitted by belladonna, Stramonium is usually the indicated drug. In the fevers, the skin is dry and burning, sweating chiefly or only on covered parts or amid thick hair. The head is nearly always hot, with a flushed face : the feet may be cold. It may be repeated that when belladonna is required the head symptoms are always prominent, often they are the first to appear (headache, etc.) and the other parts of the body are affected later. In spite of the signs of local congestions, patients who need belladonna are generally chilly and like hot applications and external heat.

Belladonna follows aconite well : the deep acting drug, calcarea carbonica, has a very close relationship to it, which has already been sufficiently emphasised, and whenever a case has responded well to belladonna, calcarea should be thought of to complete its action. It is interesting to note that belladonna grows best in dry limestone soils.

BRYONIA

Bryonia alba. Tincture of root gathered just before flowering. Bryonia dioica is the common English plant, and has been used with such success on the indications for bryonia alba that the properties of the two plants are probably nearly identical, but as the provings are of bryonia alba, it should be preferred.

Bryonia was in use in Hahnemann's day as a drastic purgative and a line or two is given to it occasionally in modern text books emphasising this use. Also it appears sometimes in drug lists with recommendations to be used for pleurisy and arthritis. As will be seen, its provings and homœopathic experience amply confirm its value in these spheres and the recommendations are probably unconscious echoes of homœopathic therapeutics. It seems to have been a favourite remedy of Hahnemann, its provings are good and clinical experience of it very wide, so that its spheres of action can be defined with confidence.

There are five characteristics of bryonia that stand out prominently. The first is the intense aggravation from any movement, even the slightest. Not only muscular movement aggravates the pains of the bryonia patient, but what may be called exercise of the nerve centres ; in other words, mental exertion is distressing to the sufferer, and in bryonia cases headache, sleeplessness, fever, will all be aggravated by any attempt to use the higher brain cells. The typical bryonia patient cannot bear to be disturbed.

This modality is so constant as to be an outstanding general symptom of the drug. Whatever the condition, movement aggravates it.

In arthritic cases, in pneumonia, in pleurisy, whenever, in fact, bryonia is indicated, it will be found that the patient instinctively shrinks from any movement and finds suffering much increased by it. This is true of involuntary movements, like those of ordinary inspiration, when the pain is in the chest. A corollary to this is a relief from pressure which tends to keep the affected part at rest. Thus in pleurisy that calls for bryonia the patient will prefer to lie on the affected side, so as to fix it as much as possible and limit its movement. Precisely the opposite condition is true of belladonna, where the patient prefers to lie on the unaffected side.

Dryness is the second characteristic. There is a dryness of the serous and mucous membrane and the secretion is scanty. The mouth is dry, the dryness of the intestinal mucosa causes hard, dry, dark stools ; in respiratory conditions the cough is hard and dry. The character of the pains are stitching, sticking pains. The times of intensity of the symptoms are about 9 p.m. and in the early morning (3 a.m.).

Lastly many of the bryonia complaints are worse or brought on from exposure to cold, dry winds, like the typical east wind in this country.

There is a very definite type of fever which calls for bryonia. Sometimes in the beginning the symptoms of it will have suggested aconite, but though this drug may have given some relief, the fever will continue and presently the typical aconite features will disappear and the choice come to be rather from among bryonia, rhus tox., arsenicum, etc. Bryonia follows aconite well and will often continue its work satisfactorily. In other cases bryonia may be indicated from the beginning. Typical influenza fever more often finds its counterpart in gelsemium or baptisia, but now and then bryonia is called for. Pneumonia cases often require it and enteric typhus cases. It will be clear from this sentence that the drug is suitable to fevers of a profounder kind than those that react to aconite, to conditions which may begin somewhat insidiously, but gradually worsen till the typical bryonia symptoms may appear early in rheumatic fever or pneumonia or pleurisy.

The typical bryonia patient is dark complexioned and dark haired. There is a tendency to bad temper and irritability is the characteristic mental state. He will not talk if he can help it, every effort annoys him. In acute complaints he is irritable and dislikes being disturbed. When well developed the condition is as follows : the patient lies like a log, avoiding the least movement ; the senses and intellect seem dulled and any attempt to rouse the mind seems to aggravate the condition. This makes the sufferer very resentful of any interference or questioning, intensely irritable and averse from talking. There may be fits of anger. The memory is weak and attempts to remember cause distress. At night there will very likely be delirium (usually of an active type) or broken sleep and both delirium and dreams are very likely to be concerned with the affairs of the day or the patient's business and immediate personal concerns. The irritability and weakness of the mind appears characteristically (especially in children) in the form of vague inconstant desires for something which the patient fails to define. He wants something, but cannot make clear what it is. Throughout, the intense aggravation of sufferings from any movement persists. Thus despondency and moroseness are keynotes of the mental condition. With this ill-humour and peevishness there is often a degree of anxiety and fear. Fear of death and despair of recovery are sometimes found in the emotional state.

The headache that indicates bryonia is a severe pain, dull and throbbing with acute sharp stabbing pains at intervals, especially after movement. It is largely felt over the eyes and is relieved by hard pressure and cool applications. The head-ache usually accompanies the fever, but there is a frontal headache characteristic of bryonia in non-febrile cases, often associated with dyspepsia, at its worst in the early morning, much aggravated by movement and especially by stooping. All exertion, even the effort of thinking, of body and mind, intensifies the pain. It is a throbbing pain and recalls in its features the headache of Natrum Muriaticum, which is to some extent a chronic counterpart of bryonia. Febrile patients are naturally thirsty, but the thirst of bryonia cases is charac-teristic, being for large quantities at fairly long intervals ; with arsenicum, on the other hand, the thirst is for small quantities frequently. There is usually profuse perspiration, often sour, after the least movement, when bryonia is called for. The mouth is dry, the tongue coated white or yellow down the middle (the edges may be clean) ; the lips are dry and cracked. Bryonia in febrile complaints comes often to be considered in pneumonia and rheumatic fever (in both of which it can claim attention on the score also of local symptoms, as will be seen), and in influenza, meningitis (rarely), enteric and typhus fever. In the last named Hahnemann valued it extremely and the bryonia type of fever is perhaps more exactly met with in that disease than in any other. The enteric cases that call for it are generally among that relatively small percentage wherein the sufferer is constipated. Typical cases with loose stools more often need arsenicum ; the char-acter of the bryonia bowel symptoms will be described presently.

The brunt of the onset of bryonia, as far as tissues are concerned, falls upon serous membranes and fibrous tissues generally. Thus bryonia may be called for in meningitis or peritonitis, but especially in pleurisy. Pains are sharp and stitching and worse from the least movement. The dry cough and general symptoms of pleurisy will often find their counter-part in bryonia provings and even if effusion has occurred it may still be the remedy needed, though it is most efficacious when given early. The patient lies on the affected side to limit the chest movement as already noted. Bryonia will also benefit many cases of pneumonia ; its characteristic general symptoms will give the clue to its use and locally the presence of any pleurisy is a strong additional indication. Usually the onset is not acute, the patient feels unwell for a few days. When the bryonia state is well developed, the patient is heavy looking and dusky in appearance. The lips become dusky, dry and cracked, with a tendency to bleed. The mouth is dry and the tongue dry with a thick white coating. Intense thirst is always present. The mental state characteristic of the drug is found. The patient desires to be let alone, he does not want to move and is averse to being disturbed. The patient may even resent having to ask for anything. Movement aggravates the patient in every way and brings on stabbing pains in the chest. The pain is relieved by pressure and the patient prefers to lie on the affected side, which is usually the right side. Cold in every form relieves the condition. He feels better in cold air and from cold applications but occasionally the reverse applies. If delirium supervenes a delusion of being away from home may accompany the condition. The sputum is the typical rusty sputum of a well-developed pneumonia. It is a remedy for lobar pneumonia, seldom for broncho-pneumonia, and for pleuro-pneumonia most of all. If the pleurisy turns to empyema the case seldom calls for bryonia ; it seems to have little power in checking suppuration.

Bryonia affects the muscles, making them sore and irritable. Probably it is upon the fibrous supporting tissue that it acts ; it also affects fascia. But in the motor system its power is chiefly shown upon the joints. It causes acute synovitis, with pain, redness, heat, swelling from effusion, all the symptoms of acute joint trouble and aggravation from any movement, as always, is marked. The great distinction between bryonia and rhus in joint and muscle disorders is that when rhus is needed, though the first movements may be painful, continued movement gives relief. In view of this definite power to affect joints (small and large, but large rather than small, on the whole), bryonia is naturally a great remedy for acute rheumatism, and the heavy, sour perspiration which it can cause forms an additional point of resemblance.

It is usually (especially when general as well as local symptoms are present) a very speedy and satisfactory remedy and shows its curative power by minimising the risk of serious heart affections. Pericarditis will often need it and respond to it. As compared with the usual salicylate treatment, homœopathists find that bryonia will relieve pain if not as quickly yet more permanently, but it is true that cases are met with wherein bryonia seems reasonably well indicated, yet fails to act. These are not, however, very common. At the same time, every case must be individualised, and there are many drugs with great power to influence joint structures (rhus, spigelia, pulsatilla, sulphur, guaiacum, etc.), so that in all cases good symptomatic grounds should exist before a confident prescription of bryonia is made.

Besides its marked action on the chest and the joints, bryonia affects notably the alimentary canal and the liver. Indeed, it has been held that its main effect is exerted here. It is often indicated in meat eaters (the so-called " gouty ") and its power to influence arthritis may conceivably be secondary to its power over metabolism, rather than directly over any associated microbic infection or virus. Both the heavy perspirations and the thirst for large quantities of water which suggest bryonia in such subjects may be indications of attempts at excretion of excessive waste products. There is no clear evidence that it inflames the gastric or intestinal mucous membrane, although it may fasten on the fibrous supporting structures. It unquestionably affects the liver, there too, probably, by the road of the fibrous capsule and interlobular supporting tissue. A certain degree of jaundice is not uncommon and pain and discomfort in the liver region are generally prominent in bryonia subjects. The general result of its action on the alimentary canal and allied glands is shown in the following symptoms. There is a foul, yellowish, coated tongue (like " wash-leather "), with an appetite often capricious and for unusual things. Bryonia patients are often coarse feeders. There is the characteristic thirst for large quantities at long intervals. Though the desire is usually for cold drinks, the stomach condition itself is relieved from warm drinks.

Although the pains of bryonia generally are relieved by pressure the opposite modality is found in gastric complaints. The epigastric region is painful to touch and pressure. The patient desires to be perfectly still with the knees drawn up in order to relax the abdominal muscle. The face is flushed after meals and a chronic frontal headache appears, aggravated

by meals (and especially also by bending forward). Food
appears to the patient to be " like a stone " at the epigastrium ;
there is nausea, water-brash, bitter and sour eructations.
Belching of flatulence relieves gastric discomfort temporarily.
Pressure and dull pain appear in the right hypochondrium and
often a yellowish tint to the conjunctivæ, though seldom any
marked jaundice. The secretions of the digestive glands in
the stomach and of the bile seem to be affected. The bile is
either increased in quantity (in which case there is diarrhœa,
worse in the morning, worse on movement, worse in hot
weather), or more frequently diminished, when there is constipation of a characteristic type, large, dry, hard, crumbling
stools, brown or black, almost as if burnt. All alimentary
canal symptoms of pain and discomfort are aggravated by any
movement. This is the unfailing characteristic of bryonia. The
symptom-picture thus outlined is one that occurs frequently
in so-called " gouty " dyspepsia, and bryonia is invaluable in
many such conditions. It is less often indicated in gastric
or duodenal ulcer, though, as already stated, its power over
enteric fever is considerable. Its action on serous tissue gives
it an influence on the peritoneum, but the varieties of peritonitis
do not very often present the typical bryonia symptom-
complex.

In the respiratory sphere its curative influence over pleurisy
and pneumonia has been commented on. It has also value in
laryngitis and tracheitis. The vocal cords are inflamed, but
bronchial mucous membranes (and nasal) escape its influence,
so that it does not come prominently forward as a remedy for
bronchitis. Typically there is hoarseness, with a dry cough,
often an inclination to draw deep breaths, then stitching pains
(worse on inspiration) commence, and the respiration grows
short and hurried. There is tickling in larynx and trachea,
often referred to a point low down behind the sternum. Expectoration is scanty and may be blood-stained ; it is raised with
some difficulty. The drug meets many influenzal and pneumococcal infections of the air passages. There is little evidence
of power over tubercle. Among other symptoms, bryonia
causes mastitis and is often valuable for this trouble. A pain
in the left ovarian region seems a genuine symptom, relieved
by lying on the affected side.

Most bryonia symptoms are aggravated by warm rooms, warm weather, or getting warm. Thus the typical dry cough will come on after entering a warm room and be relieved on going into the cold air. Phosphorus shows exactly reverse symptoms. Warm food is disliked and the large draughts of cold water craved for often seem to relieve, except in the case of dyspepsia symptoms. Joint pains are sometimes relieved by heat, but many joint conditions show the opposite modality and find amelioration from cold. The general relief from cold applies even to the mentality. The anxiety, confusion and fear of bryonia are relieved by cold air, cold applications and from being cold. There is general aggravation from eating. Sweating ameliorates all complaints and with the exception of stomach and abdominal conditions, pressure relieves. The time of intensity of symptoms are about 9 p.m. An early morning aggravation is frequently experienced. For example, a patient who has been feeling unwell for several days, wakes up in the early morning generally ill and presently develops a fever.

Natrum muriaticum is a chronic counterpart of bryonia and alumina also has many points of resemblance. Calcarea and bryonia are somewhat inimical and follow one another badly. The drug has been praised and valued in all potencies from the tincture to the highest.

CALCAREA CARBONICA

Calcarea Ostrearum. Triturations of the Carbonate of Calcium existing as the soft white substance between the hard layers of oyster shells. Higher potencies also made by tinctures.*

This is one of the greatest remedies of the homœopathic pharmacopœia, invaluable especially in the treatment of children. The effects of calc. carb. are nearly all due to its calcium, a metal well known to non-homœopathic physicians as a poison, though comparatively little therapeutic use is made of its specific properties by them.

Calcium is a normal element in the body and in bones and

* Hahnemann chose this source of lime for his preparations with the conception, so familiar to older medicine, that a mineral produced in the course of life, by a " vital " reaction, would be specially suitable to influence living bodies. It is a not quite pure carbonate of lime.

teeth it is present in quantity. It is also essential to metabolism. It is slowly absorbed from the alimentary canal and if large doses are given most of it passes away unchanged, but small quantities of even insoluble preparations are taken up. It is also slowly excreted : when there is any excess of it in the body the surplus seems to be withdrawn from the circulation in some way and gradually returned for elimination, but the calcium content of the blood may remain high for some time (e.g., after an injection of a calcium salt). It is excreted through kidney and large bowel, chiefly from the latter, in the form of insoluble phosphate. Consequently, phosphates need to be freely available if this mode of excretion is to proceed.

There is some uncertainty as to the remoter effects of calcium as far as regards the details of its action. As will be seen presently, the symptomatology that suffices the homœopathist for a prescription of the drug is full and reasonably precise : it is the interpretation of the symptoms in terms of cellular activity that is obscure. The neuro-muscular connections in striated muscle appear to be weakened by calcium and later the muscle itself. Constipation is often a sequel of its administration and is possibly due to a nerve-muscular action on the involuntary muscles of the bowel. The heart action is first strengthened and later stopped by calcium and its salts make the blood vessels contract when passed through them. It has been stated that tissue cells become less permeable under the influence of calcium, so that a tendency to œdema can thereby be lessened : this is not established yet as a fact, but homœopathists certainly find that the tendency to urticarial eruptions is a good indication for calcarea.

The effects of lime in excess are, therefore, as yet not fully explained. Those of lime starvation, however, are better known. They are most marked over young growing life and resemble the effects of rickets and osteomalacia. Less lime is deposited in the bones. Both heart muscle and skeletal muscles seem to require the presence of calcium for full efficiency and suffer in the absence of it. The ova of various organisms (e.g., frog) will not develop if there is no lime present in the water in which they are. Rennet will not coagulate milk (nor will blood coagulate) in the absence of lime salts. The action of the lime in the latter case is concerned with the fibrin ferment, which cannot be developed without it. Because of this action, lime salts (especially calcium lactate) have been given by the mouth to increase blood coagulability when the property is deficient.* It has been both asserted and denied that this practice is effective : homœopathists know hæmorrhages of certain kinds and qualities to be indications for calcarea and to be remedied by it, and it is natural to connect its controlling powers with its relation to blood-clotting. But it would be the instinct of the homœopathist only to expect calcarea to be effective as a remedy when the totality of the symptoms called for it and not only the one symptom of hæmorrhage. The divergence of opinion as to the effect of calcium lactate by the mouth may conceivably be explained by realising that if the subjects to whom it was given were in need of the drug constitutionally, they would respond to it and otherwise not. In any case, in homœopathic hands, calcarea acts in potency when well chosen and its action in such cases cannot be dependent on its mass.

Other ferment actions (*e.g.*, digestive ferments) also appear to be influenced by calcium in their efficiency. The effects of oxalates and fluorides in quantity on the body are attributed to their power to withdraw lime.

Calcium and potassium appear to neutralise one another in the body, each opposing the action of the drug. Similarly, calcium antagonises magnesium (and sodium also) according to the teaching of Loeb. Clearly, for efficient life there must be an equilibrium of inorganic substances in blood plasma and excess of any one of these named elements is harmful.

Cartilage seems to combine with lime with a special readiness. This has a bearing on the treatment of rickets with lime, as will be presently seen. The parathyroid glands seem to influence lime absorption in the body and the administration of lime salts is held to influence favourably the tetany that follows their removal.

Lewin notes that urticaria may follow the administration of calcium chloride and a similar eruption that of lime water. The latter, if given to excess, causes anorexia and impaired digestion, even vomiting.

* There is no deficiency of lime in hæmophilia.

The therapeutic value of lime to the non-homœopathist is not great, but to homœopathists (and to Hugo Schulz) it becomes a remedy of great power as soon as the provings and their symptomatology are used as the basis for its prescription. As with all great constitutional remedies, the choice of it largely depends upon the presence or absence of certain general symptoms.

Prominent among these is the mode of reaction to external temperatures. Calcarea subjects are always susceptible to cold in a high degree. There is a dread of the open air, the least cold, especially cold damp weather and cold damp wind, aggravates their symptoms. They seek warmth and are markedly relieved by it, though it is to be noted they avoid exposure to the sun. In this respect the drug differs markedly from sulphur, among whose indications relief from cold and aggravation from heat are prominent. Whereas the sulphur patient is usually quick in movement, disturbed by heat, suffers from hot sweaty feet and experiences a sinking feeling in the forenoon, the calcarea subject is slow in movement, usually has cold clammy feet and may complain of a sinking feeling at any time of the day. Thus, in those who need calcarea, cold hands and cold feet are particularly noticeable. The feet are always cold and damp with the possible exception that at night when warmly covered they begin to burn. The characteristic " calcarea hand " is a soft, moist, boneless hand which is inclined to chap. Chilblains are frequent and other evidences of deficient circulation in the extremities. This lack in the power to resist external cold is only one of the deficient reactions of the typical case for calcarea. Such a case is slow mentally and bodily, slow in movement, slow in thought, slow to learn as a child, though often painstaking and industrious, the very reverse of the precocious child who suggests lycopodium.

Nevertheless, this type of child after treatment by calcarea may be so stimulated and may so improve in health as to require later other remedies. Lycopodium, phosphorus or silica may be required to carry forward the treatment of these children who start life with indications for calcarea.

Calcarea is pre-eminently a child's remedy and often those children who call for the drug are fat with large heads. In some cases, however, there may be a degree of emaciation, especially of the extremities. This fat, flabby child, often with fair hair and blue eyes, does not give an impression of health. The condition seems to result from deficient powers of metabolism. In these children, sweating is profuse, especially about the head, wetting the child's pillow and is generally sour smelling.

The infant requiring calcarea is typical ; though the child is usually fat, this increase of tissues is associated with weakness and lethargy. The fontanelles close late and teeth are delayed in coming through. Development is slow, like speech, thought, gait and movement. Milk frequently disagrees and bone development is defective suggesting the onset of rickets.

Thus the calcarea child is sluggish both mentally and physically. Physically he may be clumsy, his movements are slow and he lacks physical stamina. A sense of organ inferiority may develop so that the child is sensitive to those around him and dislikes being laughed at. The sleep in children is often broken by night terrors and he fears the dark. The skin is pale (to call it chalky is both a true adjective and a convenient mnemonic), though the face flushes easily for a moment or two.

In the treatment of children the physician may hesitate between calcarea and calcarea phosphoricum, but, in general, whereas the calcarea child is light complexioned, blue eyed with a white skin, good natured when well, with a tendency to sweat in the head and with a craving for eggs, the type of child calling for calcarea phos., though somewhat of the same type, is a little brighter mentally. Frequently he is dark complexioned with dark eyes and swarthy skin. There is less tendency to sweat, the child is less good natured and when unwell is anxious to be left alone.

This symptom-picture of calcarea already suggests a deficiency of thyroid secretion and although calcium metabolism is generally associated with the parathyroid, even marked degrees of such conditions as are often successfully treated with thyroid extract will respond to calcarea. This applies even to symptoms such as nocturnal enuresis, which has often been cured (and occasionally caused) by thyroid extract and will often yield to calcarea when other symptoms correspond.

Seeing that lime starvation leads to a condition resembling

rickets and that in this disease there is too little lime in the bones, it would be an easy suggestion that rickets is thus accounted for and that treatment with lime should be curative. But the administration of lime has no influence on the disease which has now been shown to be due to a deficiency of vitamin D so that rickets is curable by the administration of substances rich in vitamin D irradiated ergosterol or by exposure to sunlight or ultra-violet radiation. It is thought that shortage of vitamin D may cause either deficient calcium absorption from the bowel or interference with the process of ossification. Homœopaths find in calcarea an important remedy for this disease, but as the lime acts curatively in potency it is possible that the drug is a stimulant to the natural powers that lead to bone formation and that the action of the potentised lime is similar to that of vitamin D. This view is strengthened by the fact that there is actually no evidence of lime shortage in most cases of rickets : the hypothetical deficiency does not exist, and therefore no massive doses of lime are called for.

Deficient metabolism and slow reaction are thus characteristics that call for calcarea and the pronounced " chilliness " of the pathogenesis is to be read as an integral feature of this condition. But although the patient feels the cold acutely and is made worse by it and has predominantly cold extremities, there is evidence of some vasomotor instability as well, which leads to temporary heat and burning of parts of the surface (e.g., head or feet), usually as a condition precedent to sweating. Care is needed to distinguish the temporary from the more usual condition.

The adult subject for calcarea is a fat, flabby individual (though the drug meets some emaciated states too if there was a previous stage of fatness). The patient lacks energy and shows symptoms of physical weakness frequently accompanied with palpitation and breathlessness. As in the child, there is a tendency to free sweating, especially about the head and face, this occurring even in the cold air and on the slightest exertion. The general relaxation in the tissues is seen in the liability of such subjects to develop sprains.

Mentally the general slowness is again exemplified as has already been remarked. There is an inability to sustain any prolonged mental exertion ; in extreme cases his lack of mental power leads the patient to fear the possibility of loss of reason. There is great anxiety of mind which leads to all kinds of nervous apprehensions. It is part of the mental sluggishness that these are with difficulty expressed and with great difficulty combated. The night terrors of children cannot always be coherently explained, and in older patients there are vague fears and visions of fever or delirium which cause intense apprehensiveness. *The mental inertia may progress to a condition of passivity wherein the individual can do little but brood and worry over the smallest trivialities.*

Vertigo is a prominent symptom and feeling of faintness and sinking sensations. Trembling, twitching and spasm, even convulsions call for the drug, especially if the nervous symptoms are associated with vague fear or with loss of body fluids (*e.g.*, after hæmorrhages, sweatings, profuse leucorrhœa, or seminal emissions), for the after-effects of which calcarea will compete in value with china or phosphoric acid. The worst time of the twenty-four hours for calcarea patients is 2 to 3 a.m., the hour when general vitality is apt to be at its lowest. Severe chronic diseases like epilepsy or asthma will respond to calcarea when the general symptoms-picture of the disease and drug are alike.

Calcarea can cure both sensory and motor nerve symptoms, both neuralgias and paralyses, when other symptoms call for it. It is the chronic counterpart of belladonna and whenever this drug has temporarily relieved, calcarea is very likely to produce more permanent improvement.

Homœopathic observation certainly places calcarea among the drugs which have the power to control hæmorrhage, especially menorrhagia. If the menses are too early and too profuse, that is the characteristic symptom. The general relaxation of the calcarea subject may lead to prolapse or to a profuse continuous leucorrhœa which is thick and acrid.

In the male the patient is weak sexually, sometimes impotent. In such individuals a compensatory increase of sexual desire may be present, but coition is followed by a condition of general weakness. Also clinical experience finds that small non-malignant growths (*e.g.*, papillomata or polypi or lipomata) often occur in subjects that present the general symptoms of calcarea and the drug has a considerable reputation in such cases. It is often noted that these patients are very susceptible to damp weather and the reaction of calcarea subjects to this kind of atmosphere is nearly as marked as to cold.

Apart from the general effects of the drug, it has marked local action on the digestive and respiratory systems. It tends to cause chronic catarrhs of mucous membranes which are initiated or aggravated by exposure to cold chilly weather. The secretions are considerable from the nose (muco-pus) and there is a tendency to the development of polypi and especially to overgrowth of lymphatic tissue (tonsils and adenoids). Whenever there is real obstruction from such overgrowth, or such a symptom as deafness, to remove the tissue-masses is usually imperative : when there is less urgency, proper training of the child in breathing and care and cleansing of the passages will often work wonders without drug treatment. But observation certainly shows that many cases of enlarged tonsils and adenoids occur in patients who on general grounds suggest calcarea and it is the confident belief of homœopathists that the use of it assists hygienic measures to such an extent that it should not be omitted. The phosphate of lime is the favourite preparation for these conditions.

Acuter diseases of nose and throat do not often benefit from calcarea, for just as the patients are slow in reaction, so is the drug slow to develop its power. But after these acute conditions have been temporarily relieved by the administration of some indicated remedy, calcarea may be required to prevent the tendency to such attacks. For example, Dulcamara is a remedy frequently applicable to attacks of diarrhœa brought on by exposure to wet weather. Calcarea, which has a notable tendency to aggravation from cold and wet, will often be required to reinforce the action of dulcamara and remove the tendency to recurrence.

Descending the respiratory tract, there are found symptoms of marked character, namely, tickling (as of dust) in the larynx, causing a dry irritative cough and later expectoration of muco-pus, often with blood. Pains in larynx and chest are common, and there is generally a nocturnal aggravation. Dyspnœa and oppression, wheezing and gasping, with pain and anxiety are deeper symptoms still. Taken in conjunction with the alimentary canal symptoms, presently to be described, and the profuse sweating, the picture strongly suggests early tuberculosis and clinical experience well justifies the choice of calcarea in this disease.

The symptomatology of calcarea corresponds to many pre-tubercular states, where there is gradual emaciation especially of the limbs, pallor, weariness, a tendency to take cold and marked sensitivity to cold, wet weather. Its power over early tubercle of any organ is considerable, and not the least over the form of disease in young growing subjects, which begins in the mediastinal glands. Some observers think that there is a right-sidedness in the calcarea pathogenesis worth remarking.

Among cardiac symptoms, palpitation and pain are prominent. Calcarea arsenicosa, the arseniate of lime, is particularly valuable when there is an intermittent pulse, but here no doubt the arsenic element counts for something. Chronic heart disease cases, apart from such emergencies as demand special remedies, derive much benefit in the way of strengthened compensation and improved muscular and nervous " tone " by regular courses of various iodides. Among these the iodides of arsenic, barium, gold and calcium hold the most important places and when the subjects of disease are young, growing persons, calcium iodide is very valuable.

Along the alimentary canal there are noteworthy calcarea symptoms : the tongue is dry and coated white and there is a sour taste in the mouth. The appetite is often excessive, though thirst often predominates over hunger. In young children there is sometimes a curious craving for indigestible things, and babies, if not carefully watched, will rival puppies in their desire to try the taste of anything and everything. More normal cravings of the calcarea patient are found in the desire for eggs, sweets, ice cream, salt and oysters. There may be a desire for or a dislike of milk, but milk always disagrees. There is frequently an aversion from coffee, meat and tobacco and curiously enough warm food.

After a meal there are sour eructations or even sour vomiting, with gastric pain, distension and sense of pressure. Cutting, severe pain is referred especially to the region of the gall-bladder. The catarrh which the drug causes spreads to the gall ducts and the expulsion of thick mucus from them causes pain. On symptomatic grounds calc. carb. has been used (with considerable success) in attacks of gall-stone colic. Fermentation and impaired digestion extend through the alimentary tract and the bowels are usually constipated, but the patient feels better generally when constipated ; evacuation is difficult and the stools pale and white. In children, however, there is often a sour-smelling, excoriating diarrhœa, exciting a spasm of the anus and eruptions on the buttocks. To meet disorders of the locomotor organs (nerves, muscles, joints, fascias), the pathogenesis of calcarea supplies many symptoms of pain and stiffness, cramps and neuralgias, but the choice of it will be determined by the presence of the great general symptoms of constitution and temperament rather than by the local ones.

As regards sleep, the night terrors of children are noteworthy as indication for calcarea. By day the patients are drowsy as a result of the disturbed nights.

Urticaria is a symptom that suggests calcarea. The skin itches readily and there is often an unhealthy state of nutrition, so that small injuries heal badly and suppurate readily.

To recapitulate the general indications for calcarea, the most prominent is an aggravation from cold in every form, from the least cold, from cold damp air, from cold moist winds and change from warm to cold weather. There is usually a dread of open air, consequently the patient is markedly ameliorated in dry warm weather. All exertion, either mental or physical, aggravates symptoms ; thus the calcarea subject experiences difficulty in standing for any length of time. He feels generally better when constipated and experiences comfort from touch. Rubbing, scratching or being touched or stroked by the hand is soothing to the calcarea patient.

As regards the repetition of calcarea, the homœopathic physician has found that the dose may be repeated at reasonably short intervals in children, provided it still continues to be indicated, but that it should not be repeated very frequently in adults ; its action should be allowed to continue over prolonged periods.

Calcarea is inimical to bryonia. It follows belladonna especially well, and has a close relationship to rhus. It follows sulphur well, but should not be given before that drug.

CHAMOMILLA

Matricaria Chamomilla.   Tincture of the whole fresh plant.

To the non-homœopathic physician, chamomilla is just one among many " bitters," with no distinctive virtues and hardly deserving a line in a text-book. To the homœopathist, it is a most valuable remedy, with a well-marked sphere of action, for the provings develop characteristic symptoms and these find their counterpart in practice with considerable frequency.

Chamomilla causes symptoms in various regions of the body, but those that distinguish it most clearly are in the mental group and unless the characteristic mental quality is present the drug is seldom effective. This quality is in its essence a lack of control of the power to inhibit the simpler reactions to pain or other unpleasant stimuli. It is a common observation in life that men " compound for sins they are inclined to, by damning those they have no mind to," and many of those who lament the lack of control shown by the sensualist or the quick-tempered (and incidentally pride themselves on the will power that restrains them), in reality are only less tempted, not more controlled, and succumb quickly enough to their own weaknesses. But this observation by no means implies that there are no differences in power of inhibition. Two main factors are at work in each case, relative sensitiveness (which plays the main part in deciding the strength of temptation) and relative power of control. The first is a natural inheritance of the individual, though it can be heightened or dulled by accidental or purposive experience : the second no doubt is also largely inherent in the personality, but far more than the first is at the mercy of education and conscious effort. Patients who are suitable for chamomilla are probably more sensitive than their neighbours, but certainly they lack the power of inhibition and are rightly classed as lacking in control.

This remedy is consequently often indicated in those who make overuse of stimulants and certain drugs, for all of these, from tea and coffee to alcohol, morphia, or cocaine, tend to weaken the powers of inhibition. But as chamomilla is a swiftly-acting but not very searching remedy, it is more suitable to the relief of temporary emergencies in these subjects than to the cure of the underlying disharmony which causes or complicates the emergencies. More notably still does it help the conditions wherein the poisons of disease are playing a part in the system similar to that which can be played by alcohol or opium in weakening inhibition. Here the drug is confronted with an emergency dependent on a sudden rather than on a chronic poisoning and its action is much more nearly curative.

Chamomilla, therefore, is suited to those who complain of excessive sensitiveness, who find pain all but unendurable and have no power of bearing it with fortitude. On the contrary, they are moved to ill-temper and violent irritability, e.g., to the fits of passion that recall classical scenes in novel and drama, wherein gouty old gentlemen are shown and ridiculed for their irascibility. Peevishness, anger, fury—every degree of ill-temper may appear : there is impatience, rudeness to friends, to nurse or doctor and an insistence of immediate relief to the symptoms which for the time are blackening the whole world to the unfortunate individual and hardly less to those who are around him. All this ill-temper, however, is more in the way of a violent reaction to pain than the expression of a malicious or cross-grained nature.* Between attacks the patient for whom chamomilla is suitable may be sweet-tempered and easy-going : in this respect he differs from the patient who indicates nux vomica. The anger characteristic of this latter drug is more deep-seated and more a part of the underlying character and though often better controlled outwardly, is much more dangerous and difficult. Beneath the stormy surface that suggests chamomilla there is no rancour or deep enmity. After the attack is over the patient will often show that he is really appreciative of the efforts made on his behalf, though quite unable to show his appreciation at the time of suffering. Small children, who are pre-eminently suited to chamomilla (for inevitably at a tender age great power of control cannot be expected), are soothed at once by being carried about and nursed in the mother's or nurse's arms. This is a very characteristic symptom and indicates that beneath all the peevishness and rage there is a deep desire for

---

* At the same time a fit of temper in a chamomilla case may be the starting point of a neuralgia or attack of abdominal pain.

sympathy and consolation. Though the chamomilla child obtains relief from passive movement and is momentarily quietened by being carried, the hypersensitivity characteristic of the drug is seen in its aversion to being touched, its capricious-ress in its demanding this or that, which, when offered, is pushed away and refused.

Temporary emergencies of pain leading to lack of mental control, then, are suitable for the relieving action of chamomilla, but closer analysis reveals that the cause of these pain emergencies lies nearly always in some disorder of metabolism. Gastro-intestinal symptoms are nearly always prominent when chamomilla is successful, and when they are not, there is, nevertheless, as a rule, good reason to suspect that a profounder metabolic defect is at the root of the pain, which may show as a neuralgia, dysmenorrhœa or arthritis. It is because opium and alcohol and such poisons delay and pervert metabolism that the takers of them can so often be helped by chamomilla, but while it will often relieve the symptoms due to perversion of the deeper metabolic processes, its curative action is best exerted on the more superficial emergencies, such, for instance, as may accompany gastro-intestinal catarrh.

Pre-eminently the period of dentition is a time liable to cause symptoms which yield readily to chamomilla. If a child is teething, then this drug is the drug of election for almost any temporary distress. For at the time of teething there must neccessarily be some specific adjustments of metabolism to meet the bodily demand of growth and any failures of such adjustment are precisely those likely to call for this remedy. Any toothache that exists (and chamomilla will relieve many toothaches) is characteristically brought on by warm drinks or coming into a warm atmosphere. The toothache is relieved by cold so that the child is likely to hold cold water in the mouth for a long time when drinking. An attack of toothache requiring chamomilla may be brought on by taking cold, but even here the pain itself is relieved by cold. During such an attack the hypersensitivity to pain of the chamomilla patient can be observed. The child is peevish and irritable and the pain seems intolerable. The face sweats readily (perspiration is hot), especially after food. Usually one cheek is flushed, not both (as with belladonna) : there is great thirst and sensations of heat. The tongue is heavily coated (yellowish-white) and the breath foul. Food tastes bitter and gastric pain follows eating promptly, or if not sharp pain, then weight and heaviness. Much flatulence develops, with colicky pains, which are not relieved by passage of gas, and then an offensive diarrhœa sets in. It should be noted that abdominal colic is usually ameliorated by the application of external heat. The motion feels hot and excoriates the anus ; it is usually of a yellowish-green colour and is apt to follow quickly on eating, especially if the food is warm. It is frequently applicable to the colic of infants where the child is doubled up with pain, is extremely irritable, wants to be carried, wants things which he refuses when offered, in short, the chamomilla mentality associated with colic relieved by heat.

The general sensitiveness of chamomilla is shown in the reactions to change of temperature. Most observers find that although many of the pains are relieved by heat, the patient as a whole is apt to be worsened by external warmth. On the other hand, there are individual subjects for chamomilla who feel the cold and dislike it. Therefore the physician should regard a sensitiveness to either extreme of temperature as characteristic, although for any one case the sensitiveness is not likely to vary but will remain noticeable to heat or to cold and not, as with mercurius, for instance, to both. With these symptoms the mental condition already described develops and with the ill-temper is a great sense of debility, out of proportion to the seriousness of the disease. The gastro-intestinal catarrh does not appear to be profound, and chamomilla is not often a remedy for ulceration, but many cases of infantile diarrhœa will yield quickly to it and the relation of the drug to heat makes it suitable for summer diarrhœa as well as for diarrhœas of dentition.* If both indications are present, so much the better, but chamomilla acts best when given early in the attack : it will then promptly check it in a large proportion of cases. If the catarrh spreads to the bile ducts there may be jaundice and catarrhal jaundice will yield to chamomilla if the mental condition indicates it. It seems to have some local action on the

---

* Although hot applications and heat in general worsen the symptoms in chamomilla subjects, the general sensitiveness makes them also resent damp, cold weather and especially high winds.

parotid glands and nocturnal salivation is a symptom in the pathogenesis.

Besides toothache, diarrhœa and other dentition disorders of the alimentary canal, chamomilla is suited to the skin affections of the period of teething, but the clue to its use will usually be given by the mental condition of the patient.

It is certain that the results of disordered metabolism are very variable and those that cause this peculiar irritability of the higher nerve centres with lack of control are pre-eminently the result of the conditions which chamomilla is able to relieve. Apart from rashes the skin in chamomilla cases is hot and sweating : hands and feet are hot and the feet may be thrust out of bed for coolness (cf. sulphur).

It is a frequently indicated remedy in otitis media in children, the attack coming on especially after exposure to cold. The child is intensely irritable and may scream with pain and does not want to be touched. Individuals whose ears are sensitive to exposure to cold air and cold winds may develop ear trouble where the symptom-complex calls for chamomilla.

Neuralgias and painful joint affections are quickly relieved by chamomilla, if accompanied by the characteristic mental symptoms. The pains are aggravated by heat but not ameliorated by cold (unlike Puls.) and tend to come on before midnight, often co-exist or alternate with numbness (Nash*) and are very severe, causing a restlessness that will lead the patient if an adult to get up and walk about for relief and, in the case of a child, amelioration is obtained by being carried. It is to be noted that the night hours are usually a time of increased suffering when chamomilla is indicated. The hour of maximum aggravation is 9 p.m., the pains usually abate after midnight.

Laryngeal spasm has been cured by chamomilla, but here again the general symptoms gave the clue to the remedy.

This drug influences the female pelvic organs notably. The menses are excessive, with dark clots and much pain, causing the characteristic irritability before and during the flow. Between periods there is an acrid watery leucorrhœa. The dysmenorrhœal pains are severe, unendurable, of a bearing-down character. Back and thighs are affected as well as abdomen. Occasionally chamomilla is called for in labour,

* " Leaders in Homœopathic Therapeutics," p. 158.

but here, too, the mental indications are the ones that suggest it.

CHINA

Cinchona Officinalis. Tincture of the dried bark and potencies therefrom.

China is the common term among homœopathists for tincture of cinchona bark. Its most important alkaloid, quinine, was not isolated in the days when Hahnemann proved the remedy, and although for the majority of physicians quinine has largely taken the place of cinchona, homœopathists continue to use the tincture as originally tested, since the indications for its use are clearer than those for the relatively unproved alkaloid. The greater intensity of action of quinine does not compensate the homœopathist for its smaller precision of indication : china is a drug whose sphere can be well defined and, when indicated, is sufficiently active and efficient in potencies. Nevertheless, without any doubt, the quinine in china is responsible for the larger part of its symptomatology, and the studies of the alkaloid which have been made are of the profoundest interest to the homœopathist. Besides quinine there are twenty-odd other alkaloids present in the cinchona bark. Their general effects seem to resemble those of quinine, though their presence in china probably helps to give the tincture a greater range of action.

Quinine affects the nutrition and thereby the life of nearly all protoplasm, without (like strychnine) singling out any tissue for an especially intense action. The effect of it on protoplasm is that characteristic of stimuli in general, namely, small doses (or the first action of large doses before absorption is complete) encourage life activity, larger doses depress it and doses large enough destroy it. This action is very clearly shown on many unicellular organisms : thus, the effect of the drug on the yeast cell impedes alcoholic fermentation and strong quinine solutions are antiseptic. This effect on simple organisms is paralleled by the action of quinine on white blood cells. These are hindered in their movements and ultimately killed by quite minute doses of quinine, and the accumulation of leucocytes that normally takes place in local inflammation is largely prevented by the drug. Ordinary doses of quinine cause a certain leucopenia. The power of blood to oxidise substances in certain circumstances is lessened by quinine, and ferments such as pepsin, rennet and others are hindered by its presence in moderate quantities, although their activity is increased by small quantities.

These phenomena are instances of the general effects of quinine as protoplasmic poison. They can be seen in its action on the central nervous system, where a preliminary stimulation (small dose effect) is followed by depression, and on muscle, both of heart and arteries and muscle in general : these also have their power at first increased and then weakened. Nerve trunks are very tolerant of it and peripheral nerve-ends little if at all affected.

The special senses of hearing and (less markedly) of sight are very susceptible to the action of quinine. Marked degrees of deafness and ringing in the ears are easily produced by it. Total blindness has been produced and a contracted field of vision and disturbances of the colour sense are fairly frequent. Although there is evidence of contraction by blood vessels and circulatory changes in both eye and ear, the probability is that these severe effects are caused by a direct attack of the drug on retinal nerve cells and those of the spiral cochlear ganglion.

The head after large doses feels heavy and confused : giddiness is common and some degree of ataxia. In the rare fatal cases the respiratory centre appears to have ceased action, but in spite of the ease with which some symptoms of quinine overdosing can be produced, it is not a drug that is readily fatal. Dr. Cushny quotes a case wherein the dose of an ounce produced only some confusion and noises in the ears. Presumably its effects are so universal on protoplasm that vital centres escape a fatal concentration, the poison being distributed all over the body.

The stomach is irritated by quinine and diarrhœa has been caused, but although homœopathists (see below) value china highly in certain gastro-intestinal disorders, other physicians make little use of it for these conditions. It causes the uterus to contract by direct action on the muscle : similarly the spleen contracts and (it is said) the bronchi also. The effect of the spleen contraction is temporarily to cause leucocytosis, but the characteristic leucopenia of quinine soon appears, if the drug is continuously given. Cushny * quotes Roth to the effect that a single dose causes a (splenic) leucocytosis, then follows a fall (mainly of lymphocytes), then a rise of polynuclears to the point of leucocytosis with lymphocytes remaining low.

Idiosyncrasies are frequent with regard to the action of quinine. Besides the effects already mentioned, susceptible individuals may show a variety of skin eruptions (mostly erythematous). Gastric and intestinal symptoms have been already noted. Of more importance is the appearance of hæmoglobinuria, which is undoubtedly an occasional sequel of quinine poisoning. Albuminuria may also occur. This hæmoglobinuria so resembles the blackwater fever of certain chronic malarial cases that it has been contended that blackwater fever is really quinine poisoning occurring in malarial subjects. But this view is now abandoned : the fact is that chronic malaria and quinine can both cause hæmoglobinuria (a parallel of deep significance to the homœopathist) and although quinine sometimes seems to provoke the symptom when given in chronic malaria, it can also cause it to disappear, both of these phenomena being quite in accordance with homœopathic experience with many drugs.

Any one of these more unusual effects of quinine may be accompanied with a rise of temperature and some febrile symptoms may appear without many other marked effects of the drug. That is to say, quinine has undoubtedly the power of causing a rise in temperature in many persons. It is by no means a universal effect, it is, in fact, an idiosyncrasy, but the homœopathist knows from drug experience that an idiosyncrasy is no more than *an individual exaggeration of an effect universally produced*, but usually only to an unnoticeable degree. Therefore, the idiosyncratic effects of a drug are good indications for its use in disease : although the normal healthy individual may seldom react to the extent of producing marked symptoms, yet the patient (especially the patient already affected " similarly " by disease) will be capable of reacting readily to the drug even in minute dosage, because of his heightened sensitiveness. For these reasons the fever of quinine, of little moment to the orthodox physician, is significant to the homœopathist. Furthermore, it was the febrile and

* *Loc. cit.*

other symptoms caused in his own person by cinchona bark that led Hahnemann first to conceive that *similia simillibus curentur* might be a sound generalisation. It is perhaps unnecessary to repeat that the truth or falsehood of the principle does not depend on this one experiment. It was no more than a striking experience which turned the thoughts of Hahnemann into a definite channel. Only after years of patient investigation did he become convinced that this channel led to therapeutic exactitude and success. So that if the experiment itself were to be held fallacious, it would, nevertheless, have served the purpose of suggesting a fruitful rule of practice. But other experience than that of Hahnemann is reasonably convincing that cinchona and quinine do possess the power to produce in certain susceptible persons a sequence of febrile symptoms which form a parallel to those of the malarial paroxysm. Chill, heat and sweating are the phenomena accompanied, for those who are ready to note them, by various minor subjective symptoms comparable to those of which sufferers from malaria often complain.* Lewin,† who writes fully on this matter of quinine fever, rightly notes it as an exceptional effect, but records instances of it and (though without any inclination to homœopathy) mentions and accepts Hahnemann's experience. He records temperatures of 38°, 39°, 40° Centigrade and the regular sequence of shivering, dry heat with headache and sweating, though he notes that the last symptom occasionally is wanting. In animals quinine usually causes a fall of temperature if given in large doses.

The homœopathist, therefore, has a right to maintain that this drug, which pre-eminently cures malaria, has the power to produce symptoms which run parallel to those of malaria and he finds in the hæmoglobinuria of quinine another similar symptom to set beside the febrile phenomena. With these thoughts in his mind he is inclined to doubt the explanation of the curative action of quinine in malaria as purely a parasiticidal one. Rather he would suggest that since drug and parasite stir the system to similar reactions the drug may heighten bodily resistance to the enemy and overcome it by

---

* The rigor is the rarest of the three cardinal symptoms ; heat and sweating \\more common, but a true shivering " chill " has been observed. In Hahnemann's case it was not produced.

† " Nebenwirkungen der Arzneimittel."

this means, indirectly rather than directly. Not that quinine is not directly poisonous to the plasmodium and whenever drug meets parasite in sufficient concentration no doubt it kills it : this action may supplement the indirect one. But it is by no means clear that quinine can be kept concentrated in the blood to the point lethal to the malaria organism and its affinity for body protoplasm is so great that there must be many chances of deviation of the drug. Similarly, the prophylactic virtues of quinine would seem to depend more upon the stimulation of a natural resistance and less upon the (hoped for) presence in the blood of enough parasiticide to kill the casual invader.

If the action of quinine be thus indirect, it would be reasonable to think that the natural powers of resistance would be more easily stimulated in some persons than in others. The homœopathist would say that the more closely the whole symptom-picture suggested the drug, the more likely would be the remedy to prove helpful, and would find in the fact of unlikeness between drug pathogenesis and case of disease an explanation of the undoubted failure of quinine in certain cases. But the drug will cure many and help others, and when it fails, or when its effect flags, the homœopathist at least, applying his general principle, possesses other resources. When similarity is close between drug symptoms and disease symptoms, quite small doses will probably prove effective : when similarity is not close, if there are no clear indications for another remedy, rather larger doses can be tried. During the paroxysm, the characteristics that suggest china to the homœopathist are : Relatively short chill, with long-lasting heat following ; congestion of the head with much flushed face and often delirium and desire to throw off clothing ; profuse and debilitating sweat.

There is no thirst during the stage of heat, but before the pyrexia the patient desires frequent drinks.

When the temperature begins to fall and the patient breaks into a profuse sweat he becomes intensely thirsty.

But it is needless to say that for the homœopathists all symptoms have their value, others from the pathogenesis not to be described may be present and if they exist they strongly reinforce the claims of the drug.

The profound effects of cinchona on the body lead finally to a general condition of debility so marked that none who ever realised it as caused by the drug could thenceforward think of any " tonic " power in china except as exemplifying the general homœopathic principle. When chronic diseases present similar symptoms to those about to be described, china (in small doses or potencies) will indeed prove a " tonic." In cases of debility lacking the characteristic symptoms it will do no good.

Poisoning by china results in a general torpor of bodily functions : venous congestion followed by passive hæmorrhages (nasal, uterine, etc.) ; enlargement of spleen and liver (largely congestive) ; an irritability of neuro-muscular system with considerable muscular weakness ; œdema of ankles ; vasomotor disturbances, flushings and shiverings. Physically, the china patient is debilitated and the drug is of value, should the symptom agree, after acute febrile disturbances such as influenza (cf. scutellaria and influenzinum). The subject is chilly, weak, sleepless and irritable.

The debility to which china is particularly indicated is that which follows loss of the fluids of the body, for example, after long or repeated hæmorrhages with consequent weakness and increasing anæmia. Weakness from diarrhœa, copious sweating, seminal emissions, and even long-continued suppuration are likely to produce a symptom-complex requiring china. It will often, in relation to this latter condition (i.e., suppuration), control hectic fever. Generally, the type of debility which calls for china is a condition where the debility itself is the whole illness rather than a weakness induced by some grave underlying constitutional disease.

The emotional hyperæsthesia is shown in a dislike of company and a desire to be alone : the patient will often object to being looked at, imagining all sorts of critical feelings in those around him and resenting them. There is a disposition to consider himself ill-used, which also leads to fits of temper, but these are shallow (unlike those that characterise nux. vom.) and generally mask a timid disposition, very sensitive to the judgment of others.

The rhythmic variation of symptoms which the homœopath observes can especially be noted under this drug. The over-sensitive emotional condition is frequently associated and followed by an apathetic, indifferent state of mind, where the patient experiences some failure of mental power and a shrinking from effort. There is hyperæsthesia too, in the special senses, in that the patient may be over-sensitive to noise, touch, odour and taste. The complexion is sallow or dingy yellow ; the appetite is often voracious, but digestion poor and some of the symptoms detailed below may characterise certain tissue or body-processes.

Homœopathically, three important indications for china are found in its use in certain types of debility : general hyperæsthesia, mental and physical, and in the periodicity of the occurrence of complaints.

Periodicity is a notable characteristic ; attacks that occur at regular intervals, such as febrile attacks or neuralgias, are likely to benefit by china ; an attack every other day is a not infrequent rhythm.

Headache is a severe and common symptom ; it is throbbing, hammering, congestive, often accompanied by singing in the ears and weakness of sight with sensitiveness to touch or *light* pressure ; it is aggravated by cold draughts, movement and reaches its height at night. The headache is ameliorated in a warm room and by *firm* pressure. Infra-orbital neuralgia is common and other neuralgias of head and face are more frequent than nerve pains elsewhere, the characteristic modalities are found, namely an aggravation from light touch, movement and cold. With increasing debility the patient becomes hypersensitive mentally and physically. There is sensitivity to light touch and cold so much so that even a current of air blowing on the part brings on pain. Firm pressure, however, often relieves pain, and the objection to touch is not from local tenderness, but from nervous hyperæsthesia.

The effects on sight and hearing have been already noted. In the eye there is little obvious inflammation recorded in provings, but a general weakness of sight ; photophobia and subjective sensations occur. Nerve deafness being producible by quinine is naturally a condition which suggests the curative use of it, but it needs to be used in the early stages. Ringing and humming noises in the ears are often helped by the drug. The external ear is often sensitive to touch. Venous epistaxis may occur in subjects for china, but otherwise the nose is little affected.

The genito-urinary sphere is the seat of the most frequent hæmorrhages (venous characteristically). Thus, menorrhagia or post-partum hæmorrhage and the effects of them are often helped by china and the hæmaturia of quinine is notorious. Sexual power is diminished, though the general irritability may find expression in some sexual excitement.

In the respiratory tract the symptoms recorded suggest spasm of larynx or bronchi rather than inflammation, and in practice china has some reputation in asthma if periodicity and sensitiveness to touch are marked and if bronchitis is not considerable. Asthmatic attacks are more frequent in the autumn and follow depletion of the body of fluids. Palpitation and dyspnœa are common and intercostal cramp.

The skin is generally sallow or slightly jaundiced and very sensitive to touch. Sweating is profuse and exhausting in febrile disorders and is worse at night. Rashes are erythematous usually, and œdema is not uncommon. Occasionally synovitis is relieved by china when firm pressure is grateful but touch irritates.

Apart from the general effects of china, its influence is most marked on the alimentary canal. It produces both gastric and intestinal disturbances. The tongue is flabby and coated yellowish-white. There is a bitter or saltish taste in the mouth, affecting all food and drink, even water.

Should fever be present, the patient is likely to be thirstless. Sometimes the appetite is excessive but, in spite of this, the patient does not put on weight. If food be delayed there is distress, an empty gnawing in the stomach. Yet the patient often finds that he has no appetite on beginning a meal.

Even a light meal causes oppression and pain in the stomach, feeling of weight centred about the middle of the sternum. There are some eructations and flatulence is distressing.

Eructations may proceed even to vomiting, which is sour and sometimes bile stained.

There is an aversion from butter and greasy foods. Acid and sour food and drinks aggravate his condition and may bring on an attack of diarrhœa.

Both stomach and bowels are distended with gas, but an

important modality of the condition is that no relief is experienced either by eructations or the passing of flatus.

Sometimes the appetite is capricious, and spoilt children, who clamour for dainties which they cannot digest, are often suited by china. Spleen and liver may be enlarged. A degree of jaundice is common and the milder repeated attacks of pain in the region of the gall bladder are both caused and relieved by this remedy.

Such gall bladder and liver disturbances are accompanied by excessive flatulence, but the distress of the patient is not relieved by eructations.

Should colitis develop, there is diarrhœa which comes on after eating and at night.

The characteristic state of the bowels is a sour, frothy diarrhœa, containing mucus and undigested food.

The motion is accompanied by the passing of large quantities of flatus. The abdomen is sensitive to light touch, but pain is relieved by firm pressure.

Dr. Borland makes the observation that attacks of hepatic colic, which have responded to colocynth are often benefited by subsequent doses of china.

China has a very definite effect, in substantial doses of the tincture, in allaying the craving for alcohol (especially for spirits). This was observed by Sir T. Lauder Brunton, and homœopathists find the drug useful in the dyspepsias of spirit drinkers and sometimes even in cirrhosis. Indeed, a history of alcoholism is enough to bring china into the front rank of remedies to be considered. Nux vomica vies with it for spirit drinkers, as does sulphur. For beer drinkers, kali bichrom. is generally more suitable in gastric disorders.

China is a remedy in many cases of intermittent fever accompanied by weakness and anæmia. The three stages of chill, fever and sweat are well marked. Preceding the chill there is violent thirst which subsides during the chill and recurs after. During the fever there is usually little or no thirst ; the sweat is profuse and again accompanied by great thirst.

Subjects for cinchona are chilly, loving warmth and distressed by cold and damp. Autumn is a seasonal time of aggravation for them. Most conditions are worse at night and there is a general aggravation after eating.

There is extreme sensitiveness, especially to light touch and draught of cold air.

Hard pressure ameliorates pain.

China is related botanically to ipecac. and to coffea. It is often indicated after exhausting diseases or as an intercurrent remedy during prolonged illness. For the exhausting effects of bodily fluids it competes with phosphoric acid and natr. mur.

CIMICIFUGA RACEMOSA

Actæa racemosa—an American plant of the order Ranunculaceæ. The tincture is made from the fresh root. A resinoid substance, Macrotin, has been extracted from the root and triturations of this have been used.

This remedy is one of the later additions to the Materia Medica ; it has proved to be one of considerable value, and clinical experience has made more precise the indications of the (not very extensive) provings. It is all but unknown to non-homœopathic medicine.

It has a very marked effect upon the nervous system, rendering the nerve centres (both cerebral and spinal) irritable. After the irritable stage depression follows. There is some congestion of head and face as with belladonna, but less marked. The generative organs are notably influenced, especially in the female sex, and it is conceivable that the nervous symptoms are secondary to some alteration in the quantity or quality of the internal secretions arising from these tissues. It is at least a fact that symptoms referable to the pelvic organs are generally prominent when actæa is well indicated.

The mental symptoms are in the main those of depression, anxiety and fear. Fear of death is nearly as prominent a manifestation as with aconite. But the prevailing mood of gloom is yet an unstable one ; an unbalanced hysterical condition with a tolerably constant reversion to melancholy is a fair description of the usual and characteristic mental state. The depressed emotional condition of the patient tends to alternate with physical states so that should any physical complaint improve, there is a deterioration of the emotional state with a return of gloom and dejection. The melancholy is largely associated with fears of the nature and extent of the illness, a hypochondriacal melancholy, though Hahnemann's shrewd dictum with regard to hypochondriasis holds good, that the sufferer exaggerates his sufferings but does not invent them ; they are therefore to be noted with due care.

Actæa is one of the " loquacious " remedies, like lachesis ; incessant rambling speech is a good symptom. There is inability to fix attention.

Emotional causes, such as disappointment, anxiety, fear, are often responsible for symptoms, especially disappointments in the affections.

Actæa patients are extremely sensitive to cold and damp weather and all complaints with the exception of the head pain are intensified by cold.

The headache of actæa is a characteristic and prominent symptom. It is one frequently encountered when pelvic lesions are present. In its most distinct form it appears as intense pain felt simultaneously behind the eyes (relieved by pressure on eyeballs), on the vertex and in the nape of the neck, but one or other of these spots of maximum intensity may fail to be affected. The nape of the neck is a specially characteristic site of pain, which, when present, may extend into the occiput, or cause stiffness of the neck muscles with retraction of the head, or sensitiveness of the spine with shooting pains. The intense pain in the eyes has caused the drug to be used in iritis, especially the so-called " rheumatic " variety, but there is no pathological evidence (as yet) of the power of the drug to affect the iris deeply. The pains in eyes or head are always worse from the slightest movement (as with bryonia), but relieved in the open air and worse in warm rooms. This is the more noteworthy as the patient on the whole is very sensitive to cold air. A similar inversion of reaction of head and general symptoms to cold air is found with arsenicum ; like arsenicum also, actæa symptoms are worse at night.

Actæa is characterised by pains elsewhere. As a rule they are sudden, lancinating and sharp, though often there is a general bruised feeling that persists. They are of the kind usually called " rheumatic " and the drug is often indicated in those who have had typical attacks of rheumatism. The areas more frequently attacked (besides the head and neck) are the loins and vertebral joints and the cardiac region and the inside of the left arm. With this last there is often palpitation

or feeling as though the heart stopped. Numbness may follow
this pain down the arm. Touch and movement worsen ;
warmth as a rule relieves. The pains and headaches of actæa
are apt to be associated with the passage of profuse pale urine
(*cf.* ignatia). An allied remedy, Actæa Spicata, has a special
influence over the wrists and small joints of hands and feet. In
recent cases where osteo-arthritis is associated with disease of
the pelvic organs, the actæas have great value. In more
chronic cases they are rather palliative than curative. It has
a real value in chorea, which again marks its relation to rheumatism. Trembling and jerking of muscles are prominent
symptoms and aggravated by cold. It is noteworthy that such
jerking is excited in any muscles under pressure, *e.g.*, lying on
one side brings on the characteristic jerking and twitching.

In the digestive sphere there are symptoms of dyspepsia :
coated tongue, sticky saliva, unpleasant taste in the mouth.
Sinking sensations at the epigastrium are marked. On the
whole, the symptoms referable to the alimentary tract are
rather of secondary value.

There is a very characteristic cough, not resulting from any
obvious catarrh, but suggestive rather of reflex irritability.
It is a dry, teasing cough, worse at night and worse at every
attempt to speak. This has proved a valuable indication for
the use of the remedy, naturally more valuable when accompanied by other characteristic symptoms.

In the sphere covered by the generative organs, the symptoms of actæa become numerous and important, though much
more so for the female than the male sex. Pains are sharp and
definite : inframammary pain and pain also in the ovarian
(left side chiefly) and uterine regions, with tenderness on
pressure. Painful and *irregular* menstruation, more often
scanty than excessive : leucorrhœa with a sense of weight and
pressure in the pelvis are marked. The dysmenorrhœal pains
are apt to be like those of labour, at their worst *during* the flow.
The whole condition of the cimicifuga patient is aggravated
during the menstrual flow.

The actual pains of childbirth are often rendered more
regular and effective by actæa. It seems also to have some
power in overcoming rigidity of the os uteri in labour. Naturally the claims for prescription of actæa are enhanced by the

presence of others of its symptoms, especially in the mental sphere. Puerperal mental disturbances, even puerperal manias, have been benefited by it.

Actæa is a very useful remedy at the menopause in restless, irritable patients, gloomy but often voluble about their ailments ; flushes frequently suffuse the otherwise pale face, with dark rings under the eyes. Twitchings and cramps disturb the sleep and palpitation and quick pulse may be present, as also increased blood pressure, especially in thin single women of " rheumatic " tendencies.

Finally, the symptom of insomnia is prominent in the actæa pathogenesis, and given anything like a characteristic actæa temperament, the use of the drug will be found satisfactory for the condition.

Macrotin in the lower potencies has been praised for lumbago.

COCA

This drug is prepared from the leaves of a South American plant, Erythroxylon coca. The main source of its activity is the alkaloid cocaine and potencies of this have also been used. Probably the leaf tincture is preferable, but in the symptomatology that follows no distinction has been attempted between the two sources of our information through provings and clinical use.

General Considerations

Cocaine has proved one of the greatest curses to so-called civilisation in spite of its medicinal value, and " doping " with it is far too frequent. There was for a time an unfortunate belief (now abandoned) that cocaine would combat the morphia habit, and it was then given rather recklessly for this purpose. But to-day it is disastrously established as one of the fashionable vices, and a false air of romance hangs about it which may lead foolish people to experiment with it, whereupon it very quickly takes a sinister grip on the unhappy experimenter.

The only cure for the cocaine habit is deprivation of the drug. A period of intense physical and mental suffering has then to be endured. It is possible that high (thirty and upwards) potencies of the drug might help at this stage.

There is a certain amount of evidence that the potentised drug can, for a time at least, lessen the desire for the crude poison. Thus potencies of *tabaccum* will in some cases lessen or remove the desire for cigarettes. One thing can be confidently asserted, that if the drug be indicated and given in potency there is no fear whatever of inducing a habit or of causing any of the harmful symptoms that follow larger doses. With cocaine as with any other agent, the dictum " the greater the poison, the greater the remedy " holds good. But of course the symptoms must match for true effectiveness because, as Dr. Julian has well said, when symptoms appear which resemble those of a drug it is safe to assume a susceptibility to that drug and no large quantities are necessary.

When Conan Doyle made his famous character Sherlock Holmes take cocaine as a substitute for his specialised brain activities when these were not in demand, he was speaking more as a romancer than as a physician. For cocaine taken as as a " dope " does not seem often, if ever, to produce effects such as opium and hashish can bring. These do on occasion cause subjective visions and illusions that can be enjoyable, however great the risks are in other ways, though the experiences are not always pleasant. Also, as De Quincey and Coleridge found, they may stimulate the imagination or, more likely, make it easier to influence in certain directions, not necessarily the highest.

The whole problem of the imagination and what we call inspiration and its relation to drug stimuli is of the greatest importance. It might seem more suitable to discuss it in reference to a drug which has more power in this direction than has cocaine, but on the other hand there may be an advantage in treating the subject free of the necessity to consider any one relationship.

Inspiration, as its name implies, has been held to be an influence from without, generally divine, using the inspired mind merely as a channel.*

That one mind can influence another directly (telepathy) is now generally accepted but there is no clear evidence that such an influence can be continuous and persistent enough to be

* Though we do not dispute the possibility of divine inspiration, as physicians, we are only concerned with the factors and mechanisms within the human framework that function when creative activity occurs. To pass into the region of metaphysical speculation is a temptation to be avoided when reflecting upon the structure of the human personality.

responsible for creative work through the medium of another brain.

There is, of course, the phenomenon of automatic writing in trance, and some " spirit " messages written in this way are difficult to explain away.* But of these phenomena no one as yet is in a position to dogmatise, and judgment on them must be reserved. If they ultimately are accepted as genuine, there will arise the interesting question as to whether any drug can make the automist more or less permeable to an outside influence, but at the moment that thought cannot be pursued fruitfully.

All the recent psychological work makes it probable, almost to the point of certainty, that it is to the unconscious that we must look for an understanding of imaginative creative work. We think of this mainly in the kingdoms of art, but science too has recorded flashes of insight that must be called inspiration. Indeed Einstein has testified to this. The interesting point is the feeling that is experienced that the work is in some ways beyond the direct control of the worker. The line " Das Lied das aus der kehle *drängt* " (the song that *forces its way out* of the throat), for instance, expresses in the final word that sense of something that forces itself into recognition.

We are not overlooking the fact that the behaviourists place a very different interpretation on these phenomena. Let Mr. H. G. Wells outline this doctrine simply :—

" The right-out Behaviourist does not see man as a simple unified mind or psyche at all. He sees him as a neuro-sensitive apparatus. This neuro-sensitive apparatus extends all over our bodies : it includes not only ganglia but the circulation, glandular secretions, anything with excitability in it. . . . It is the body that holds the mind together says the complete Behaviourist and not the mind the body. The body has to go where the dominant system in the neuro-sensitive apparatus takes it, but all the time an immense variety of other reaction systems are going on and either depleting or replacing the dominant system." Wells continues and explains that the behaviourist conceives each person as consisting of " a col-

* Particularly these messages purporting to come from Dr. Verrall and Frederich Myars wherein two automatic writers having no relation to one another, these record each a half of the whole message at about the same time.

lection of mutually replaceable individual systems held together in a common habitation. One ascends ; another fades before it. If the systems vary, you call John Smith moody or inconstant, and if they vary widely you may have such contradiction that at last you have a double personality. . . . This description of a man as a sort of armoury of selves like a bag of golf clubs, first this one and then that going into play with its body owner, is supported by a thousand phenomena of forgetting and remembering, of double personality, of the changes of what we call character that appear under different stimuli and at different phases of life." (Extract from *Babes in the Darkling Wood*, H. G. Wells.)

A great novelist speaking of the work he put into his novels added, " But when it comes to dialogue between my characters in moments of passion not a word is my own." That is to say, his characters seemed to be beyond his power of direction.*

Dramatists also have recorded similar experiences as though their imagined characters took on a life of their own. At least two plays in our time have been based on this phenomenon, and a notable writer of drama, describing his way of work, said that he devised his story ; fitted characters to it ; planned its acts and scenes and then tried to live with the creatures of his imagination until they began to " talk of themselves " and only then would he put pen to paper to write his play.

Any physician who is familiar with the writings of Jung who has described his clinical observations on this matter will realise how these experiences can be related to the workings of the unconscious which appears to dominate creative work in a way heretofore unexplained. That the conscious mind assimilates and transmutes into artistic form impulses from the unconscious, is one of the postulates of these studies. Our principal object is to consider the mode by which the potentised drug may modify this conscious-unconscious relationship.

Into the region of the unconscious pass memories trivial and intense at the time. It can hardly be doubted that much of what seems to the artist to be beyond his control is actually

* It is important to note that he elsewhere defined " Passion " as " Noble strength on fire." He did not use the word as often for ungovernable anger or desire. For him it connoted both strength and nobility with the added quality of burning vital energy.

an uprush from subliminal regions not only of things long
forgotten but also from the inherited racial layers of the
unconscious.*

Though it is probably the revival of things long forgotten
that supply words and descriptions that have the vividness of
reality, for once they or something like them were real. There
naturally comes in the effect of culture and knowledge. The
well stored brain has not only more to draw on in experience
(second-hand in so far as it is drawn from the writings of
others but made personal when deep affinity exists between
the reader and the writer), but colours from its cultivated taste
and conscious knowledge the thoughts and images that derive
from the unconscious. Here comes in the "labour of the
file " : the " capacity for taking pains " ; but neither of these
alone will awake the thrill which makes the recipient cry
" Genius." It is by a realisation of all the factors that we are
able to form valid judgments, if only for ourselves, as to the
relative worth of works of art.†

It is doubtful if any such work can appeal profoundly to
anyone unless there is a sense of participation, as of one unconscious reaching out to another, and unless the unconscious
has played a part in the creation, that appeal cannot be made.
We can be entertained, interested by works deliberately and
consciously constructed but we shall not feel any thrill if that
be the whole matter. Yet we have to confess that a genuine
thrill is experienced by many from works of art which to us
seem tawdry, commonplace and trivial. But here comes in
the background of culture.‡

It is a fact that many undistinguished minds have had the
faculty of drawing on their unconscious and so giving to their
works that quality that can appeal. But since they have little

---

* " As the body is a sort of museum of its phylogenetic history, so is the
mind. There is no reason for believing that the psyche, with its peculiar
structure, is the only thing in the world that has no history beyond its individual manifestation . . . the unconscious psyche is immensely old . . . it
is part of the human species just as much as the body, which is also indi-
vidually ephemeral, yet collectively of immeasurable duration. . . ." (JUNG.)

† Works of science can be dispassionately tested.

‡ There are many untrained listeners and observers whose innate appreciative faculties are subtle as well as spontaneous. These will often surpass in
judgment more highly trained and learned critics. This must depend on a
close instinctive correlation of the senses, the conscious brain and the unconscious, which many of us have to acquire, if at all, by long and painful effort.

or no culture, what comes from the unconscious is not enriched
or shaped. Their appeal may be (often is) widespread and is
genuine in that it arises from the unconscious element which
we postulate as essential, but it will only be an appeal to
similar minds with similarly limited backgrounds. For them
something is expressed which they would have gladly expressed
themselves and they pay their tribute of admiration. Those
minds at a higher level of development have passed beyond
(though they may have passed through) this stage and the
expression of it has nothing to give them but boredom or
nausea. Criticism far too often fails to realise its essential
" relativity " and the only valid kind is that given to works
which the critic values and admires. Dislike may depend as
much on the critic as on the criticised and is comparatively
valueless, though it may be illuminating as to the critic himself. But liking implies sympathy and understanding and
can throw genuine light for others on the work that is thus
appreciated. This has a reference to the antipathy some
physicians show to the study of the (as yet embryo) science of
psychology.

Returning now to the possible effects of drugs on the creative
faculty, they will probably be most evident in their influence
first on the relative encouragement or inhibition which they
may produce in the way of letting " unconscious " influences
rise into consciousness, and secondly on any particular
" colour " which they may encourage in these messages.
This last will depend to a great extent on the subject's constitutional make-up, and that again to modern conceptions is
interpreted largely in terms of hormone balance. That some
natures are more prone than others to emotions like jealousy,
suspicion, fear, on the one hand and altruism, confidence,
courage, on the other is familiar enough. Even granting that
finally " man is master of his fate " in this respect and that
persistent effort can modify or encourage these tendencies,
this education is much more difficult for some than others.*

Excessive taking of drugs tends to lessen control, encourages
tumultuous and incoherent subliminal messages and is no help

---

* There is of course the belief held by some that men are automata and
that free will is a delusion. As the question cannot possibly be determined
finally we lean to the alternative that control and guidance are possible for
human beings however difficult it may often be to practise them.

to any fine work. All the " dopes " do more or less what alcohol does, confer a sense of power which is illusory, mainly through loosening bonds of normal inhibitions. Work done in such circumstances seems satisfactory to the worker but is actually poorer in quality. But since the massive doses thus diminish good judgment and mental power, small doses should help both when disease is imitating the effects of the poisonous quantities and that is the finding of the homœopathist. There are a few interesting observations as to the effects of drugs on brain workers. It remains true that the finest quality of imaginative work is seldom if ever aided by any kind of doping. But there are brain workers whose work is not of the highest quality who seem to be capable of stimulation to fancy if not to imagination by small doses of either drug or disease toxin. In the case of drugs the taker seldom if ever has control enough to limit his dose. Habituation demands increasing quantities and before long the gross effects of the drug appear and any stimulant becomes too fugitive to have any value.

With disease, during the early stages and even later, fluctuating quantities of toxins may at times encourage mental activity (cf. Tuberculosis). At least one case is known to us wherein a sufferer from chronic bowel toxæmia was cured of his physical symptoms by an appropriate vaccine but lost entirely for a considerable time his ability to invent the lighter literature (stories and so on) by which till then he had made a comfortable living. A final point of interest is concerned with the fact that the messages from the unconscious that are allowed to come through by drug influence are so much more often unpleasant, horrifying and morbid than pleasant and cheerful. Even the pleasure-giving ones, those of cannabis (often though not always) are almost entirely sensual. This is no doubt explained by the fact that the tissues are also affected and therefore mould stimuli from the unconscious in a disordered way.

High imaginative messages or flashes of deep insight rarely if ever come from drugs. It may be that the explanation lies in the fact that the " dope " taker being deficient in will and resolution has faced up less well to the more difficult life experiences and has repressed many more than he has sublimated. Furthermore, the probability is that the quality of the mind in such individuals is inferior, bodily tissues will be adversely affected, so that the brain does not function adequately. Hence the individual is unable to interpret and fashion the unconscious contents which reach awareness.

The really great creators have always been men of character and moral courage. The saying " Great wits to madness are near allied " is not true for the really great, though it has a relative validity for some minds of more than average power.

General Action of Coca on the Body

Returning now to coca, its stimulating effects are nearly all exerted in the nerve-muscular sphere. It does remove fatigue and increase ability for exertion, deepens respiration and gives a sense of well-being. The medullary centres are certainly affected so that heart and respiration are first stimulated. Following this action elimination might well be (at least temporarily) forwarded and some of the effects of lessening fatigue would thus be accounted for, while the effect in the respiratory centre would counteract the tendency to breathlessness following muscular exertion and high altitudes. Whatever be the explanation, coca has been found of value in complaints such as dyspnœa or attacks of fainting or even anginal attacks following mountain climbing or occurring in certain individuals who become distressed when exposed to life at great altitudes.

Here it may be noted that coca assists the dyspnœa and asthmatic attacks in the aged.

But while the neuro-muscular activities are helped, on the higher centres the stimulating effect is very fugitive indeed. For a time perhaps more mental work can be done, but for a short time only and it is by no means of a high quality because of other mental effects to be presently described. The order of stimulation is cerebrum first, the midbrain and then medulla, and the effects last longer in the loser brain region. This confirms the finding that physical fatigue is more easily relieved and for a longer time than mental.

These effects on the body have guided the physician to administer coca to patients who are suffering from the results of overstrain either mental or physical. The final effects on the muscular system is to produce exhaustion and so the drug may be indicated in cases of extreme physical weariness and, especially, weakness of the legs.

Depression follows stimulation and this appears in both cardiac and respiratory systems. Blood pressure rises at first from contraction of the vessels and later falls. There is little evidence from massive doses of much effect on metabolism. Under massive doses the brain degenerates, will-power is lessened and moral control almost to extinction. Sleeplessness is common. Hallucinations and delirium begin to appear and mental disturbances to the region of insanity. On the neuro-muscular side there are tremors and convulsions.

Patients in the earlier stages may be restless and talkative or anxious and confused. But a calm languor is not infrequently observed and this is one of the effects that the cocaine lovers enjoy. It is not really restful or followed by any stimulation of mental activity.

Homœopathic Indications

The effects on the sensory nerves of cocaine locally are, of course, well known and often employed surgically. It is a local anæsthetic, paralysing the ends of the sensory nerves. Pain and tactile sensations are abolished, those of heat and cold less affected. In the matter of taste, salt can be perceived, bitterness not at all and sweetness partially. But when the drug is habitually taken there develops a sensory symptom affecting the skin which is very characteristic. The sufferer describes it as resembling the feeling of small foreign bodies like grains of sand under the skin, or more commonly as though a living organism (worms or insects) were crawling there. The feeling is so intense that the sufferer thinks that he can see the organism crawling on his skin. If touched, they disappear momentarily but quickly return. Now sensations such as these do not occur very frequently as a result of disease. If they do, their appearance makes a strong call for coca. But short of the full sensation picture, lesser degrees of formication will be controlled by the drug and it should be remembered. Skin cases frequently lack distinguishing features, it is rather as though, since the skin is an excretory organ, when it is notably affected by disease the rest of the organism remains relatively free from trouble. Therefore the local symptoms in such patients often take on a greater importance and this one of exaggerated formication is worth remembering. Erythema has been recorded as a result of cocaine but the sensation symptom is more valuable than the rash.

There is some evidence that coca affects the gonads. Desire in both sexes is increased and may be excessive. Sexual power is finally diminished. Probably the chief effect on the gland is one of depression and the increased desire may be a transference to the mental sphere of the unconscious apprehension that sexual power is diminished.

The candidates for the drug are generally bashful and timid and that fact again suggests that the sex hormones are, to say the least, not increased in quantity. The mental preoccupation with sex often leads to self-abuse and dissipation and when weakly nervous patients complain of fatigue and confess to sexual excess, coca is a good remedy to remember. In such cases there is usually melancholy, great preoccupation with the health. Solitude and darkness are preferred.

Conditions of mental prostration, depression and confusion, sometimes alternating with periods of mental activity, at times even excitement and loquacity, may call for coca. Recently it has been found useful in cases of this kind which have arisen from deferred shock following war experiences (air raids, etc.).

We note here an interesting symptom recorded by one prover of cocaine. Following a large dose (8 mg.) of the hydrochlorate of cocaine, there followed a condition where all brain work became impossible. The sufferer could not undertake the smallest sum in arithmetic.

There has been noted a headache with frontal tension as though from an elastic band or a dull feeling in the occiput or both. The last may be relieved by lying face downwards.

Taste effects have been described : sense of smell is much diminished and now and then the drug helps post-influenzal cases where taste and smell are largely lost. Small doses of the drug given to the healthy retard both hunger and thirst. In patients, loss of appetite and craving for spirits and tobacco are common : salt appears to disagree. This is real but much aggravated by hypochondria. The patient is always thinking about it and worrying about it even when it is not severe.

There is a considerable amount of distension of the abdomen and stomach which may bring on violent palpitation.

A peculiar sensation recorded is that the flatus rises from the stomach with such force that it seems as if the œsophagus would be rent with it.

The cardiac symptoms are important. Susceptible subjects experience cardiac crises, precordial oppression, thready pulse, palpitation and pain. The pulse is usually rapid at first and later slowed and intermittent. The cardiac symptoms are frequently accompanied by excessive sweating. The effects are produced by action through the nerves though the power of coca to relieve muscular fatigue applies also to heart muscle and it can supplement arnica in heart strain. But while arnica can deal with chronic conditions, it is better to use coca for emergencies.

Finally it has a value for some forms of sleeplessness, particularly when the patient feels inclined to sleep yet cannot find rest. He may be overpoweringly drowsy and yet cannot pass over into slumber.

Subjects indicating coca are aggravated generally by mental exertion. Their symptoms are worsened by cold and during rest and many complaints are brought on when ascending high altitudes.

There is a general amelioration from the open air, especially rapid motion in the open air such as walking or riding. Symptoms tend to improve after sunset.

Coca is a drug of great interest and it may be that it is less used in potency than it deserves.

Appendix to the Study of the Three Drugs :
Anacardium, Argentum and Coca

Homœopathy is concerned primarily with practice. If a symptom can be held to be the result of a drug effect on the human body, then that symptom appearing in disease is an indication for the remedy. We may explain symptoms in various ways, but their worth as pointers to a good prescription remains unaltered.

But to attempt to explain the possible "mechanism" of symptoms has value in that it may show relationship that makes possible symptom groupings. Thus memory is aided and it is even conceivable if (or when) fuller knowledge is available that a realisation of relationship will take the place of much more laborious symptom matching by enabling one or two observations to imply the whole picture.

But while that day is far off, no apology is needed for an attempt to explain the why and wherefore of characteristic drug symptoms.

In the three articles on anacardium, silver and coca, we have tried to approach the characteristic mental effects of each drug from the standpoint of modern psychology and endeavoured to show that these effects can be expressed in terms of psychological conceptions.

We repeat that this neither adds to nor detracts from their value as indications for a prescription, but we have thought it of interest to attempt the task.

The psychological conceptions that are the background to our suggested explanations are (chiefly) that individuality * is a real entity but subject to possible division and confusion and that the unconscious mind is a part of it and an important one responsible for many phenomena both in disease and health. But another view has been put forward which may be summarised as maintaining that individuality is a delusion and what is held to be that elusive entity is the expression in human beings of a variety of strains of tendency made of experienced memories and deductions therefrom and that power of will and choice are incomplete. The strains of tendency are largely independent and sense of division is due not to a splitting of an entity but to the co-existence of two (or more) strains whereof neither is wholly dominant. In other words, the race may be in process of developing real personality but as yet the elements to make it are not fused or controlled enough to warrant the word. The ego on which we pride ourselves is no more than a realisation of a dominant strain of tendency.

---

* We are employing this term according to the concept of Jung who uses it to embrace the peculiarity and singularity of the individual in every psychological respect.

If future investigation should find this (or any other) conception closer to the facts of observation, suggestions as to symptom mechanism based on other views will naturally fail. The prescriber will be left with the value of symptoms unaltered for his purpose and the student of " mechanism " will have to look elsewhere for his explanation.

It appears to us that so many varying interpretations of psychological mechanisms have been formulated because the subject has been approached, in every case, from a different angle. What each man beholds depends upon his orientation. The essence of the psyche remains a mysterious thing and certainly its depths have not yet been probed. While we have used principally the concepts of Jung to essay an explanation of the action of drugs on alterations of personality, we realise that other systems are of value both in the elucidation of the mechanisms of the mind and in the problem we have undertaken.

The theories of the behaviourists, for example (which we have mentioned), though we do not feel able to accept them as a complete exegesis of the individuality, clearly throw light on one facet of this fascinating subject.

Again, we consider that we could have incorporated with advantage an outline of the Gestalt psychology in this study, a conception which is especially congenial to the homœopathist who, above all, puts emphasis on form (isomorphism) and views his patient as a whole.

But just as various aspects of the human body can be expounded in terms of the anatomist, the physiologist and so forth, so the psyche can be described within the content of different psychological systems. All contain part but none the whole exposition of the problem. From this point of view we think that we are justified in not having attempted to embody the concepts of every psychological school of thought in these studies. " Concepts really are organs, that is, for us the better to understand reality." So we have used one organ of mental vision only in our thesis.

" *It is not the eye that sees, we see by means of the eye.*"

(PLATO.)

FERRUM

Ferrum Metallicum.   Triturations of the pure metal for lower potencies.

There are several salts of iron available for the physician, but, as far as the homœopathist is concerned, ferrum metallicum suffices for most cases when iron is indicated. Ferrum phosphoricum (phosphate of iron), though presenting resemblances to the metal, demands separate mention and has its own important spheres of action.

Iron is an element essential to life, entering as it does into the composition of hæmoglobin. It is a material essential for the proper production of the mature fully hæmoglobinised erythrocyte, and a deficiency of iron causes an anæmia at that stage of erythropoiesis at which hæmoglobin is being absorbed by the developing red cells. The anæmia is one in which the cells are deficient in hæmoglobin though the number of cells produced may, in some cases, be almost normal. The utilisation of iron is dependent on several factors, the most important of which is an efficient gastric function. Gastric acidity appears to be one of the main factors in promoting an adequate iron absorption, and the massive doses of iron which are usually administered may be reduced if HCl or bile pigment be given at the same time.

Given in excess ferrum causes gastric pain, nausea, vomiting and purging, and for the homœopathist has a definite remedial power over certain gastro-enteric cases with diarrhœa. Smaller doses if persisted in tend to cause constipation and when chronic cases call for iron they are usually constipated. One observer (Buzdygan) quoted by Cushny maintains that the secretion of gastric HCl is increased : homœopathists on clinical grounds would be inclined to endorse this observation.

Local congestion of the upper air passages with fullness and heat in the head, and hæmorrhages from throat, nose, and lungs are symptoms of the over-use of iron, with which the provings have made homœopathists familiar, and they are (with qualification to be noted later) good indications for the remedial use of the metal. Dr. Cushny holds such symptoms to be either imaginary or the result of gastro-intestinal reflex action. It is at any rate difficult for those who have used the drug homœopathically to adopt the first alternative, but it is true that there is no evidence of much direct action on heart or vessels. The central nervous system is depressed and finally paralysed. The kidney is irritated, casts and albumen appearing in urine. It is the action of iron upon the blood constituents that is of the most direct significance when the metal is regarded as a remedy. It is said to cause leucocytosis (Pohl, quoted by Cushny *).

Much argument has been expended and many experiments made to determine the problems of iron absorption and metabolism. Iron is taken in the food in an ordinary dietary to the extent of $\frac{1}{12}$ to $\frac{1}{6}$ of a grain per day and about the same amount is excreted in fæces (chiefly) and urine. Since iron is excreted by the large bowel, the measurement of the amount found in the fæces throws little light on the previous adventures of the metal given by the mouth. It seems clear that it is slowly absorbed from the small intestine, stored for a time in liver, spleen and bone marrow, then gradually removed from these tissues and finally excreted by cæcum and colon. Its course appears to be from duodenum to spleen, later to liver, and finally into the blood, and gradually back to the alimentary canal (cæcum) for excretion. There is iron in the bile, but this secretion does not seem to be used as a means of disposing of any excess of the metal : whether iron be absorbed in solution or in solid form is as yet a doubtful point, but of any ordinary dose swallowed, only a fraction is absorbed at all. That which is absorbed, however, increases the hæmoglobin content of the blood in certain anæmias. It may act by supplementing the food iron when a deficiency of this has been the cause of the anæmia, for food iron follows the same course in absorption as does inorganic iron : in these cases to increase the food without adding inorganic iron is successful.† But iron deficiency

* " Pharmacology and Therapeutics," p. 662.

† Recent investigations on over 1,000 unemployed families (3,500 individuals) showed that anæmia was present in 50 per cent. of women and absent in men. Analysis of the diets showed that they contained, in some instances, less than half the normally accepted standard amount of iron requisite. Though it was adequate for the men who maintained a satisfactory hæmoglobin level, this figure was not sufficient if any increased demands for iron were made on the individual. The increased demands in women are presumably those made by menstrual loss, repeated pregnancies and lactation.

The conclusions drawn from these investigations were that the prevention of idiopathic hypochromic anæmia is largely an economic one. If the population received an adequate diet, this disease would rarely occur. (Dr. J. M. Vaughan, " The Anæmias.)

anæmias occur also when food iron is not deficient and then to increase the food iron is not a procedure that cures.   Yet inorganic iron in these cases will cure, and the most reasonable explanation is Van Noorden's that the medicinal iron is a stimulant to the blood-forming tissues and enables them (thus stimulated) to take up again their task of elaborating hæmoglobin and making red blood corpuscles when previously they had flagged in the performance of both functions.   It has also been suggested that the quantity of iron given medicinally is a factor in the stimulation, for to increase food iron to the amount of several grains would involve giving more food than the body could digest.   Yet if the mechanism is one of stimulation it is at least equally likely (if not more likely) that the difference in quality of the inorganic iron as against food iron counts for something, and if this were so large quantities might be quite unnecessary.

There has grown up a practice in recent years of administering iron in anæmia in very large doses.   A generation ago doses were substantial, then there was a period when smaller quantities tended to be used, and now the dosage is very large indeed.   In many cases demonstrably rapid increase of red cells and hæmoglobin follows the use of this method.   It is further claimed that small doses are virtually useless, and that it is impossible to exhaust the bone marrow activities by over-stimulation.   On the other hand, only a small fraction of the iron given can be deemed to be used constructively, and if the massive doses are necessary some other factor must be at work. In most cases that show anæmia there is evidence of greater or less chronic intestinal infection especially by organisms of the non-lactose fermenting groups.   Possibly the course that iron follows in the body with its conclusion in the colon may have some inhibiting influence here on bacterial growth and so indirectly help towards recovery.

Although in the iron pathogenesis there appears a type of anæmia, to be presently described, yet the blood count and hæmoglobin ratio in our experience is seldom notably influenced by iron in high potencies.   In such cases the drug would be regarded as a stimulus to bone marrow activity and the actual supply of the metal obtained from a suitable diet.   In theory this should avail, but in practice the results are disappointing, so that from the angle of experiments also there appears to be a factor in these anæmias for which an appreciable quantity of the element is necessary. But if the lower triturations of the metal are used, involving a dosage of only fractions of a grain finely divided and spread out as it were in surface, then we find a satisfactory response in the hæmoglobin level. It is this practice to which homœopathists incline rather than to the massive dosage now fashionable. The late Dr. Galley Blackley introduced the protoxalate of iron for anæmia and it has proved itself a very useful remedy. He usually employed the 1x trituration or a grain or two of the substance.

Iron is of little or no value in pernicious anæmia and the hyperchromic types generally, nor do its symptoms as accepted by homœopathists tend to appear in these conditions.

The attitude of the homœopathist to iron as a remedy for anæmia is, therefore, that it can produce an anæmia of a definite type and can cure cases of that type, when they occur, in potencies high or low.

The general symptoms that suggest its use are debility even after slight exertion, easy fatigue and lack of endurance, general sensitiveness to cold, vaso-motor instability and tendency to hæmorrhages. The vaso-motor instability leads to local flushings : thus the cheeks are characteristically flushed, though there is pallor of the lips and mucous membranes. There may be pallor of the face when at rest, but the least excitement induces flushing of the cheeks.

Throbbing headache, pulsation of arteries, which is sensible to the patient, throbbing neuralgic pains (especially if aggravated by cold water), swelling of the feet and obstinate constipation, all these are common symptoms of many anæmias and are also symptoms that suggest iron as a remedy. The pulse is full, but the tension low : the hæmorrhages come from nasal or gastric mucous membranes or from hæmorrhoids or from (previously) diseased lungs,* or from the uterus. They tend to recurrence and they aggravate any anæmia that may be present.

The easy fatigue and breathlessness of patients who need

_____
* Ferrum aceticum in low potencies is one of the best remedies for hæmoptysis.

iron is often out of proportion to their actual anæmia and suggests a cause in a weakened nervous system. Mentally, patients who indicate the drug are very restless and irritable, changeable in mood and impulsive.

So essential is the relation of iron to the blood that it is possible that any case that requires it will have some degree of anæmia, but there are certain symptom-groups that suggest it that have no obvious derivation from anæmia. Thus in the alimentary canal there is a peculiar irritable diarrhœa that occurs now and then, especially in young people, which meets a ready remedy in ferrum. It seems to be due to an exaggeration of the gastro-colic reflex, for its great characteristic is that it is brought on by beginning to eat. The first mouthfuls cause a call to stool. Lientery also is a ferrum symptom. Another feature is an immediate aggravation of all digestive symptoms from attempting to eat eggs. Gastralgia, hæmatemesis (suggesting gastrostaxis rather than gastric ulcer), periodic vomiting, which may occur immediately after eating or about midnight, are all ferrum symptoms. It is unusual for these to be accompanied by the sensation of nausea.

In the genito-urinary sphere the menorrhagia has been already mentioned : miscarriage has been caused by iron and it seems to affect sexual power adversely. It may also be required in the vomiting of pregnancy where the patient is typically weak and flabby, with a flushed face. The characteristic modality here is the absence of nausea.

There is a peculiar irritability of the bladder comparable to that of the bowel which causes diarrhœa : it leads to incontinence of urine, for there is also a weakness of the sphincter and the irritable sudden contraction of the bladder easily overcomes the guarding muscle.

Another form of symptom is a spurting of urine which comes from sudden motion such as walking or coughing and the incontinence is more common in women than in men.

It is noteworthy that it is more marked by day than by night, the spasm being largely reflex and the erect position being an unfavourable one for the patient. Cramps of all kinds are common in the pathogenesis of iron. The irritability of the mind, in fact, as with arsen. and china, is accompanied by an irritability of the body : ferrum antidotes both china and arsenicum, so that the arseniate of iron is not a very useful preparation.

Ferrum phosphoricum is the only iron preparation that is often indicated in respiratory diseases, except for the use of ferr. acet. already alluded to for hæmoptysis. But occasionally asthma is helped by iron when the general symptoms agree, and especially if there is relief from moving about.

Iron develops in its provings very definite pains both aching and more acute, especially in the region of the shoulder joint and deltoid muscle, and has proved a good remedy when the pains are relieved by moving about slowly. Sudden movement or exertion aggravates symptoms. The right side seems more readily affected than the left.

The principal time. of acute aggravation when ferrum is called for is about midnight, but for many symptoms (e.g., joint pains, eneuresis, etc.) the day is a time of greater suffering than the night. The subjects suitable to it are chilly and worse in winter, but also resent extremes of heat. This is another expression of the temperamental and bodily irritability. The patient is often restless when keeping still, his symptoms being ameliorated when moving about quietly and gently. When the general symptoms suggested it, Dr. R. T. Cooper found iron very useful in chronic deafness.

FERRUM PHOSPHORICUM

Pure Phosphate of Iron prepared by trituration.

Ferrum phosphoricum was introduced into the Materia Medica by Schüssler, when he published his "Twelve Tissue Salts," and it is from his work that the knowledge of its uses was first obtained.

Schüssler considered the drug to be indicated in and capable of curing the first stage of all inflammatory processes before any exudation sets in, and the early stages of infective and febrile disturbance. He also used it in cases of hyperæmia following contusion, sprain or wounds. Thus ferrum phos. came to be regarded as largely confined to acute conditions, notably acute febrile disease. Incidentally it is interesting to note that it is prominent among the mineral constituents of tinc. of aconite.

Since the first introduction of the drug, some partial provings have been made and a considerable amount of clinical observations have been accumulated with the result that its value therapeutically has been found to extend much beyond the range of its earlier practice.

Certainly, ferrum phos. has a first place among the list of remedies employed in the treatment of acute illness. Schüssler, regarding his tissue salts essentially as foods, administered them in the lower potencies, but the homœopathist uses these " tissue remedies " when similar symptoms are present in the patient, and rather than regarding these drugs as substitution therapy is prepared to employ any potency, even the very high ones.

The characteristic appearance of the ferrum phos. patient is one of habitual pallor, often with delicate texture of the skin. But the unstable circulation renders him liable to flush easily on excitement or exertion.

In acute conditions, the clear delicate pallor of the patient is accompanied by a malar flush which tends to disappear when the patient sits up (in very severe cases, the face becomes dusky).

The typical ferrum phos. patient is of a delicate physical constitution and with the bodily debility is associated a mental weakness. He is unable to concentrate his mind and deal with the various difficulties in his life. The memory is notably impaired, especially is there a difficulty in recalling names. The mental sluggishness of the patient causes him to experience considerable irritability over his own defects. When in this state he feels better when alone. He has an aversion from the presence of other persons who may upset him, causing an outbreak of violent anger. The patient experiences many fears, fear of a crowd ; of death ; that some misfortune may befall him.

Ferrum phos. is often indicated in patients suffering from an Iron Deficiency Anæmia, especially when associated with varicose veins.

Physical exertion tires the patient. His low vitality is sometimes associated with a tubercular inheritance, and the drug has proved helpful in phthisis (Cooper). The pulse as generally with ferrum is full but of low tension.

Headaches of ferrum phos. are often located in the right supra-orbital region and are usually worse in the morning on waking ; stooping, excitement, and heat aggravate the headaches ; cold applications and pressure relieve.

These blinding headaches are sometimes associated with hemianopia.

Acute conjunctivitis in the early stages of otitis may be controlled by ferrum phos., and in the initial stages of all inflammatory infections of the respiratory tract the drug should be considered.

The ferrum phos. patient has a predisposition to acute catarrh of the nose and attacks of epistaxis are liable to occur in children. The drug is indicated in many cases of acute tonsillitis, where the throat is red and swollen (even in first stages of diphtheria). It is valuable too, for the treatment of laryngitis, when hoarseness or even loss of voice is brought on by exposure.

It is one of the commonly indicated remedies required in the early stages of pneumonia and pleurisy. There is usually a history of exposure to cold followed by sudden onset of infection. The face is pallid with a malar flush. Though the patient is distressed and restless, the condition is not so intense as in aconite, nor is much physical and mental tension present. The tongue is dark red and there is thirst for large quantities of water and for sour things. He resents interference and prefers to be left alone. The attacks of coughing are aggravated by cold air ; the time of aggravation is in the early morning. The appetite is poor and the patient has an aversion from meat and milk, and a desire for sour foods and sometimes for stimulants.

In gastritis, the patient develops intermittent attacks of vomiting of undigested food, which may also appear in the stool. Should hæmatemesis occur, the blood is bright red.

It may be indicated in the first stages of peritonitis, where there is general abdominal enlargement, accompanied with extreme sensitiveness of the abdomen, so that even the touch of the clothes may be painful. The ferrum phos. patient is often constipated, but in acute conditions, attacks of diarrhœa, with blood-stained mucus may occur.

Ferrum phos. produces acute inflammatory condition of the bladder, so that the patient has a frequent desire to urinate, with pain and sometimes incontinence of urine either during the day or night. There may be a tendency for the urine to spurt, should the patient cough.

It is a valuable remedy in rheumatic fever, accompanied by pyrexia, attacking one joint after another. The joints are swollen, intensely painful but not reddened. The pain is aggravated by the slightest movement. The joints selected for the attack are more usually the wrists and hands but later on, other joints become involved.

Sub-acute rheumatism also comes within the sphere of ferrum phos., but here modalities are different and resemble those of ferrum met. The pain is ameliorated by gentle, and aggravated by violent, motion : site of the rheumatism is frequently the right shoulder and upper arm.

In general, symptoms are worse at night and early morning, and are aggravated by touch, jar and movement. The right side of the body is more likely to be selected for attack. The patient, in general, is sensitive to cold, though many of his symptoms are relieved by cold applications e.g., the headaches and acute attacks of toothache are relieved by cold water, and aggravated by warm drinks.

GELSEMIUM

Gelsemium Sempervirens.   Tincture of the bark of the root.

Gelsemium owes its place in the Materia Medica chiefly to the work of Dr. Hale. It is not unknown to non-homœopathic medicine (mainly to relieve symptoms of headache and pain and for these a good deal of " similarity " can be claimed), but there are apt to be great variations in susceptibility to its action, and the ordinary doses of the " orthodox " are not unaccompanied by danger to the patient. Consequently it has no wide popularity.

Gelsemium (or at least its alkaloid, gelsemine) has a certain relationship to strychnine, but it does not seem a very close one, and homœopathic provings at least give little warrant to the claim of close resemblances between gelsemium and nux vomica. Its effects on tissue as a poison point to the much closer likeness of it to Conium and this statement homœopathic research tends to confirm, though there are differences in the two symptom-pictures easily recognised in practice. Like coniine (the alkaloid of conium), gelsemium appears mainly to paralyse motor nerves peripherally, though an action is probable at least on the respiratory medullary centre which seems to account for death after excessive doses. The sympathetic ganglia are also paralysed.

The provings and homœopathic experience in the use of gelsemium give a definite symptom-complex of which the keynote is paralysis. There is a stage of irritation shown in twitchings and spasms, but paralysis sets in early and some degree at least of paresis is characteristic of any case that strongly suggests gelsemium ; while spasm is the predominating element in the nux vomica picture, 'paralysis is conspicuous in that of gelsemium.

Various groups of muscles about the eye or throat may be affected producing such conditions as ptosis, diplopia or dysphagia.

It is a paralysis less central than peripheral and therefore the drug is very suitable, for instance, to post-diphtheritic paralysis. But while its effect on neuro-muscular action is due to a gross poisoning of tissue the paresis is much enhanced by the effect of the drug in the mental sphere. Here, too, it may be said to paralyse ; the mind is sluggish, and lassitude, mental as well as bodily, is pronounced ; the underlying condition of the sluggishness is not so much a stupor of indifference (as with baptisia) but a neurotic " hysterical " mental state which is none the less real for being but dimly expressed. Thus the mental state exaggerates the physical : the patient is so sure of the gravity of his condition that he tends to worsen all the appearances of it. For this reason the drug is particularly well indicated homœopathically in neurotic excitable subjects and for conditions aggravated by mental causes. Thus a lassitude and prostration that set in after the effects of anger or grief, or bad news, or the kind of fear that often precedes an examination, or of " stage fright," find a frequent remedy in gelsemium.

Anticipation also induces a state of nervous excitement in the subject for the drug and may even initiate an attack of diarrhœa.

It is noteworthy that alcohol seems to relieve such symptoms as call for gelsemium and that not only temporarily. Alcohol is seldom of lasting benefit in real and important illnesses, however valuable occasionally as a temporary measure, and the relief it gives to those cases is largely the result of the " suggestive " power of it and of its immediate effects on the mind—and this in spite of the fact that some provers of gelsemium have experienced symptoms very like those of alcoholic intoxication. Thus, given a state of lassitude and paresis, mental and bodily, as a result of acute or sub-acute disease, or of some emotional assault on the nerves, gelsemium is invaluable. Actual paralyses are common ; ptosis frequently appears on diplopia, partial œsophageal or anal paralysis, or paralysis of the tongue may be noted, or all the limbs may be moved with difficulty. The pupils are widely dilated. But gelsemium is also indicated by the irritation of nerve tissue that shows in general tremor, a condition precedent to paresis. Quivering of eyelids or tongue, or of groups of muscles, indicate it, tremor or twitchings of single muscles is a strong keynote of this remedy. When nerve symptoms (convulsions with lassitude supervening) are prominent in measles or scarlet fever, gelsemium may be most useful.

Headache is a very common symptom : it is of sudden onset, often it begins with blurring of the sight or double vision. It is usually worse in the morning and is relieved after copious urination. The headache may be so severe that the patient cannot stand up, but lies exhausted, preferably with the head high in bed. The headache may be the result of masturbation or follow seminal emissions, especially when any " sexual " experiences are brooded over, or foolishly and ignorantly considered. The headache is often felt first in the occiput or lower, then on the vertex, and may culminate over one eye (usually the right) ; with it go vertigo, faintness, drowsiness, and a sense of throbbing. Such headaches often occur with influenza, for which gelsemium is a remedy frequently indicated.

There are two curious effects of the drug on the nervous system which have been observed. First, a strong desire for expression in speech and writing, with a sense of increased power, especially of memory.

This may be regarded as the stage of stimulation preceding the characteristic lassitude. The other " odd " symptom is a " desire to throw herself from a height," which was experienced quite definitely by two independent (female) provers. This goes with the excitable neurotic condition which so often suggests a patient suitable for the action of the drug.

There is a very definite coryza caused by gelsemium, with sneezing in the early morning and a profuse rather watery discharge. It helps hay fever in neurotic subjects, and when influenza is accompanied by nasal catarrh gelsemium is generally to be preferred to baptisia.

As gelsemium is the remedy for such a large proportion of ordinary influenza cases, the symptomatology should be considered in some detail.

The onset is usually slow, the patient feels indefinitely unwell, complaining of vague pains, headache accompanied by a degree of pyrexia.

After some hours the typical gelsemium influenza has developed. The patient is weary and heavy, mentally and physically. He does not want to be disturbed, and is upset by having to make an effort.

If he has to be moved, his symptoms are aggravated : he is extremely sensitive to cold draughts and his extremities feel cold. (N.B. The gels. patient in general is aggravated by heat.)

There is general aching in the muscles and a characteristic stiffness in the cervical region. This latter is associated with severe headache, which is intensified by any motion : the patient feels better when propped up in bed. The headache may be relieved by passing large quantities of urine.

The face is somewhat flushed, the lips slightly dusky and the eyes injected.

There is an acute coryza and the accompanying conjunctivitis is aggravated by light, although the patient may want light as he fears the dark.

There is a tendency to tremor or tremulousness, when the hands may become unsteady and shaky.

Both gelsemium and baptisia are suited to drowsy patients, but the baptisia symptoms are the more profound in this respect and the consciousness more clouded ; gelsemium belongs more to the neurotic and "highly-strung." On the whole, the baptisia patient seems the graver case to the physician and the gelsemium patient to the sufferer and his friends, for the characteristic neurotic temperament causes some exaggeration of feeling and of expression.

In enteric or typhoid it will be but seldom that gelsemium is to be preferred to baptisia, arsenicum, or bryonia, but occasionally a sensitive neurotic patient obtains great relief from it. In such cases of enteric as call for gelsemium the characteristic sluggishness of mind and body is found. The mind is sluggish, the muscles are relaxed, the patient experiences a sensation of heaviness in the limbs and so lies quietly. The face is flushed, dusky and hot. As a rule the gelsemium patient is thirstless. Tremor or paralysis of the tongue is a suggestive symptom for its use.

As is usual with remedies that affect the neurotic particularly, there is evidence that the sexual glands do not escape the influence of the drug. But it is useful rather for subjective symptoms than for objective ones. Thus dysmenorrhœa (with headaches or neuralgias) in sensitive subjects often benefits exceedingly wherever the pain happens most to be felt. In the male it has a value for symptoms of pain referred to the sexual organs, especially when the starting point of them is overmuch brooding on some excess or sexual misconduct.

In nervous conditions palpitation is experienced, the pulse is soft, feeble and irregular. A similar condition may occur during febrile states. All kinds of symptoms of peripheral nerves will benefit from it in suitable cases. It produces neuritis and will help recent cases (e.g., diphtheritic), but sensory nerves come well into its sphere of action also and will respond favourably to it. Professional neuroses (e.g., writers' cramp) are particularly likely to suggest the use of gelsemium.

Motion aggravates most symptoms and the patient's desire is to lie down and rest. But as an exception to this rule there is a nervous heart condition that suggests the remedy when the patient feels as though if he did not move about the heart would stop. Muscular pains also are relieved by movement. Excess of tobacco may cause conditions of this kind and nervous symptoms generally in heavy smokers often find help from gelsemium.

The symptoms are made worse by heat of rooms or sun, especially when thunder is approaching, but local heat often relieves the headache or dysmenorrhœa. Damp weather especially damp warm weather is harmful to the cases that need the drug.

IGNATIA

Ignatia Amara. Tincture of seeds of St. Ignatius Bean.

The seeds of ignatia contain more strychnine than those of nux vomica and the presence of this alkaloid in quantity naturally implies a considerable resemblance between the two drugs. But the provings nevertheless develop noteworthy differences and the two are by no means interchangeable. Thus again is illustrated the phenomenon so familiar to homœopathists that the effects of the most striking and poisonous of active principles in a medicine are greatly modified by the presence of other substances which seem at first almost negligible. The symptoms produced by tincture of ignatia differ notably from those caused by tincture of nux vomica and both complexes again differ from that which ensues on the administration of strychnine.

The first characteristic of the symptoms of ignatia is the unexpectedness of their nature. The ignatia patient presents a symptom, but the manifestation of it is contradictory and unexpected. There is a kind of perversity about the condition that can be caused and cured by ignatia. For example, if the patient is in the chilly stage of a fever and is cold, he wants to be uncovered, but when he is feverish and hot he wants to be warm. He is thirsty when cold and chilly, but when feverish he is not thirsty. Again, pharyngeal irritation causes him to cough, but the more he coughs the more there is irritation to make him go on coughing. The contradictory unexpectedness is seen in certain headaches which are relieved by stopping and are ameliorated by lying on the painful part.

It is usual for an inflamed surface to be painful to touch, but the inflamed part indicates ignatia when it is possibly relieved by hard pressure ; when suffering from an inflamed throat the patient states that he gets his greatest relief from swallowing solids.   In stomach complaints, it is often the simple unirritating foods that trouble him while he is able to take foods that one would expect to disagree.

The symptoms of ignatia are parodoxical, unexpected and perverse.

Hypersensitivity is the second marked characteristic of ignatia.   It is a drug to be considered for patients who are over-sensitive to pain.

There is here to be noted a peculiar modality of ignatia. The pains and symptoms generally tend to pass off after profuse urination.

Hahnemann pointed out that the emotional disposition of patients for whom ignatia is serviceable differs widely from those for whom nux is of use.   He said that ignatia is not suitable for persons in whom anger, eagerness and violence is predominant.   The ignatia patient tends to be highly emotional, capricious, moody and changeful.

Thus the type of patient to whom ignatia is particularly adapted is the sensitive, refined though excitable woman— often of dark hair and skin.   A marked emotional reaction is that of intuitive perception, for she is quick to perceive, rapid in action.   Ignatia symptoms are less likely to occur in the sluggish individual than in the sensitive intuitive girl disposed to concentrate on the arts.

The mental symptoms of ignatia are important.   The drug is seldom indicated unless the mental condition corresponds as between that produced by disease and that caused by drug proving—and when the mental symptoms are strongly marked many diverse diseases may be benefited.   The great mental characteristic of ignatia is rapid alternation of moods, recalling in this respect pulsatilla and crocus.   There is little or none of the anger and irritable violence that suggests nux vomica, although the patient is not quite so soft and pliable as when pulsatilla is required. Gaiety alternates rapidly with melancholy, which is notably tearful, but there is this feature that helps to distinguish the need for ignatia from that for pulsatilla, that the latter is more likely to show a kind of self-pity, little concerned with the sufferings of others ; while the emotional state that calls for ignatia, however unbalanced, is less selfish : there may even be some attempt to conceal grief, and while symptoms often take rise in sorrow from actual loss of friends or other mental suffering, they may also come from sympathy with the troubles of others. The effects of grief in general on sensitive natures are very likely to suggest ignatia and there is no single remedy so likely to be of value for the symptoms arising from recent sorrow. Under its influence patients sleep better, wake more calm in spirit and with more courage and endurance. The effects of mental anxiety or of worry, no less than those of grief, may give rise to a condition which ignatia can help : but although there is so much melancholy and depression in the drug pathogenesis, it must be remembered that violent hilarity with uncontrollable laughter from slight causes may alternate with the mood of sadness. Changes take place without any warning and swiftly : thus the picture of an unbalanced, exaggerated emotional state is completed and the resemblance of the drug pathogenesis to some hysterical conditions is manifest. But anger and violence are seldom if ever prominent among the symptoms ; there is often love of solitude, but no resentment at attempts at consolation, as with sepia or nat. mur.

Not only mental but all physical symptoms change character swiftly and unexpectedly ; changefulness is nearly as marked in the effects of this drug as in those of pulsatilla, but the cause of the symptoms in the latter drug arise less from the nervous system as is the case with ignatia. Suddenness, especially a sudden and unlooked-for loss of function, make it again suitable for the hysterical type of reaction.

It is not wonderful in view of the presence of strychnine in the drug that the ignatia complex should show many spasmodic symptoms. A spasm of the œsophagus occurs which exactly parallels the globus hystericus, the sense of a lump in the throat which rises from the stomach, and if swallowed down constantly returns. This symptom is made worse by drinking water. Twitches and spasms of muscles (marked often in the facial muscles) are common. Hiccough and hysterical vomiting occur and very painful spasm of the anus ; convulsions and spasms from physical causes (fright, fear, etc.) are noteworthy. Ignatia affects the female generative organs considerably (see below), and therefore is indicated in puerperal convulsions when the mental condition corresponds to that producible by the drug. Laryngismus stridulus is another affection that often suggests it. On the other hand, it will often succeed in hysterical aphonia. It affects sensory as well as motor nerves, and is often a remedy for painful conditions. Characteristically the pain is concentrated in small spots, there is a headache that is met by ignatia, described as though a nail were being driven into the head. The fact that the headache often vanishes after copious urination suggests some acute toxæmia. Pains are apt to change their locality suddenly and also are badly endured, so that they seem severe. Pains appear suddenly and cover small circumscribed spots (cf. kali bic. : oxalic acid).

Ignatia, like nux vomica, is one of the remedies suited to persons who feel the cold very much, whose complaints are made worse by cold weather and are worse out of doors, while relieved by heat of sun, or fire, or clothing. Rest relieves symptoms of pain, and movement worsens them. Hard pressure also relieves many pains, but the hypersensitiveness often makes light touch irritating. Cramps and spasms are excited or aggravated by touch. Any strong sensory stimuli are apt to worsen symptoms. Coffee and alcohol disagree with the patient and mental excitement or strong emotion is the cause of many symptoms of distress. There is a great aversion from tobacco which is noteworthy in the pathogenesis.

Turning now to the effects of the drug upon particular regions, it is to be noted that not only do the eyes react subjectively with photophobia and symptoms of flashes and flickerings of light, but that where these symptoms are accompanied with conjunctivitis and lachrymation and inflammation of the edges of the lids, ignatia will cure the objective signs as well as the subjective.

The headaches appear suddenly and are severe. They are aggravated by noise and light and are also brought on by odour, especially tobacco. They are always ameliorated by warmth, rest : lying on the painful side and sometimes by stooping. The patient may describe the pain as if there were a nail being driven into the head (cf. thuja : coffea). The headaches frequently terminate with the passage of a copious flow of urine (cf. aconite, gelsemium, silica).

The appearance is characteristically pale and wan and drawn. Twitches of the facial muscles are common. The throat feels sore and may present an appearance of redness, though not of deeper inflammation or ulceration. Swallowing is very difficult from tendency to choke (spasm, globus hystericus), but the actual soreness of the pharynx is often relieved by the acts of deglutition, showing it to be much more a nervous than an inflammatory symptom.

The appetite is capricious. There may be a complete loss of appetite or a craving for food. Alcohol, coffee, meat are often disliked, and cold food is, as a rule, preferred to hot—an exception to the general rule for this remedy of preference for heat over cold. There is often a craving for sour things. Sensations of weakness and emptiness in the stomach are marked ; the surface is very sensitive to touch and to pressure which relieves neuralgia pains generally with this drug and aggravates the cramps and colic that occur. Hiccough and nausea, even vomiting, may be prominent and much flatulence is complained of, but all these symptoms may be relieved for a time after eating, and are markedly influenced by nervous and emotional causes.

In the genito-urinary sphere the copious urination (of clear and pale fluid) that often relieves the headaches should be noted. The male genital organs are little affected though the drug is often suitable for the nervous results of sexual excesses. In women there is a characteristic dysmenorrhœa, for which ignatia is very valuable, if the mental type of the patient approximates to that of the drug. Its characters are very severe cramping, labour-like pains, relieved by rest and by hard pressure, and the flow is excessive, clotted and venous. All the physical signs in fact are those of uterine spasm.

The respiratory organs and the heart are again affected as regards their nerve supply rather than their structure. Palpitation and throbbing and precordial anxiety brought on by grief or emotion will often yield to ignatia. There is little coryza or bronchial catarrh, but a dry, hacking, spasmodic cough, when the paroxysm gets worse and worse up to a climax, with a tickling referred to low down behind the sternum. Such a cough will often respond to ignatia, either when physical signs are few or none, or when the cough is the result of the irritation of disease, though in this latter case the drug will be a palliative only. It should not be forgotten in whooping cough.

The limbs show many symptoms of pain : violent and sudden neuralgias with cramps and spasms of muscles. Particularly sciatica is to be noted when every movement causes pain, when startings in the muscles are common and sense of weakness in the whole limb. Heat relieves, and hard pressure and rest ; usually some of the mental symptoms will be present to suggest the remedy, and if these appear, spasmodic affections, like chorea, hysteria, and even recent epilepsy, will benefit from it. As with nux vom., there is a tendency to violent itching of the skin. Sleep is generally profound, but dreams may be troublesome. In febrile conditions the odd symptom has already been noted that there is little or no thirst except during the rigor (malaria). Coffee and tobacco are inimical to the action of ignatia.

The symptomatology of ignatia seldom arises from organic lesion, but in functional conditions the patient may become progressively worse and develop symptoms requiring drugs of a deeper acting power. Natrum muriaticum and sepia are the most probable followers of ignatia. But should profound depression of the nervous system develop, phosphoric acid may have to be considered.

IPECACUANHA

Cephælis Ipecacuanha. Tincture and trituration of the dried root.

This is a well-known remedy, and its most salient characteristic of producing nausea and vomiting is familiar. This symptom is nearly always present in greater or less degree when ipecacuanha is likely to be useful, but it has certain qualities which enable the homœopathist to distinguish the nausea it causes and cures from that of other drugs. The distinguishing quality is the persistence of the nausea which accompanies all complaints. There may be a constant desire to vomit, while vomiting, nevertheless, does not take place : or if the nausea ends in vomiting it is not thereby relieved, even for a short time, and there is often a desire to vomit again. The nausea and vomiting are due to the local effect of the drug on the gastric mucous membrane and the medullary centre is unaffected. Consequently, from the homoeopathic point of view, its value is proportionate to the local causation of its characteristic symptom. There is a profuse secretion of saliva, but the tongue is not markedly coated and may even be clean. This is at once a distinction between the effects of ipecacuanha and antim. tart.* This nausea characteristic of ipecacuanha is naturally often associated with disorders of the alimentary canal, but occurs also with respiratory diseases and in febrile complaints (e.g., malaria). Whenever it is present the drug should at once be thought of and confirmatory symptoms looked for. With the nausea not unnaturally goes a disgust for food, and it is noteworthy that the starting point of the milder conditions that call for ipecac. is often indulgence in rich food, pork, pastry, ice cream, etc. The patient often complains that the stomach feels as if it were " hanging relaxed."

This emetic quality of the drug has always to be reckoned with and colours the whole symptom-picture. The condition of the alimentary canal is largely due to an inflammation of the mucous membrane which lines it, and nausea and vomiting are followed or accompanied by frequent loose stools, generally greenish or yellow (the bile secretion seems to be increased) and containing much mucus and generally blood. The stools, in fact, that ipecac. in poisonous doses produces can justly be called dysenteric. There is constant urging to stool with tenesmus with the passage of bright red blood. The patient is pale and prostrate and the whole condition is accompanied by continuous nausea. Consequently the long-standing use of the drug as a cure for amoebic dysentery is of great interest to the homoeopathist. Characteristically the haemorrhages of ipecac. are of bright arterial blood and the power to cause haemorrhage is one of its noteworthy symptoms, but associated with the bleeding there is nausea. The respiratory and the female genital tracts show the tendency as well as the alimentary.

Of late years the alkaloid of ipecac., † emetin, has been used with great success for amoebic dysentery, but its use has been accompanied by warnings, from sources untouched by any interest in homoeopathy, that care is needed to avoid over-

* The vomit may contain bright arterial blood.
† The active principle of ipecac, is actually made up of three distinct alkaloids—cephaeline, emetin and psychotine.

dosing because the symptoms of emetin excess resemble so closely those of the disease that a patient may be gravely poisoned under the impression that his disease is specially refractory.

The orthodox explanation of the unquestionable curative power of emetin (and ipecac.) in amœbic dysentery and its sequel, hepatic abscess, is that the drug has a specific parasiticidal power exerted on the entamœba histolytica. It must be pointed out that the quantity of the drug that reaches the parasites must be uncommonly small at the best. The dose is injected subcutaneously and is presumed to reach the parasites in the process of being excreted. Its power in large doses to cause gastro-enteritis, however introduced into the body, is certain and therefore there is little doubt that, given medicinally, it finds its way to the affected places. But the homœopathist may be pardoned, perhaps, if he speculates whether the curative effect be not reached by arousing a reaction in the mucous membrane rather than by directly killing the parasite. Surely this explanation would render more explicable the danger of over-dosing, for if the first and foremost effect of the drug be on the tissues, then it is clearly easy to poison them instead of merely stimulating them, but if its primary action be on the parasites, then a little too much ought not to be very harmful, as only the excess over and above whatever is taken up by the amœbæ will be available for the mucous membrane. The homœopathist, it is needless to say, welcomes the emetin treatment, and will welcome it even if its pure parasiticidal action be finally established, for it is undeniably effective ; but he retains at present his doubt whether there is not here another instance of the use of a " similar drug," and while he inclines to the view that it acts on tissue rather than on parasite, he is not likely to overdose his patients. It should be added that (presuming that the drug acts indirectly) the evidence points to a local tissue action rather than to a stimulus being given to any kind of general blood resistance such as so often combats bacilli : this consideration again would incline the homœopathist to the use of lower potencies. It is quite possible that triturations of emetin would be effective by the mouth, but more clinical experience is required here.

Before leaving the subject of the orthodox uses of emetin, it may be noted that the drug has been considerably praised recently for controlling hæmorrhages (not only intestinal, but respiratory and other) in cases where there is no question of the entamœba, and therefore no question either of a parasiticidal action. The homœopathist may fairly point out that he has known for a century that ipecac. will control hœmorrhage of a definite type and that this " discovery," therefore, is no novelty to him, but it is difficult to explain save as an instance of his basic generalisation.

The central feature of the ipecac. symptom-complex is this instant action on the alimentary canal. Non-homœopathic observers regard the increased bronchial secretion which it produces as reflex, an effect of the gastric irritation and not the result of direct action upon the tissue of the bronchi (œdema of the lungs has been noted in animal poisonings). This is a point of considerable interest. Provings develop many symptoms of bronchial catarrh. The characteristic cough is dry, spasmodic, asthmatic : there may be dyspnœa with wheezing : or at a later stage there may be accumulations of mucus and inability to get rid of it. It is occasionally valuable in the early stages of pneumonia. The cough is paroxysmal with difficult expectoration of tenacious mucus intermingled with bright red blood, and accompanying the cough there is the characteristic persistent nausea. Usually some gastric disturbance is present, but in spite of this the tongue is clean and moist. The patient is irritable, even bad-tempered and difficult to please (cf. bryonia, the patient wants to be left alone). The most intense paroxysms of asthma have been produced when susceptible subjects are exposed to the drug in the course of preparing it for medicinal purposes. Both epitaxis and hæmoptysis are common. The drug is most often indicated to the homœopathist in bronchitis and asthma among respiratory diseases and frequently appears to act satisfactorily in potencies. On the other hand, it is true that unless there is some degree of gastro-intestinal disturbance and the characteristic nausea, the prescription of the drug is seldom successful. It is a very familiar experience that patients who suffer from one or other of the metabolic disorders which are named " gout " or " gouty," are subject to asthma and bronchitis and their frequent high arterial tension often results in hæmorrhages. The starting point of their disorder is usually the alimentary canal and accessory glands. If, then, the main action of ipecac. is upon this region, it might, by causing improvement there, influence favourably the secondary symptoms and it may well be that it is in respiratory complaints of this kind that it succeeds.

The principle of prescribing on the total symptom-complex is thus justified once more : the bronchitis may appear the most urgent call for assistance, but the accompanying persistent nausea may be the symptom that points conclusively to the ipecac., which will act indirectly through the alimentary canal. However, though orthodox research inclines to the view that ipecac. acts almost exclusively on the gastro-intestinal tract, it must be remembered that the repeated small doses of the provers are a better road to the development of the refinements of the drug action. Therefore, homœopathists may be justified in believing that other tissues than those of the alimentary canal are susceptible to ipecac., and that it is an error to explain all its other effects as reflexes from the main site of action, or only brought about by local irritation. Thus, there is no doubt that ipecac. is intensely irritating locally to the conjunctiva and to the skin : applied to the latter it may cause a pustular eruption, yet when taken internally no such symptoms are readily seen, nor is conjunctivitis a sequel of a large dose. But although no prover developed a pustular eruption, intense irritation of the skin, with uncontrollable desire to scratch it, does appear, and has proved a guiding symptom to the successful use of the drug. Similarly, conjunctivitis, with intense photophobia, lachrymation and neuralgic pain, has appeared in the pathogenesis and the drug helps recent inflammation of this character considerably.

In the genito-urinary sphere its chief use is for uterine hæmorrhages. It controls best those that come as a steady flow of bright arterial blood, and nausea with the hæmorrhage is a determining symptom. The menses are too early as well as too profuse, and the hæmorrhage of threatened abortion, if presenting the characteristics of ipecac., will yield to it. Thick leucorrhœa has been reported as a symptom, and vaginal irritation.

Throughout the ipecac. complex there are a good many

symptoms of pain, generally dull, bruised pains, headaches and neuralgias and such as cause or are accompanied by nausea. They are best read as the concomitants of alimentary toxæmias and are relieved most likely by the influence of the drug upon the alimentary tract.

In considering most remedies, the mental symptoms rank high in importance. But with ipecac. they, too, seem to depend upon the gastric effects of the drug. They are just such as would be expected from the intense irritation and discomfort of the abdominal region. Patients show a morose irritability, the face is pale and drawn and the eyes hollowed, with dark circles round them : children cry and scream readily and (as with bryonia subjects) have desires which they cannot properly express—vague, indefinite longings.

The joints are not much, if at all, affected.

The good subjects for ipecac. are sensitive (as are those who are suited to mercury) to every change in the weather, so that any extremes both of heat and of cold aggravate their symptoms.

Finally, ipecac. in its symptom-complex shows a marked periodicity. Botanically, it is related to cinchona, and it may be that this may have a bearing upon its usefulness in intermittent fever. Whatever the mode of action, homœopathists have found it of great value in obstinate malaria cases, especially when nausea is persistently present, when bone pains are marked and distressing and when the stages of an attack are not regularly defined, but chill and heat vary much in length and severity from one paroxysm to another. Such cases are not uncommon when much quinine has been administered without care, and there may be truth in Dr. J. H. Clarke's suggestion that ipecac. is antidotal to quinine and owes some at least of its virtue in these cases to that fact. Be that as it may, the rule of Jahr to use ipecac. for intermittent fever if no other remedy were clearly indicated is a sound one. If it does not itself cure, it often clears the symptom-complex to a recognisable type and this points the way to the remedy required. The characteristic ipecac. nausea is a good broad hint, whenever present, that the drug is indicated.

Ipecac. does not go well with arsenicum and this fact must be remembered in treating respiratory diseases.

KALI CARBONICUM

Carbonate of Potassium.   Solutions and Triturations.

Sodium, as an element, belongs characteristically to body fluids, while Potassium is associated with body cells. Both elements are absolutely essential to life. Of the sodium salts, the chloride (natrum mur.) is to the homœopathist the most useful remedially, and the potassium salts, the carbonate now under discussion and the hydrate (causticum). To the non-homœopathist it must seem at first almost absurd to expect remedial virtue from either chloride of sodium or carbonate of potassium, since relatively large quantities of them both have so little obvious effect on the body. But as with nat. mur., so with kali carb., the process of potentisation develops unexpected powers and no homœopathist would willingly dispense with either in treating chronic diseases. Each, rightly chosen, is an agent of extraordinary efficacy.

The effects of kali carb. depend for the homœopathist mainly on the potassium it contains. Potassium is well known to physiologists as a poison acting chiefly on the central nervous system and the heart. Muscular weakness sets in early and general sluggishness and apathy. Cushny quotes Mathison as maintaining that spinal centres are first stimulated and then paralysed as the dosage increases, an instance of the familiar rule of Arndt with regard to stimuli. Respiration is difficult and quickened. The heart swiftly responds to the poison, its power is lessened, the beats become weak and irregular and the pulse rate is usually lowered. Heart block and auricular fibrillation may appear. It seems that the main action of the drug is on the cardiac muscle. Peripheral nerves lose irritability under the influence of potassium and other muscles than that of the heart are weakened by it. Potassium salts taken into the alimentary canal pass very rapidly into the urine, so that the poisonous effects of the metal are not observed even after large doses of most compounds of it : but homœopathists have grounds clinically for their belief that the potentised drug has a much more profound effect, principally upon the regions mentioned above and also in other more detailed ways to which the provings give the clue.

To the non-homœopathist the non-metallic ion in both

hydrates and carbonates is more powerful than the metal, but the alkalinity which is the source of the power has little influence in potencies and shows its effects only when acting in some quantity. The hydroxyl (OH) ion is then very poisonous. The therapeutics of alkalies as such do not much concern the homœopathist. They are given to reduce gastric acidity (it is no longer believed that small quantities of them increase it) and improve the gastric circulation : prolonged administration of them has caused gastro-enteritis. It has also been shown that their supposed direct effect on the bile is illusory and that any that seems to appear follows the action on the duodenum. Even after large doses of alkalies the alkalinity of the blood is not increased to litmus, but for a short time there is more alkali in the system available for the neutralisation of any excess of acid and this may be the explanation of the success of very large doses of carbonate of soda, for instance, in some cases of persistent vomiting from acidosis (pregnancy, etc.).

Homœopathic experience results in giving kali carb. a high place among remedies for deep-seated chronic diseases. It will often relieve acute conditions, but best when these are manifestations of some underlying disorder (e.g., tuberculosis). It is valued most by those who use high potencies and infrequent doses, but Professor Schulz, whose provings of the drug confirm those of avowed homœopathists in broad outline and in many details (though less elaborately worked out), finds valuable employment for the remedy in solutions of the strength of 1 per cent.

The symptomatology of kali carb. is particularly clear in regard to involvement of fibrous tissues. Thus, ligaments and structures in the neighbourhood of joints are much affected and in the direction of loss of elasticity and power. In this way characteristic signs appear of slackness, weakness, strengthlessness : there is a chronic, weary aching of the back, a general sagging of tissues, a tendency to give way physically. The muscles are weak or even partly paralysed, the joints are painful and tired, and there is a general lack of energy to keep the bodily machine going.

There are several characteristic modalities presented by the patient requiring kali carbonicum. The pains which may be

felt in any part of the body and found in connection with any
ailment are of a stitching, cutting nature. They occur during
either rest or motion. All these pains are made worse by
lying on the affected side and are aggravated by cold (cf.
Bryonia, which has the opposite modalities). The region
between the right hip and right knee on the outer side of the
thigh is a particularly characteristic place for pain, and the
existence of pain there has often been the clue to the successful
use of kali carb. The patients who need kali carb. feel the
cold, are worse for cold air, cold winds or cold applications
and are gratified by warmth of the sun or fire. They catch
cold readily : catarrhs are prominent among kali carb. local
symptoms, for the general powers of resistance to germs are
low. The subject for kali carb. displays both emotional and
physical hypersensitivity. He is sensitive to noise and pain
and physically this is shown by the easy aggravation of his
symptoms from exposure to all atmospheric changes, to cold
air, touch and pressure. There is one very characteristic time
of symptom-aggravation for kali carb. and that is between
2 a.m. and 4 a.m. That is the time when, after more or less
sleep, the patient wakes, feeling pains and discomforts worse,
and to elicit this particular symptom is to obtain a strong hint
for the use of the remedy. Secretions from mucous membranes
are often scanty, especially when the patient is exposed to cold
air, but in the warmth a copious secretion is set up.

The tissues of the skin lose their elasticity ; relaxation of
tissues is a general symptom of kali carb., but it is often most
readily seen in a sagging of the tissues between the eyebrows
and upper eyelids, giving a kind of puffy appearance which is
not œdema. Patients suited to this remedy are often fat, for
combustion proceeds ineffectively with them and metabolism
is apt to be incomplete.

These physical signs correspond to and are enhanced by
the mental condition. Not only is the body slack, but the
mind also : there is an enfeebled reaction to the circumstances
of life, an inability to stand up courageously to the needs of
the hour, a general failure of will and a tendency to throw
individual burdens on to anyone who will undertake them, to
disclaim responsibility and let events take their course. No
one could be less the " captain of his soul " than the typical

candidate for kali carb. This condition may be reached as the result of chronic illness, overwork, sexual excess, but usually when kali carb. is indicated there is in the patient a root of feebleness, a " defeatism " of the soul that readily exaggerates genuine symptoms into intolerable burdens and makes a great ado about comparatively little suffering. There is a characteristic solicitude over physical complaints. It is often necessary to choose between Sepia and Kali Carb., but there is usually about the patient who requires sepia, however broken down and feeble, a fibre of endurance, a remnant of strength that finds expression in resentment and ill-temper, if no other way. The temper when kali carb. comes in question is rather peevish than angry, irascible rather than passionate, timid and fearful, with apprehensions that have little reason for existing. Fear is a very prominent symptom indeed. He fears to be alone and is easily startled by any noise, especially if it be unexpected. Digestion, as will be presently seen, is seldom very good, but apart from definite gastric morbid conditions fear of any kind is usually accompanied by subjective gastric discomfort.

The mind is weak like the body : mental effort is shunned and is badly performed : the memory is weak. But there is a good deal of sensitiveness : slight external stimuli are regarded as severe : the patients often resent being touched, especially unexpectedly.

The circulation is feeble, blood pressure usually low, the pulse poor—it may be intermittent. The drug finds its chief sphere in affections of the heart muscle that are the sequel to general toxæmia rather than to failing compensation in valvular disease, for it affects heart muscles as well as skeletal ones. One result of this feeble circulation is a general chilliness. With the feeble circulation and low tension goes some vasomotor instability so that localities readily become congested. There is characteristic headache with congestion, generally one-sided (right side), affecting forehead and temple and often ending in vomiting. The pain is severe and shooting and regarded by the patient as nearly unbearable. Headache may alternate with catarrh of the nose, the former being relieved when the discharge commences. Severe headaches, accompanied by epistaxis where the condition is aggravated by washing the face have been cured by the use of this drug (cf. ammon. carb.). Many of the pains of kali carb. are made worse by the act of eating, but some symptoms are ameliorated. Backache or headache, or general tiredness and weariness, sharp pains or dull chronic pains—all are felt more during the actual time of taking food and for a short while after. The sense of fatigue may also be so increased as to lead to a drowsiness almost irresistible. The characteristic sign is that it should come at once on beginning to eat, as though the mere efforts of mastication and deglutition and the early secretion of digestive juices put an extra strain on the system which is resented. Interestingly enough, the effects of carbonate of soda are exactly opposite, for with this drug there is, for a time, marked relief from eating.

The pains (especially the backache) are often made worse by firm pressure. In spite of the disinclination of the patient to make any exertion, to move about sometimes relieves the pains and the daytime is usually more endurable than the night. During the day there are things to be done that distract the invalid slightly from the thought of his pains and possibly long-suffering friends and relatives to be grumbled at and complained to, and there is no doubt that these complaints and grumblings give a certain (unacknowledged) relief. But at night these resources are unavailable : night brings vague fears to these timid souls and, with no distractions, the pains seem to become worse. In this way relief from movement and worsening from rest both come into the pathogenesis, but they need to be interpreted in the sense given above.

Kali carb. affects the respiratory organs prominently (see below) and an asthma that habitually chooses those hours (2 a.m. to 4 a.m.) for its paroxysms will often yield to this drug. The patient cannot lie down, but must sit up and bend forward.

There are no marked skin symptoms, but the sweat glands are readily stimulated. Sweating, backache, weariness form a triad of characteristic symptoms (Farrington). Not only the back, but many other joints may be chronically affected with pain and inability to perform their duties well. Large joints rather than small are attacked and the outer fibrous tissues rather than the synovial membranes. The right-sidedness of kali carb. is definitely marked and appears in joint and neuralgic affections. The nerve pains are due, at least partly, to affections of the nerve sheaths.

Kali carb. is often of great value in the chronic pelvic disorders of women. Schulz reports that in parts of Germany it is taken as an abortifacient. Its profound effect upon fibrous and muscular tissues makes it, in homœopathic experience, appropriate to illnesses the result of difficult or repeated parturition, subinvolution, prolapse, with all their accompanying symptoms of backache, weariness and depression. The periods are usually excessive (where sepia is needed scanty) and a profuse leucorrhœa of mucus and pus is a common symptom.

It has often proved of value in uterine complaints (e.g., fibroid) when the menstrual periods are profuse and prolonged for some days, and followed by a constant intermenstrual oozing until the copious flow of the next period begins.

All kinds of aches and pains from head to foot are apt to be associated with these conditions. Sexual intercourse aggravates all symptoms, both in the male and female. In the male, the drug is often useful for the nervous effects of sexual excesses. In both sexes pelvic diseases that call for kali carb. are often accompanied by that pain between right hip and knee that has been already mentioned as characteristic.

The alimentary canal symptoms are those of chronic rather than of acute disease. They suggest an impaired efficiency of the digestive factors in metabolism, which both reacts unfavourably on the nervous system and is unfavourably influenced by it, so making up the too familiar " vicious circle " of neurasthenia. The face looks haggard, slack and puffy and the cheeks flush easily : the teeth and gums are sore and pyorrhœa is common. The tongue is flabby and pale, sometimes feels swollen. The base is thickly coated, but the tip is sensitive and raw. The appetite is capricious. There may be complete loss with discomfort after taking food, even a small meal, but should the patient refrain from eating, he experiences a sinking, empty feeling. On the other hand, the appetite may be increased. In these cases there is then a desire for food at frequent intervals, nevertheless, after eating there comes discomfort or even sharp stitching pain in the epigastrium, made worse by moving about.

In addition there are frequent and sour eructations, nausea which produces faintness, epigastric sinking and ill-defined abdominal pains and discomfort. There is often a strong desire for sweets and sour things, but an aversion for meat. Flatulence in the bowels is considerable, with a feeling of bloating in the abdomen and throbbing in the epigastrium. Such attacks of flatulence and abdominal distension tend to occur in the early hours of the morning. Mucus is freely secreted from the rectum and constipation is the rule. The stool is expelled with difficulty and pains in rectum and anus are usual. Large painful hæmorrhoids are frequent and a contradictory modality appears in this connection : the burning pains are relieved by application of cold water.

It is interesting at this point to compare the indications in abdominal conditions of another potassium salt. Kali bichromicum is one of the most valued remedies for acute intestinal complaints, especially for the treatment of gastric ulcer and ulcerative colitis.

In catarrhal gastritis, the tongue is thickly coated, the saliva is sticky and stringy. There is a strong aversion from food, especially in the morning, so that breakfast especially is repugnant. There may be attacks of nausea and a sour vomit of stringy mucus. The appetite is always poor, though the patient feels faint when hungry and craves sour bitter things, which aggravate the trouble. The effects of gastritis following excessive beer drinking have been helped by this drug. It is also a valued remedy for ulceration of the pyloric end of the stomach. In addition to the above symptoms, in the latter cases the patient develops pain two to three hours after meals, usually accompanied by the vomiting of stringy mucus.

A clinical examination reveals the fact that the patient has developed a small area of tenderness in the region of the epigastrium.

Kali bichromati influences ulceration in the colon. Ulcerative colitis, where there is a severely painful, watery diarrhœa, together with an offensive discharge of stringy mucus tinged with blood is helped by this remedy.

In the respiratory sphere the tendency to profuse catarrh of the nose has been mentioned. The secretion is purulent and after cleansing the nose for a time often feels dry and uncomfortable. Hoarseness, aphonia and a dry, tickling cough, especially at night (3 a.m. to 4 a.m.) indicate laryngeal and tracheal irritation.

Kali carb. is a drug to be considered in the later stages of pneumonia, where the patient has partially responded to other drugs, but the lung condition has not cleared up (cf. lycopodium : stannum). The patient looks and is exhausted and weary. His most comfortable position is sitting up and leaning forwards, but after a severe bout of coughing, he is so exhausted that he is compelled to lie back. He is intensely chilly and aggravated by cold air. The cough is hard and dry, but in warm air a copious expectoration of tough mucopurulent sputum is expelled after spasmodic attacks of coughing. The secretion is apt to come away suddenly after two or three ineffectual coughs. Stitching pains in the chest are common, worse on inspiration and on lying on the affected side. There is almost always a degree of digestive disturbance accompanying the respiratory trouble. In a large number of cases, it is the lower lobes of the lungs which are involved, though the condition may spread upwards. In addition, the heart is affected. Cardiac exhaustion is an accompanying symptom.

Pleural adhesions are often found and the drug since the days of Hahnemann has been found to have a special value for tuberculous cases where the tuberculosis shows first after pneumonia or pleurisy, or is accompanied by formation of fibrous tissue, while the disease smoulders on in spite of these efforts to heal. Spasmodic asthma, emphysema and bronchiectasis are all conditions that may make up a symptom-picture that suggests kali carb. The early morning aggravation has a great value as an indication in these cases.

On the whole, this drug is most often called for in persons past the prime of life, who have come badly out of the struggle, either through disease or overstrain, or through deficient powers of will and mental energy. The subjects for it are often fat, suggest slackness and nervelessness, and belong to the class of patients who between their physical and emotional sufferings are difficult to handle or to relieve.

The drug has a close relationship to arsenicum, the carbons and sepia, and is not inimical to any important drug.

LACHESIS

The poison of the South American serpent, Trigonocephalus Lachesis.

The lance-headed viper whose poison glands supply this drug is one of the most feared, being one of the most deadly of the serpents. Constantine Hering first (and principally) proved the poison, and knowledge of its effect on provers is supplemented by knowledge of the effects of the actual bite of the snake. Clinical use for some ninety years has again defined the outline of the symptom-complex and added features to it, and the indications for the prescription of this most valuable remedy are to-day recognised with little difficulty.

The serpent poisons resemble one another in their action on the body : they kill by their effect on the nervous mechanism of the heart and their power here can be used medicinally in treating disease. But if death is delayed or avoided through smallness of dose other effects appear. There is a local action on the blood, leading to lowered coagulability and destruction of the red blood corpuscles, with extravasations of blood under the skin. These two marked effects on the heart and on the blood are both shown by all the serpent poisons used homœo-pathically, but the degrees of them vary with different venoms. Thus Naja, the cobra venom, affects the heart exceedingly and the blood but little, while Crotalus, the rattlesnake poison, causes marked effects on the blood and less on the heart, at any rate in the human subject. Lachesis acts intensely in both ways and largely for this reason is the most used and most valuable of them all.

The powers of lachesis over the different elements of the blood need defining in terms of laboratory experiment, but the symptoms that call for the drug clinically are usually clear enough. There is lowered coagulability with liability to sub-cutaneous hæmorrhages : great destruction of red blood corpuscles which may give rise to (hæmotogenous) jaundice (this is a very marked symptom of crotalus) and apparently a lowered power of resistance to septic invasions, so that unhealthy ulcers develop, wounds are slow to heal, inflam-mations readily suppurate and signs of septicæmia appear. There is marked engorgement of veins and venules, so that blueness and lividity are characteristic appearances when lachesis is called for. Whenever sepsis attacks a case and resistance to it is poor, either lachesis or crotalus may prove invaluable. Similarly, when an epidemic disease occurs in a specially virulent form, overwhelming the body resistance, whether it be enteric, small-pox or a streptococcal infection, symptoms often appear suggesting the use of a serpent poison and lachesis or another can then be used with confidence. The lachesis pathogenesis, though symptoms predominantly affect the left side, show, nevertheless, a relation of the drug to the appendix region, and when cases are not seen till suppuration has begun, then if after operation there are signs of septicæmia, this remedy or crotalus should be given. In acute tuberculosis or acute exacerbations of the chronic form of the disease, these poisons are invaluable, but on the whole Crotalus and Elaps are preferable here to lachesis. For severe diphtheria cases again lachesis is one of the most frequently used remedies and its characteristic general symptoms often appear, apart from the fact that the pharynx is a notable region for its local action. In all these profound bacterial poisonings the effects of the serpent poisons can best be explained by conceiving them as powerful stimulants to resistance processes. They follow baptisia and bryonia well, act even more profoundly and are therefore suited to more desperate cases. They are powerful aids given in minute quantities, because they are powerful and overwhelming poisons to body resistance in larger or long-continued doses.

From the general relationship of lachesis to virulent infections, it is time to turn to the specific symptoms which guide to the choice of it in these or other diseases. There are three very characteristic general symptoms (as distinguished from local ones) that belong to all serpent poisons more or less (and all in high degree to lachesis) and a fourth which helps to distinguish lachesis from crotalus or elaps. The first three are : (A) aggravation of all distressing symptoms (pain, delirium, etc.) after sleep ; (B) very marked sensitiveness of the body surface, so that even touch is intolerable and especially the slightest tendency to constriction ; (C) relief to distressing symptoms from the onset of a discharge : *e.g.,* dysmenorrhœal pains come before the flow and are at once relieved when it appears, or severe headache is relieved when a nasal catarrh begins. It is also true that if an expected discharge (e.g., menstruation) does not appear normally, symptoms of pain or discomfort begin or are aggravated if already present. The fourth symptom belonging to lachesis itself (though not to crotalus, elaps or naja), is a predominant left-sidedness of symptoms (except as already noted for the appendix region) and especially a tendency for pains to pass from left to right. Thus in diphtheria, the left tonsil will show disease first and then the right. The exact opposite is characteristic of Lycopodium which supplements the action of lachesis in many ways.

Symptoms A, B and C demand a little more discussion. The aggravation of distress after sleep is in itself, if well marked, enough to make a claim for the use of lachesis. The physiological differences between sleeping and waking are no doubt numerous and their interaction probably complex, but it is virtually certain that during sleep the waste products of active life are eliminated. To be eliminated they must pass, for however brief a time, into the circulation, and it is easily conceivable that certain constitutions and states of disease should be peculiarly sensitive to their presence in the blood. If this sensitiveness is enough to cause aggravation of symptoms (i.e., a further breakdown in the regions already affected by disease), it will produce this lachesis symptom of aggravation from sleep. On the other hand, patients who are notably better for sleep suggest nux vomica ; but aggravation of distress after sleep is a more important symptom than amelioration, just because it is a more striking and unusual occurrence. The symptom manifests in a multitude of ways ; thus an asthmatic subject may wake to a violent paroxysm (it is characteristic that the patient sleeps into the aggravation, there is no interval between sleep and increase of distress) ; pains of all kinds may become so acute that they wake the patient ; palpitation or vertigo may increase even at the first onset of drowsiness and effectually banish sleep. In such cases as this last example, if sleep does come on, the patient will be the better for it, because sleep is impossible until there is a change in the body condition, thus the power to sleep is the indication of the change and the improvement after sleep the evidence that the change for the better has so far endured.* The aggravation from sleep of the serpent poisons concerns physical rather than mental symptoms. Thus the night terrors of children more often find their remedy in stramonium or belladonna or its chronic counterpart, calcarea.

Symptom B, the intolerance of pressure or constriction, often stands out prominently in a symptom-complex. The patient desires all clothing to be loose and cannot endure collars or corsets to be in the least tight. Even the slightest pressure round the neck is particularly resented, and headache, if present, is worse for wearing a hat (as with lycopodium). If the larynx is affected, merely to touch it externally will bring on a paroxysm of coughing or spasm and dyspnœa. Patients who suggest lachesis as their remedy often suffer much from flatulence, but the desire to loosen clothing which they show is not a result of this only. Indeed, the cause of the intolerance of any touch or constriction is not so much fear of pain as a kind of nervous uneasiness, quite uncontrollable as a rule. This points to the fact (confirmed in many ways) that nervous, unbalanced, hysterical subjects are very likely to come into the sphere of action of the drug and the intolerance of pressure is to be read mainly as tactile hypersensitiveness. This sensitivity of the body surface is part of a general hypersensitivity produced by the drug. Thus the patient is susceptible to his surroundings and all the special senses unusually responsive to external stimuli, for example hearing is acute, the patient being distressed by slight noises. Associated with it is a strong desire for air ; patients who feel suffocated when windows are shut, who cannot endure heat or exposure to the sun and long for cool, fresh breezes, whose symptoms are worse in spring and summer—these are often found to call for lachesis by other indications. Lachesis (as are serpent poisons generally) is emphatically a remedy for those who are distressed by heat both physically and mentally. Hot drinks aggravate many of the symptoms ; a hot bath may induce a faint. Even if the patient is cold, a warm room will intensify his symptoms.

* The following symptom is very trustworthy ; a sense of confusion on waking ; patient at first is unable to recognise surroundings and wonders where he is.

This is the very reverse of the chilliness of subjects who need arsenicum or nux vomica or calcarea.

Symptom C, relief from the onset of a discharge, is sufficiently clear as an indication. The explanation of it probably lies in the fact that great vaso-motor instability is a characteristic effect of the serpent poisons. Consequently local congestions and hyperæmias are common and possibly the onset of a free discharge relieves these. The vaso-motor instability is expressed in the provings by local flushings, rushes of blood to the head and face. These and allied nervous symptoms make lachesis a remedy of great value at the climacteric, especially at the onset of that period when the menses are becoming delayed and when the non-appearance of the monthly discharge results in symptoms of discomfort and distress.

The " left-sidedness " of symptoms characteristic of lachesis is one of the most marked of these preferences of certain remedies for one side or the other of the body. It is impossible at present fully to account for them, but clinical observation will soon show that a predominance of such a symptom as pain or skin eruption on one side is a common phenomenon, quite independently of obvious disease of a special organ. If the spleen or heart or gall bladder is the seat of disease, it is, of course, easy to understand that symptoms should be referred to left or right, but apart from such simple explanations a right-sidedness or a left-sidedness of symptoms is often met with. Similarly it appears in drug provings and when well marked, alike in case and in pathogenesis, it is a symptom worth noting. Lachesis markedly affects the left side (although for symptoms to proceed from left to right is also characteristic) and this feature of the remedy is often a helpful guide to the use of it.

The mental characteristics that suggest lachesis have been determined for the most part clinically, by observing the types of individuals who respond best to the use of it. They somewhat resemble those of Arsenicum in being a mingling of melancholy with anger. In spite of the greatly increased physical sensitiveness and nervous irritability which is shown in the intolerance of constriction or pressure, the subjects that indicate lachesis are often not obviously excitable, but their melancholy breaks easily into fits of anger, however lazy an

sad they may be between the outbursts. The egocentricity
of the lachesis subject may be seen in outbursts of unreasonable
suspicion or unwarranted jealousy. The state of sensitiveness
and tendency to suspicion may proceed to paranoia with
delusions of persecution ("believes that they are trying to
poison her"). The cyclothymic personality in the depressive
phase, accusing herself of having committed the unpardonable
sin, also suggests the exhibition of lachesis. It is said that
women with red hair and freckled complexions often conform
to this type. Thin rather than fat people suggest the drug,
and it is more often needed for children or those past the prime
of life than for men or women between twenty-five and forty-
five. Although melancholy, the patient who requires lachesis
is the very reverse of silent. Loquacity is a characteristic
symptom which becomes very marked indeed if the patient is
delirious. It is a frantic loquacity, striving to express one
thought after another with no apparent connection between
them, while the mental powers now seem exalted, now depressed
and a swift succession of ideas sinks into incoherent confusion.
Even apart from delirious states there is volubility and hastiness
of speech wherein the patient passes from one subject to
another with little sequence of thought or expression. The
sense of time is frequently more or less disturbed in acute
cases that call for lachesis (cf. mercurius to which lachesis is
an antidote). Hysterical subjects who talk interminably will
often show other symptoms of the serpent poisons.

The delirium that suggests the drug after its stages of
loquacity and deranged time sense, sinks, in severe cases,
into a low muttering condition with marked tremor ; tremor
of the tongue is characteristic (cf. gelsemium, but lachesis is
suitable to more severe illness than is gelsemium). Tremors
and trembling readily occur in lachesis subjects apart from
delirium, and cramps and spasms and even convulsions are
often prominent. Spasms of the throat muscles are particularly characteristic and the drug has been used for rabies on
this and other indications.

Fainting is a prominent symptom in the pathogenesis and
attacks of faintness are generally accompanied by other
troubles, e.g., cardiac pain or nausea or vertigo. It is to be
regarded as a symptom of the nervous system and should be

read in relation to the real value that serpent poisons often have in recent epilepsy, especially in *petit mal*. Subjective disturbances of sight and hearing are common complaints of lachesis subjects and headache is apt to be a marked and persistent symptom. Characteristically it will be predominant on the left side and show intolerance of pressure and aggravation after sleep.

The head pains indicating lachesis are of a pulsating hammering character, and these pains are accompanied by a purplish face and engorged eyes. The headaches show the distinctive modalities of lachesis. They are worse after sleep and on waking in the morning but often wear off after moving about. Such headaches may accompany cardiac condition, the pulse is weak and there are violent pulsations over the body.

The alimentary canal is the site of many symptoms. Mouth and tongue may be inflamed, swollen and painful, the tongue trembling, dry, red and cracked, or brown or even blackish. Thirst is excessive. There is a constant tickling in the throat with dryness and burning. Lachesis affects predominantly the mind and throat and affections of the latter illustrate the peculiar modalities of the drug. The throat may be very painful though only apparently slightly inflamed, or ulceration may develop (lachesis is often needed in diphtheria). There is a sense of constriction with a constant desire to swallow, but swallowing is difficult and very painful. Spasms often check it, but solids are managed better than fluids and empty swallowing is most painful of all. The hypersensitivity of the drug is seen in the intolerance to touch or any external constriction or pressure near the throat. The saliva is copious and tenacious. The left tonsil is first affected. After eating, the throat is temporarily relieved and there is often a desire for food and increased appetite. Gastric symptoms are those of pain with convulsive vomiting, cramps and eructations. The pressure of clothing is intolerable ; flatulence is excessive, making the abdomen hard and sensitive. The lachesis patient often has a craving for oysters. There is sometimes obstinate constipation, but more often violent and painful diarrhœa, watery or pasty, offensive or bloody. Spasm of the anus occurs and hæmorrhoids are apt to appear, large and bleeding freely (venous blood).

The effect of Crotalus on the liver is very marked, producing a parallel to the effect of yellow fever, for which it is a most valuable remedy. Lachesis has no such profound influence, but provers experienced pains in both hepatic and splenic regions. The value of serpent poisons in appendicitis has been mentioned.

In the urinary sphere there are symptoms of difficult and painful micturition and violent pains in the urethra, but nothing that can be translated very clearly into morbid anatomy. For the male sexual system its use in obstinate ulceration (syphilitic or malignant) is of value, but on the testicles and prostate there is little evidence of profound action. But its relation to the climacteric makes it one of the most important of remedies for women. The drug can match all the general symptoms of the " change of life," the flushes, the nervous sensibilities, the multiple aches and pains, many of the mental and moral perturbations. It does excellent service also in dysmenorrhœa when menses are delayed, scanty (black blood and clotted), and when the pains and headache and discomfort precede the flow and are at once relieved by it. Pains in the left ovarian region are especially characteristic. Sexual desire is usually increased and some troublesome cases of abnormal desire at the climacteric may find a remedy in this drug, whenever general symptoms of it are also present.

Sensitiveness and reflex spasms are also found among respiratory symptoms. The larynx feels constricted and touching it externally brings on cough or spasm. Tickling sensations are usually referred to the trachea or lower, with a fatiguing dry cough. Subjective sensations of discomfort and pain are prominent. Asthma (with little bronchitis as a rule) is well within the lachesis sphere if general symptoms agree, e.g., heightened reflex sensibility and aggravation after sleep. Pneumonia (especially of the left side) in its later stages, especially septic or post-influenzal or post-enteric pneumonia, with an enfeebled subject, a failing heart and a persistent temperature will often find a remedy in lachesis. If the disease is right-sided, crotalus or elaps is to be preferred. When chronic or latent pulmonary tuberculosis becomes infected with subsidiary organisms (streptococci particularly) and an acute exacerbation occurs with profuse (often blood-stained) expectoration, debility, sweats and hectic temperature, there are no remedies so likely to help as the serpent poisons. Here they follow Baptisia well. Also in miliary tuberculosis they are of great value, reinforcing the power of potencies of tuberculin, which avails as a rule most in that most intractable and dangerous form of the disease. · In all these conditions the indications are to be looked for in some or other of the well-known general symptoms accompanying cases obviously labouring under profoundly poisonous infections and lowered resistance thereto.

From much that has been already said, the use of all serpent poisons for any septicæmic state will be frequently suggested. Just as poisonous doses of them lower coagulability (causing hæmorrhages and extravasation of blood) and diminish resistance to septic invasions, so medicinal doses heighten resistance and enable the body to combat sepsis. No remedies surpass the serpent poisons for helping profound systemic bacterial poisonings. Arsenic, carbon, nitric acid compete with them, but while arsenic presents the general symptom of aggravation from cold, nitric acid, like mercury, affects most those to whom both extremes (heat and cold) are unpleasant. The serpent poisons, on the other hand, find their subjects most readily among those to whom cold is grateful and heat distressing. Such diseases as bubonic plague would in general suggest to the homœopathist the application of lachesis or one of its congeners, and, as has already been indicated, symptoms calling for one of these remedies are likely to present themselves in the grave cases of many acute diseases, enteric, pneumonia, scarlet fever, etc.

Seeing that these poisons kill through their action on the nerve mechanism of the heart, it is no wonder that homœopathists prize them for the relief of certain cases of morbus cordis wherein that mechanism is affected. Palpitation with fainting, cramp-like pains and dyspnœa, quickened and irregular pulse, sense of constriction and intolerance of the least pressure—these are the most prominent symptoms that suggest it. It will help functional as well as organic diseases if the symptoms correspond. When marked valvular disease is present, possibly naja is the serpent poison of election, but lachesis has much to advocate its use. Malignant endocarditis, on symptomatic grounds, calls for it frequently. In this deadly disease vaccine treatment has had some striking successes and lachesis or naja should be given between the vaccine doses, as they seem to tend to heighten the response of the body.

The effects of the drug on the skin are secondary to its influence on the blood. Thus ulcers and wounds bleed readily, heal badly and are very sensitive. Petechiæ are common and a variety of eruptions have been recorded. Lymphatic glands swell. Particularly do ulcers and wounds show a bluish margin and unhealthy granulations when lachesis is indicated. Even gangrene or the tendency thereto may be notably helped by it. A purple bloated face in heart disease draws the attention of the physician to lachesis.

Since sleep so often causes an aggravation of symptoms in patients who require lachesis, the rest is apt to be much broken and consequently the day is often a period of great drowsiness. When asleep dreams are frequent and unusually detailed ; they are generally horrible and terrifying.

Lachesis is a remedy which has been hardly, if at all, used in potencies lower than the sixth centesimal. Crotalus and naja can be obtained in lower potencies and there is some evidence that when sepsis is marked and threatening the lower potencies are preferable. Given, however, characteristic general symptoms, the highest potencies of lachesis, with infrequent repetition, seldom fail to give good results. Lycopodium is complementary in its action to lachesis and to a less extent hepar sulph. and nitric acid. Iodine precedes or follows it well, especially in pulmonary complaints.

LUETICUM

Lueticum or syphilinum is prepared directly from the primary sore of syphilis. It is one of the early nosodes and one of the most valuable. As with Medorrhinum, repugnance at the thought of the origin of the remedy disappears when it is realised that it is only used in potency and usually not below the 30th, so that any perceptible quantity of the morbid material has long since vanished.

Syphilis, like gonorrhœa, follows so regular a symptomatic course and causes such definite tissue changes that it is relatively easy to use these symptoms as indications for the remedy when they occur in the course of other diseases. The drug was also proved by Swan in potency, and clinical use over nearly a century has added many valuable indications. Therefore, a clear drug picture can be drawn and the remedy will seldom fail to give satisfaction.

Since the indications for it are reasonably precise, the general rule to repeat rarely with similiar drugs, and never without good reason to think the effects of the last dose exhausted, *applies with redoubled force to all nosodes and should be even further emphasised for lueticum*. Syphilis is so penetrating and persistent a poison that, as a remedy, it suits some of the most chronic cases, but just as it is slow in its harmful action, it requires time to develop its remedial power.

In recent sub-acute cases, we have seen weekly repetition of the 30th helpful, but in any chronic case much longer intervals are desirable, particularly if high potencies are employed.

In the acuter stages of syphilis, other remedies are preferable, though lueticum has more claims than some nosodes to be thought of even here, since the poison of syphilis is so relatively slow in developing its action that an early dose of the nosode might well hasten the process of resistance. In the more chronic stages, there is more call for it, particularly in neuro-syphilis, to make other remedies more effective. In congenital syphilis, and also where the symptoms and signs of the patient suggest a remote specific taint, even though the biochemical examinations reveal no evidence of infection, it has great value. A history of syphilis apparently cured, or in a parent, should bring it to serious consideration. In every other respect, the ordinary rule holds that the drug must be well indicated before results can be expected, and to the indications for it we may turn.

A very well marked and most important general symptom of lueticum is a definite worsening of the condition (pain, etc.,) at night. Sunset to sunrise is the bad time for a lueticum patient, while sunrise to sunset is the troublesome period for medor-rhinum. We have known this indication crucial for the success-ful use of lueticum, even when no other noteworthy one was present, and the drug seldom succeeds if this symptom is entirely absent, although it may not always be underlined in the case. So whenever the symptoms of a case are aggravated at night, we must consider lueticum and its allied remedies. That life energy is rhythmical is a very well known fact. Broadly speaking, it consists in preparation for activity, and then activity itself and the rhythm varies with different tissues, according to their functions. But in the space of 24 hours we have the rhythm of sleep and waking, rest and display of varied energy. The monthly cycle in women gives them another obvious life rhythm and seasonal rhythms throughout the year can be noted and are at times, with certain individuals, very marked.

The daily rhythm of sleep and waking is the one we are concerned with in this modality of lueticum. The general metabolism of the body must differ in the two states, and there is a gradual passing from one to the other which introduces possibilities of symptomatic stresses or relaxations in disease, according as the metabolic condition of the moment helps or hinders body resistance. With the disease syphilis, and correspondingly with all the similar remedies that can influence it, arsenic, mercury, hepar, nitric acid, gold etc., the metabolism of the night hours, which normally conduces to repose, appears to be favourable to the disease, rather than to the resistance, and the patient is worse at this period. To the homœopathist, all well marked modalities of daily (or larger) rhythms are most important symptoms. They are " general " in a deep sense, depending on general body metabolism and displaying individual differences therein.

Next to the time modality in general importance comes the indication of lowering of resistance to pus germs, so that ulcerations, abscesses with free discharges of pus (which is notably foul smelling), appear. A gumma has, in any case, a tendency to break down, but if lueticum be incautiously given an abscess will almost certainly develop. Inflammation of bone, particularly in the nose, with breaking down of foul discharges is especially noteworthy.

One of the interesting general qualities of lueticum is its frequent suitability for inveterate alcoholics, particularly if their tendency is inherited. Dr. Clarke points out that Bacchus and Venus have ever been close allies. Naturally the drug is more confidently given when other lueticum symptoms are present, but if the case be not clear, and no other remedy is obviously similar, lueticum should have the preference, for as usual with " clearing up " remedies like the nosodes, it will probably not only help but point the way to subsequent medicines.

Patients who have suffered from syphilis in years gone by often remain in an unsatisfactory state of general health, even though no obvious symptoms or signs of the disease remain.

Should such a subject develop an acute infection, (e.g., typhoid or even influenza), the patient may resist it badly. In such instances a single dose of lueticum in high potency will augment his powers of resistance and set him on the road to recovery. Furthermore, it will lay the way open for the more efficacious action of allied and indicated drugs.

Apart from the attack of acute diseases in such subjects, the general lowered vitality which is a not infrequent sequel to massive doses of anti-syphilitic drugs, is revived by the administration of lueticum.

When little but mercury was used in the treament of the early stages of syphilis, there was a fairly high risk of the administration of too much of it. Today, even thinking as homœopathists, there is much to be said for giving first arsenic and then mercury.*

The final test of all treatment of syphilis, and it is probably too early yet to apply it, will be to decide whether or no neurosyphilis in its grave form diminishes.

If our colleagues are curing syphilis, tabes and G.P.I. should be on the downgrade.

Claims are already made that this is, in fact, happening and, if the claims are substantiated, the efficacy of modern methods will be a hard thing to contest. The homœopathist will rejoice as a citizen ; exercise his private judgment for the cases that consult him and be gratified and remember that arsenic and mercury (if not bismuth) are drugs that have great similarity to the disease in its primary and secondary manifestations very often. With modern treatment secondary symptoms are often absent or negligible. As such manifestations can be very pain-

---

* The homœopathist would prefer in syphilis, as in every other disease, to look for the individual simillimum, but a large number of cases of primary syphilis would work out to arsenic whereas secondary manifestations of this disease would call for mercury.

ful and distressing, the patient is naturally very pleased. But they have such an obvious appearance of a marked system reaction that the homœopathist may have a doubt whether to eliminate (possibly suppress) them altogether is entirely a good thing

Similar remedies (chiefly mercury) usually prevent the symptoms from being very troublesome and it may be that a secondary stage thus modified is of final advantage.

Dr. Kent stresses the observation mentioned above that when lueticum is given in these unsatisfactory cases, although general malaise will improve there is a tendency to skin eruptions.

The symptoms complained of by sufferers from the remote effects of syphilitic infection are generally those of pain. They may be felt in nerves, joints or periosteum.

The nocturnal aggravation appears and as a result the patient is sleepless and very prostrate in the morning on waking from a short spell of sleep which most likely comes to him late.

Sometimes heat, sometimes cold, relieves the pains, there is no regular modality here. Extremes of heat and cold are badly borne. Here is another point of resemblance with mercury. For epilepsy has been found to respond to lueticum on many occasions. As the mental state (presently to be described), shows, the drug has the profoundest effect on the brain in both its higher and lower centres. So a condition like epilepsy may well be influenced. A hint here for the use of lueticum in female epileptics is that there is a tendency for attacks to occur after the menses.

Badly healing ulcerations, fistulæ, exostoses, warts as well as obvious broken down gummata respond to the drug. There are cases where sulphur has been the selected remedy and given in high potency for such troubles. If then an aggravation has been produced, lueticum is likely to encourage proper repair of tissues.

Another valuable pointer is that remedies *apparently well chosen fail to act or only help for a short time*. This is a reminder that a nosode may be needed whenever cases are not reacting to the well chosen remedy, whatever the trouble may be. But the choice of the nosode clearly depends on the background of symptoms and the history of the case. The mental symptoms are of supreme significance. The brain power weakens to the point of imbecility. It is not only when senile dementia seems to be approaching that the drug is valuable, for no remedy surpasses lueticum for the mentally deficient infant, child or adolescent. After the administration of the remedy, brain power will often develop to an extent that, at the first taking of the case, would seem all but incredible.

The treatment of obsessional neuroses always presents a problem which the psychiatrist regards as difficult and sometimes resistant to the most skilled psychological treatment.

However, it is recorded of certain drugs (e.g., lueticum, silica, thuja) that compulsive acts have occurred in provers. The following symptom is recorded of lueticum : " always washing her hands." The psychologist would doubtless find it difficult to believe that symptoms of a " guilt complex " as seen in compulsions can be controlled by the giving of a remedy. Our personal experience is that lueticum has, in fact, influenced beneficially a " washing neurosis " and other compulsive acts. in certain young adults. This observation has been made over only a few cases, and we must confess that personally we have had no success in the homœopathic treatment of compulsion neuroses in the middle aged.

With loss of mental power goes melancholy and despair of recovery. Thus it is indicated when such a state of mind is the result of realisation of brain failure in older people who have been able to work competently and now feel their power slipping.

A peculiar symptom should be recorded here. The patient says that he has a feeling as if he were going insane, and this peculiar phobia has been associated with the presence of a positive Wassermann reaction. Treatment by lueticum and allied drugs resulting in a negative Wassermann blood examination was followed by disappearance of the symptom.

The effect of syphilis on blood vessels is so well marked that many of this group of symptoms are no doubt due to degenerative processes consequent on interference with the local blood supply.

The patient dreads the night and dreads the morning. These are his worst times but he takes little or no pleasure in anything at any time. He laments his helplessness but has no power to struggle against it.

Many remedies cause headaches, but the head pains of lueticum are quite outstanding features of the drug.

The pains are violent, sometimes almost unbearable, seeming to go through the head from side to side or from back to front. The occiput is often the site of the worst pain but the supraorbital region, too, is a common point of attack.

Sometimes the pain follows a well defined line but not invariably.

Warmth frequently relieves the pain and the nocturnal aggravation is always clear and well marked. The pain is worse until midnight after which it improves, often ceasing by daylight.

Hair tends to fall out and exostoses of the cranium may be present and painful.

All kinds of eye troubles are in the sphere of lueticum. The eye muscles suffer causing squint, diplopia or ptosis. Iritis is often helped by the drug, also inflammation of the cornea and retinitis. Again, the nocturnal aggravation is a guiding symptom and the ophthalmic pains are relieved by cold bathing. Eye troubles in hereditary syphilis frequently need an occasional dose of the nosode to supplement other remedies.

The power of late syphilis to cause deep ulcerations, slow to heal, eating even into bone, is well known, and many obstinate affections of this kind find a remedy here, especially when it is the region of the nose and face that are attacked.

It is worth remembering in lupus and rodent ulcer.

Certain physicians have considered that there is a close relationship between syphilis and tuberculosis. Certainly antisyphilitic drugs like Aurum can avail considerably to help tuberculosis and the use of lueticum in lupus is another illustration of this possible relationship. The homœopathist, taking the symptoms as his guide, does not pay overmuch attention in prescribing to the name he gives the disease, but in chronic non-reacting cases the physician is often glad of any suggestion that may give him a valuable hint.

Chronic ulceration anywhere may benefit from lueticum as an intercurrent remedy, but the two ends of the alimentary canal, the throat and rectum, are particularly favourite sites for its action on ulcers, swellings, fissures, condylomata and so forth. The appetite is capricious. There may be an aversion from meat and a craving for spiritous liquors. Constipation is the rule with these cases and, as always, the aggravation at night gives a useful clue.

Naturally the generative organs offer a wide field for the remedy. Nodules, ulcerations, testicular or ovarian or uterine inflammation have all been helped by it. Menses are often excessive and foul leucorrhœa is common. Recurrent miscarriages always arouse a suspicion of syphilis. Whether or no this can be proven, lueticum is very likely to be the remedy to ensure that the next pregnancy will proceed normally.

Chronic arthritis usually requires one or more of the nosodes. The intestinal group are often very indicated, but apart from them Tuberculinum, Medorrhinum and Lueticum are all but indispensable. A chronic case often needs one only, but they in no way quarrel with one another, and at different times, there may be need of two or even three.

The case of arthritis requiring lueticum presents the usual modalities of the drug. The stiffness and pain is worse at night, especially when warm in bed.

Hot applications aggravate and cold, especially bathing, relieves.

The time of aggravation, day or night, settles the choice for medorrhinum or lueticum, either will do well with tuberculinum. In any case, whichever is used, the dose if high potency should be well spaced.

Asthma more often comes into the medorrhinum sphere, but lueticum may be indicated when the attacks are nocturnal, occurring between 1 to 4 a.m., and are worse on lying down. Aggravation during a thunderstorm and relief from attacks in mountain air are additional indications.

The skin symptoms are numerous :—eruptions which ulcerate and which occur principally where bones are near the surface : pigmented patches, or bullæ ; these would bring the drug to mind. They do not itch at all.

The " syphilitic type " can be recognised even in cases where the blood tests are negative in a patient. It appears well established that the infection of syphilis leaves its marks on subsequent generations, even though all active signs of the disease have disappeared.

Dr. Vannier recognises many abnormalities in structure and degenerative processes which he describes as the stigmata of degeneration. He regards such malformations and degenerative processes as belonging to the syphilitic type in which there is a remote history of syphilis in ancestors. This, he considers, should draw attention to the use of lueticum and other antisyphilitic remedies, provided as always that the drug symptoms of the remedy are present.

As mentioned above, repeated abortions or a history of premature labours in women would direct one's mind to the consideration of lueticum : so also asymmetry of various organs of the body, e.g., one ear higher than the other ; six fingers on one hand ; the irregularity of teeth implantation and excessive separation of the incisors. Skeletal deformities, such as achondroplasia, Dr. Vannier would include in the syphilitic type.

Degenerative processes in the nervous system, such as Disseminated Sclerosis and Paralysis Agitans should also be added to this list.

Persons who have a definite artistic capacity, for example in the musical or literary spheres, but whose works show a morbid tendency come under this heading. Dr. Vannier believes that children with remote syphilitic inheritance suffer from a disturbance of mental equilibrium. It is not only in slow and backward children that lueticum should be thought of, but also in certain very precocious children.

The syphilitic type of child may thus be slow in learning to talk and walk or, on the other hand, be unusually brilliant, but perhaps showing disturbing abnormal characteristics in his behaviour, such as cruelty to other children.

The intercurrent use of other drugs beside the nosode will almost certainly be required in the treatment of the " syphilitic type." The French school believes that frequently the prescriber cannot obtain the full advantage of lueticum without the use, sooner or later, of other anti-syphilitic remedies, notably Phytolacca.

If lueticum does not give the satisfactory results anticipated, very frequently symptoms of Phytolacca are found to present themselves.

To recapitulate the general modalities of the lueticum

patient : all symptoms are worse at night, from sundown to sunrise. He may even fear the night and the suffering and exhaustion that he knows he will experience on waking.

His sufferings are aggravated at the seashore (*opp.* medorrhinum) and in damp warm weather. Generally he experiences amelioration during the day and when he is moving about slowly and in mountainous districts.

From this most terrible of poisons thus emerges a sovereign remedy, and those who have grasped the principles of " similarity " look upon it as one of their most important weapons.

LYCOPODIUM

Lycopodium clavatum (Club Moss). Trituration of Spores or Ethereal Tincture of Spores.

The spores of lycopodium when collected form a light dry powder, which is used as a coating to pills and as a dusting powder for excoriated surfaces and is generally held to be quite inert. A century or so ago it had a regular place in medicine, being prized for certain conditions which suggest that an unconscious homœopathy had found its way into the uses of it. Hahnemann found it in use, and by his method of trituration quickly made it one of the most valuable of all remedies. Within the outer coating of the spore is an oily layer wherein seem to reside most of the medicinal virtues of the drug and trituration, by rupturing the spore, sets this free. Ether will extract the oil and an ethereal tincture is therefore another method of pharmacy, but there are also mineral salts in the spores which are included in the trituration and it is probable that they count for something in the pathogenesis. Particularly prominent are the elements silica and aluminium and resemblances to the symptoms of the first named are significant in the provings. The use therefore of trituration seems desirable for lower potencies and tinctures (colloidal solutions) or triturations for the higher ones.

Lycopodium is very highly valued in chronic diseases, being chosen very largely on general constitutional symptoms, but it has also a very marked relation to the alimentary canal and the liver, and is frequently indicated in disorders of that tract by the local symptoms. It will be well, however, to master first the general characteristics and peculiar symptoms. They are so definite that lycopodium is one of the drugs most readily selected on a homœopathic basis.

It is particularly well adapted to patients in whom the mental powers have, as it were, outrun the physical, where the intellectual faculties and interests count for much, but the bodily strength is deficient, the muscles weak and the fundamental processes (digestion, excretion, etc.) apt to be faulty. There is a feeble body with an active brain that has become overtired. This relation of drug to patient is true at any age, precocious weakly children respond to it wonderfully. Dr. Kent instances Paul Dombey as a lycopodium subject and that is a convenient instance to fix the type in the mind. The lycopodium child is usually thin, rather dark with sallow skin. Such a child is sensitive, shy, nervous and a difficult subject to his parents. He is likely to be irritable and demanding, always complaining of some bodily trouble and showing a tendency to develop into a hypochondriac. Older people become mistrustful of themselves and of others, hypochondriacal, complaining (often with reason) of failing memory and slowness of mental reaction, and this generally when they have been accustomed to consider their brain power above the average. The physical strength is nearly always below the average also, but usually the complaint is of failure of mental powers, for the typical candidate for lycopodium has probably never rejoiced much in bodily activity or cared for athletics. He is apt to be a brooding, sedentary person, mentally absorbed, physically indifferent. He is a taciturn individual and though he wants to be let alone, he does not want to be entirely alone because of his fear of solitude. If he is in a room in the house, he likes to feel that there is someone nearby, perhaps in the next room. Lycopodium has been called the " miser's " remedy : the hint is valuable if interpreted to mean (as it does) that the saving and meanness come out of a real gnawing anxiety for the future and undue sense of responsibility. It is not so much love of money as such, but anxiety as to the possible lack of all that money means for the individual and his dependents, that make up the " miserliness " that calls for lycopodium. This sense of responsibility developed into a positive burden to life is characteristically shown also in a constant fear of breaking down under stress (*e.g.*, the barrister fears he will lose the thread of argument in court), a fear which is constantly falsified, but nevertheless persists. This symptom is very marked also under silica and possibly in lycopodium the silica is responsible for this characteristic. The state of mental weariness and incapacity for undertaking new work and a general impairment of intellectual powers that follow some acute illnesses may be met by lycopodium.

A good deal of depression and irritability is likely to accompany a condition calling for this remedy. Undernourished states, especially those due to chronic dyspepsia or threatening tubercle or congenital syphilis, will often suggest its use. The skin is often dry and reacts poorly, the hair falls readily : vasomotor disturbances (flushings and sensations of sinking and emptiness are common, especially at the characteristic time of aggravation of lycopodium, to be presently noted), and with them a consciousness of pulsation of arteries that has led to some special uses of the drug.

Among the general symptoms there are some very characteristic and easily recognised. Thus, symptoms are worse from 4 p.m. to 8 p.m. (occasionally the aggravation endures longer, though commencing at about 4 p.m.) : if the disease is characterised by paroxysms (*e.g.*, asthma, neuralgia, etc.) the worst attacks will fall into this part of the twenty-four hours. Times of aggravation point generally to an alteration of the normal rhythm of life. In health there is a curve of the general vital activities which has a relatively constant maximum and minimum : in disease this curve is apt to be altered (the inverse type of temperature in tuberculosis is familiar) and alternation of rhythm, if shown by fairly constant times of worsening and of amelioration, have great value as general symptoms. The lycopodium symptom is rather an intensification of the normal rhythm than an alteration of it, but is very characteristic. Hellebore and Chelidonium are the only other drugs that show the symptom in so marked a degree (for the twilight aggravation of pulsatilla and phosphorus seems rather a reaction of the mind), and whenever it is clearly marked it should always bring the thought of lycopodium to the mind of the prescriber. Typically (though variations occur frequently), the aggravation begins at 4 p.m., continues till 6 p.m., then tends to lessen till

8 p.m. After this it may disappear or begin again after a period of amelioration. There is also a morning aggravation of symptoms, especially emotional symptoms. The lycopodium patient is a despondent individual and his depression is at its worst in the morning.

The symptoms of pain, etc., that indicate lycopodium characteristically begin on the right side and then travel to the left. Drugs that notably influence the liver, as lycopodium does, have always a certain " right-sidedness " in the incidence of their symptoms, a predominance of right-sided aches and pains and inflammations. It is difficult to explain the phenomenon ; but it certainly comes out clearly in drug provings and equally is often prominent in disease and the homœopathist finds it, when well marked (and no symptom is of much value unless well marked), a good indication for the remedy. With lycopodium it might show as a tonsillitis beginning in the right tonsil and then attacking the left, or it may be a headache or pain in the ovarian region, but if the symptom takes the direction right to left that is so far an indication for lycopodium. Lycopodium is a complementary drug to lachesis often completing a cure which lachesis has begun and with lachesis the direction of symptoms is the exact opposite, being left to right, and lachesis symptoms are as predominantly left-sided as lycopodium symptoms are right-sided.

Relief to pain and discomfort from uncovering is a lycopodium symptom. Thus in headache, to remove the hat relieves, in abdominal pain the clothing is loosened. It is not only a desire for cool air to the head (although the candidate for the drug prefers the open air, is better out of doors and worse in a stuffy atmosphere), but also a dislike of pressure that is thus exemplified. It is interesting to note in view of the presence of silica in lycopodium and the hint above mentioned that silica makes its presence felt in some symptoms, that the headache of silica is relieved by wrapping up the head warmly, the exact reverse of the condition sought for when lycopodium is the indicated remedy.

Although the open air and general coolness are preferred, there is a general amelioration from warm drinks, any abdominal pains and discomfort are aggravated by cold food and drink and relieved by swallowing warm things, but this applies to other symptoms, *e.g.*, tonsillitis is relieved by warmth. Phosphorus patients are chilly in type, but their gastric symptoms lead them to desire cold food. It should be added that with lycopodium patients the aggravation from cold food and relief from warm extend also to the sore throat. Though the lycopodium patient finds relief from open air and is distressed by the heat of a room he is a chilly patient. He is generally better for warm things, warm drinks and the warmth of the bed. The pains with the exception of the head and spine pains are relieved by heat. Two curious lycopodium symptoms may be noted here : the first is the frequency of to-and-fro movements of the *alæ nasi* in patients requiring it. These are not (as has mistakenly been maintained) the movements of dyspnœa : they are not synchronous with respiration, but are of the nature of twitchings, occurring with some rapidity. Spasm is not infrequent when lycopodium is required, spasm, for instance, of the tongue and of the facial muscles, movements of the head, constriction of the throat (globus). The other curious symptom is that the right foot may be hot and the left foot cold. Much derision has been poured on this statement and it has been attributed to thrombosis of one side and so explained away, but it is a subjective symptom which unquestionably occurs every now and then in chronic disease, independently of any blocking of circulation. Its explanation is impossible at this stage of knowledge, but without a doubt it depends on some definite pathology and there is ample evidence that on the (not very frequent) occasions when it is complained of it is an excellent indication for lycopodium.

Other general symptoms are restlessness leading to desire to move about, which generally removes pain, as with rhus tox., dryness of the skin, especially of palms of the hands, dryness of mucous membranes, falling of the hair. The fear and apprehensiveness noted among the mental characteristics are apt to have a profound effect on symptoms affecting the body (*e.g.*, gastric and liver symptoms), making the drug suitable for obviously hypochrondriacal persons : crossness and irritability are frequent concomitants of these groups of symptoms and form in themselves additional indications for lycopodium.

Apart from general characteristics, lycopodium has a very definite relation to diseases of the alimentary tract. When it is needed there will usually be present several of the general symptoms already noted. The patient is frequently underweight, and with it there is associated the mental weariness, timidity and apprehension that has previously been described. The local symptoms indicate catarrh, chiefly of stomach and duodenum, with extension to the bile ducts. In appearance, the patient is sallow and a yellow discoloration of the teeth may be observed : the tongue is usually coated and characteristically dry, saliva being tough and scanty.

The throat is sore and dry : ulceration or tonsillitis (diphtheria will react well to lycopodium if the general symptoms to it are marked) will be on the right side with a tendency to spread to the left.

The appetite is capricious, being sometimes lost and sometimes excessive in spite of discomfort. The patient may feel hungry when he sits down to a meal, but after a few mouthfuls he feels replete. Characteristic is hunger with sudden satiety after a mouthful or two. A sour taste in the mouth, nausea with sour risings, a general tendency to acidity are noted. The patient often complains of a "sour stomach," with water-brash and hiccough which is worse in the late afternoon. Craving for sweet things is common and for oysters, both of which upset him.

He is also worse for cold and relieved by warm foods.

Patients who are labelled " gouty " are often candidates for lycopodium. Without doubt there are several disorders of incomplete metabolism confounded often under one heading of gout and each with its own particular excess of this or that waste product. There is a metabolic disorder of the vegetarian, as well as of the meat-eater, and other cases may incline predominantly to one type or the other. Lycopodium seems generally more suitable to patients who eat little meat (or may even dislike it) : they are liable to pass an excess of oxalates in the urine, though the characteristic excretion of lycopodium contains also urates in quantity and uric acid. Nausea, vomiting, water-brash and gastric pain are relieved by heat locally ; these all testify to the involvement of the stomach. Flatulence is a very marked symptom of the remedy, but affects the bowels more than the stomach and is passed more by the anus. The result of the fermentation and distension is a

sense of acute discomfort felt especially in the right hypochondrium and, leading to a characteristic desire to loosen the
clothing or to intolerance of any pressure. The liver may be
felt enlarged and the patient may be jaundiced : the drug
seems to have power to cause catarrh of the bile-ducts and as
this is a precedent condition to gall-stone formation, lycopodium
may be useful in that disease, in the intervals between attacks.
Cramping pains point to irregular peristalsis and rumbling and
gurgling to the fermentative quality of the disturbed digestion.
The patients are usually constipated. As with Alumina and
silica (both of which are prominent among the mineral compo-
nents of lycopodium) the constipation arises from an inertia of
the bowel, the motions are only passed with considerable
straining, hæmorrhoids are common and there is often pain and
bleeding from evacuation. The constipation of infants is often
much helped by lycopodium.

All these abdominal and alimentary canal symptoms are to
be read as signs of a general failure of the tract to function
normally, with consequent incomplete metabolism. Invariably
with such cases, symptoms (conveniently though summarily
labelled as " toxic ") are apt to occur, such as headaches,
neuralgias of this or that nerve, joint pains and chronic swelling,
to say nothing of mental symptoms such as have already been
described, which lead to a diagnosis of " neurasthenia " or
" hypochondriasis." *   Sometimes these (really) subsidiary
symptoms are more prominent than the alimentary canal
symptoms and mask them, but whenever they are such as to
call for lycopodium they will have some of the characteristic
features of the drug. The pains will be worse from 4 p.m. to
8 p.m., the headache will be relieved by open air and made
worse by pressure (as of the hat), the sciatica will be worse from
pressure (lying on the affected side), and so on. The symptom-
complex is to be read as a whole, but if the abdominal symptoms are clear and are recognised early, then lycopodium will
clear up the case and these later evidences of uncured trouble
will not appear.

Joint pains are often accompanied by cramps and spasms of

* In lycopodium subjects, cultures from the bowel frequently show the
presence of a non-lactose-fermenting bacillus intermediate between *B. Morgan*
and *B. Gaertner.*

muscles. External heat gradually relieves the pains, so as a rule does movement. Wasting of muscles is common (lycopodium patients are often emaciated), less from organic nerve disease than from general malnutrition and inability or unwillingness to exercise. The skin is not very characteristically affected by lycopodium. Urticarial eruptions are perhaps the most generally seen, though chronic ulcers, if lycopodium symptoms are present, do well on it. The dryness of the skin, even degrees of psoriasis, especially of the palms, should be remembered.

In the genito-urinary sphere the drug is often called for. There is some evidence that it affects the prostate gland, and chronic disorders of that organ may be benefited (baryta and digitalis are more often helpful in enlarged prostate than any other remedies). Especially is lycopodium valuable in premature or temporary loss of sexual power either following masturbation or excess. Characteristic is sexual desire without sexual power. Gleet remaining after gonorrhoea is often helped by it. In the female the periods are irregular, apt to be excessive (though not always) and there is generally increase of desire and local burning and itching.

The urine is increased in quantity, sometimes clear on being passed, but containing as a rule both urates and uric acid in excess. Oxalates are often increased in quantity. The urine is generally markedly acid and thus causes pain on urination in sensitive subjects. Renal calculus and gravel may be helped by lycopodium.

The air passages and respiratory organs are (next to the alimentary canal) an important site of action of this drug. The voice is apt to be husky rather from tracheitis than from laryngitis : the cough is typically obstinate, dry and tickling, but there is also a condition met with in late phthisis or bronchiectasis that is helped by lycopodium, where the sputum is copious and purulent. It has great value in chronic lung affections, tuberculous or pneumococcal, when any general symptoms are present, but the evidence seems to point to its power being exerted less against tubercle specifically and more against the secondary infections (catarrhalis, streptococcus, etc.) that so often are added to tubercle. The dry cough which it benefits is more likely to be pneumococcic or influenzal than early tuberculous and for chronic pneumococcal cases (pneumonias that resolve badly) it has great power. In such conditions, many general characteristics of lycopodium are seen. The patient is often thin and looks worried and distressed. There is often extensive involvement of the right side. Frequently this condition has commenced in the right lower lobe and spread to the left side. Mentally the patient is irritable and difficult to nurse. He experiences considerable anxiety about his condition and is fearful if left alone. There is a tendency to muscular twitching which may be seen in the fan-like movements of the *alæ nasi* which are not synchronous with respiration,* or there may be twitchings of the facial or other muscles of the body. He may or may not be thirsty, but he gets discomfort from cold drinks and prefers warm fluids. The skin is usually harsh, the sputum scanty and expectoration difficult. It may be noted that pneumonic involvement requiring lycopodium is usually accompanied by some degree of digestive disturbance. Chronic nasal catarrhs (catarrhalis, pneumococcus) will often benefit. There is often noted a tendency to slight capillary bleeding (not the big hæmorrhages of tubercle, but the oozing of surfaces) and the taste of blood in the mouth is often complained of. Asthma may be relieved by lycopodium (the time of the paroxysm frequently gives the indication).

As regards the heart-pain, palpitation and anxiety are often complained of, but they appear to be secondary to the metabolic disorders and not due to primary heart lesions. Nevertheless, if they are notably caused or aggravated by abdominal flatulent distension lycopodium should not be forgotten. More important, however, is the effect of the drug in producing a great increase in consciousness of arterial pulsations, throbbing of arteries anywhere and arterial excitement. This symptom has led to the use of lycopodium for inoperable aneurysm and so much success has followed it, at any rate as a reliever of symptoms, that it is difficult not to credit the drug with some influence on arterial tissues. Remembering its relation to alimentary " toxæmias " and how often gout in all its forms affects arterial degeneration, it is probably from this side of its

---

* Dyspnœa in a lycopodium case will certainly show very marked movement of the *alæ nasi*.

power that lycopodium achieves any results : it is in any case well worth remembering, competing in this disease with barium and adrenalin. In Graves' disease, if the vascular symptoms are prominent, lycopodium has a place, though perhaps natrum muriaticum is here more often called for and belladonna for the ready relief of symptoms.

Lycopodium patients often sleep badly, as the four to eight aggravation may be continued through the early night and so conduce to restlessness. In febrile cases the time aggravation should be marked if lycopodium is indicated.

It is not too much to say that the physician who learns to use lycopodium has at his disposal a most potent remedy for many chronic disorders, especially those common to civilised communities and the classes who use up nervous tissue rather than muscular. High potencies and infrequent repetition give the best results, but diseases of the alimentary canal will often be helped by low and medium potencies at any rate for a time.

When joint and limb symptoms are prominent Lycopodium frequently takes up and completes the work of Rhus. Iodine and especially chelidonium are complementary to it in action. If lycopodium seems indicated, yet fails, the case will often respond to chelidonium and *vice versâ*. Graphites, too, especially in its abdominal symptoms, is a drug to be remembered in its helpful relation to lycopodium.

MANGANUM

Manganum Aceticum—Acetate of Manganese Solution.
Manganum Carbonicum—Carbonate of Manganese Trituration.

Both the preparations of manganese were proved by Hahnemann. Their symptomatologies are similar and either may be used on the indications which follow.

Physiologically manganese appears to resemble iron in its tissue reactions. Like copper and certain other metals, it appears to promote the utilisation of iron in hæmoglobin formation. Its provings show that it causes anæmia of a definite type with destruction of red blood corpuscles. When other symptoms confirm the choice, it is a valuable remedy for anæmia : the varying results obtained in non-homœopathic hands arise no doubt from its being used in cases for which it is not suited. Individualisation is the only road to success with drugs, and "anæmia" is a name covering a large variety of conditions : only a proportion will be covered in their symptom-totality by manganese and only those will be relieved by it.

Chronic manganese poisoning (seen in workmen exposed to the dust of it) presents symptoms predominantly in the nervous system : psychical (of the nature of hysteria) and physical, affecting motor centres with spastic gait and increased tendon reflexes. Epileptiform convulsions have been seen in rabbits and depression of the vaso-motor centre with falling blood pressure as a result of large doses. More chronic poisonings cause jaundice, with destruction of red blood corpuscles and nephritis with albuminuria. The alimentary tract is irritated but not ulcerated.

Professor Hugo Schulz regards manganese as a remedial agent of considerable importance. His observations confirm in general those of homœopathists. He uses the drug for some cases of anæmia and disorders of the liver : to the jaundice noted above as an effect of the metal he adds fatty degeneration of the liver.

Mr. McDonagh points out that in the vegetable kingdom manganese plays a part comparable to that of iron among vertebrates. He uses colloidal manganese (often with copper and antimony) to increase resistance to certain bacterial diseases (notably gonorrhœa) and claims good results.

Permanganate of potash is a very familiar disinfecting and deodorising (oxidising) agent and is used in this way as gargle and lotion. It antidotes opium. A proving of it made by Dr. H. C. Allen brought out some very marked symptoms of the upper respiratory tract and pharynx : swollen uvula, intense irritation of nose, pharynx and larynx with free discharge of pus and blood. The other salts of manganese influence the larynx especially, but their effects on pharynx and nose (though observable) are not so marked as those of the permanganate. These symptoms have led to some use of the permanganate for diphtheria and considerable success has been claimed: great prostration is said to be a confirming symptom. Permanganate is a favourite gargle and its value may be more than that of a simple antiseptic.

The profound effects of manganese on the nervous system have been already alluded to as revealed in poisonings. The provings confirm these and add details. The prevailing mood is one of depression, it may be described as a taciturn peevishness and fretfulness with occasional outbursts of hysterical mirth. Great anxiety and fear may be experienced or apprehensiveness, with the fear that " something is going to happen." The restlessness and anxiety of the manganum patient is more pronounced during the daytime when he is moving about. There is a marked amelioration of his fear when at rest lying down (cf. arsenicum : rhus). The mind appears abstracted from daily life and the senses dulled. The paralysis is of a spastic type with increased reflexes and later symptoms that suggest degeneration of the cells of the anterior horn of the cord : progressive muscular atrophy appears. The paralytic symptoms tend to begin below and extend upwards. The symptom of inclination to run forward on trying to walk is recorded. Muscular cramps and twitchings are observed. Sensory symptoms are also caused : particularly noteworthy is a general feeling of soreness all over the body. The bones become very sensitive to touch and neuralgic pains are common. The hands and feet (apart from the joint symptoms to be presently noted) feel swollen and tactile sensation is diminished. Cases of disseminated sclerosis may recall the symptom-picture of manganese and it is a drug to be considered in relation to this disease.

Of other important spheres of action of the drug, the joints take a prominent place and manganese is often a remedy for chronic arthritis. The general soreness and sensitiveness and aching of bones (probably due to periostitis) are accompanied by pain and swelling of joints, especially of the ankles. Every part of the body feels sore when touched. Red spots like those of erythema nodosum are noted and an unhealthy state of the skin, particularly in the neighbourhood of the joints, when small injuries suppurate and ulcers are sluggish and slow to heal, with bluish unhealthy margins.* The drug is often needed for joint and bone affections in syphilitic or tuber-

* The ability of the remedy to increase resistance to staphylococcal infections is well known, but as it is not by any means universally successful it is more than likely that only when a general similarity exists between drug and patient can it be given with confidence.

culous subjects. The alimentary canal is irritated : the tongue often furred and notably sore, developing little ulcers or papillomata or vesicles, the throat dry and sore and heat and burning in the stomach ; flatulence and griping pain in the stomach usually with constipation. On the whole, however, the alimentary canal symptoms are secondary, though the drug has a profound effect on the liver (fatty degeneration and some degree of jaundice) and has a value in syphilitic cases. It may, however, be indicated in early cases of tabes mesenterica when the patient is anæmic, the face characteristically pale, waxy and sunken ; the appetite is poor, diarrhœa may occur, and as the patient emaciates, abdominal glands are palpable.

The effects on the respiratory tract are more important, at least in its upper part. There is chronic catarrh of the nose, with, as a rule, dryness and scanty secretion and the middle ear is notably affected with thickening of the tympanum. Much shooting pain is experienced in the ears, with tinnitus (whistling tinnitus is said to be characteristic) and deafness. Chronic otorrhœa has been benefited by it. The drug's relationship is to middle ear disease of rather a chronic type. The throat feels dry, the larynx dry and painful ; dry painful cough, worse from talking but relieved by lying down and aggravated in damp weather. It resembles dulcamara in that cold damp weather tends to bring on attacks of bronchitis ; the voice is hoarse and speech often painful. Tuberculous or syphilitic laryngitis may call for it. The influence of the drug does not seem to extend to the lungs.

The red blood corpuscles are destroyed by over-doses of manganese with resulting anæmia, and for anæmia with chronic gastric symptoms, loss of appetite, general body soreness, an unhealthy skin and weakness of the joints, such anæmia as is frequently seen in commencing tuberculosis, manganese has a well-deserved reputation. It suits young and growing patients : in women the periods are typically too frequent but scanty : hæmorrhage is not often a symptom of manganese as it is of iron or china.

Symptoms are generally worse at night, worse from motion, worse from cold, especially cold and wet before a storm. Rest and warmth relieve most symptoms.

MEDORRHINUM

A trituration of the urethral discharge containing gonococci.

One hundred and twenty years ago, Hahnemann formulated the concept that all chronic diseases are the sequelæ of three miasms, psora, syphilis and sycosis. For the word miasm the more familiar term infection might be substituted and the condition called a chronic toxæmia.

The orthodox physician certainly recognises the remote effects of tuberculosis and syphilis, though he might not be so ready to concede a similar hereditary potency to other venereal, notably to gonorrhœal, infections apart from occasional arthritis. Nevertheless, the homœopathist believes that the results of gonorrhœal infections are not only acute, but also remote. A series of manifestations and symptoms in patients have been observed and collected, by which the effects of remote gonorrhœal infection may be recognised. To these manifestations, and the morbid state which slowly develops after a venereal but non-syphilitic infection, the term sycosis has been applied. Even more important is the concept that venereal non-syphilitic infection can influence detrimentally the progeny of an infected person in much the same way as can syphilis itself. Whether the theory of remote transmission of non-syphilitic venereal infection approximates to the true state of affairs or not, the homœopathist recognises an hereditary sycotic type by certain clinical signs and symptoms in the patient and, for the treatment of these, the nosode medorrhinum and allied drugs are used. Thus the sycotic type in his mind is analogous to the syphilitic and tubercular types.

There is almost certainly much yet to be learned about the after effects of many acute illnesses. It seems reasonable that sometimes there should be deep changes concerned with the mechanism of resistance to infections that should leave a patient less than a hundred per cent. recovered from an acute attack which has proved severe, either through the virulence of the invader or the poor defence of the organism. In so far as such effects might tell on blood-forming tissues or on endocrine balance, it is again conceivable at least that a mother suffering in this way might hand on to her offspring a defect. The time is not in any way ripe for confident statements, but homœopathists have found it useful to take note of many points in family histories generally regarded as negligible, and the hints so obtained are often confirmed by a symptomatology suggestive of a nosode.

There are other groups of coccal organisms besides the gonococcus, which appear capable of acting as foci of chronic infection, and of producing a symptom-picture that would fall under the heading of sycosis. A coccus frequently found in the lower bowel and a similar one that appears in chronic respiratory affections are associated notably with the sycotic type, but it is, as always, the symptom-picture that suggests the remedy, rather than the organism found, and the nosode should be prescribed strictly according to its indications.

Medorrhinum was introduced into the homœopathic Materia Medica by Dr. Swan over a hundred years ago, since when it has been extensively proved. The provings on the healthy have elicited many symptoms, both in the emotional sphere and the physical. The characteristics of the remedy are marked on both the psychic and emotional side and, on the physical side, all parts of the body are affected and, in particular, the sensorial nervous system : and disturbances appear in the respiratory, genital and cutaneous systems. Mucous membranes particularly are apt to show chronic catarrhs and free discharges of muco-pus. This deep acting remedy has a profound influence on the psychic and mental state of the patient. Firstly, there is often a nervousness and weakness experienced, especially during the daytime and the early hours of the morning and on waking up (cf. lachesis : thuja). He becomes quickly fatigued and is distressingly aware of his easy liability to experience weariness. Therefore, he endeavours to hurry through his occupations because he fears that his mental and emotional depression will overtake him before he has completed his work. This is the explanation of the recorded symptom that " he is in a great hurry." He is agitated and anxious to do things as quickly as possible. Therefore, scarcely has he begun one thing than he wants to start on another. This precipitous anxiety produces confusion of mind so that, for example, the patient has difficulty in relating his symptoms.

In spite of this, a very important characteristic modality of the medorrhinum patient is that he feels that time passes too slowly (*cf.* arg. nit. patient who fears that he will be unable to undertake his work because time passes too quickly). Thus he becomes indisposed to work, disinclined to make any exertion, and may be exhausted on the least effort, as though nothing were worth the effort of doing it, yet is often unable to keep still.

The subject for medorrhinum is hypersensitive, both mentally and physically. He easily develops anxiety regarding future events. He has difficulty in expressing himself, both in writing and speaking. In conversation he will hesitate because he cannot find the appropriate word to use. Thus he replies slowly to the questions put to him by the physician, and experiences difficulty in describing his symptoms, frequently appearing to be unable to grasp the gist of the enquiry. In a more advanced condition, the memory becomes definitely feeble, as much for the written as for the spoken word. In like manner, the sycotic child has difficulty in the studies at school, particularly from an inability to spell correctly. He also finds it hard to memorise words or a phrase, though he may apprehend well enough the meaning of the question.

The medorrhinum patient has an aversion from being touched and an aversion from people around him.* Generally he is nervous, hypersensitive to noise, and fearful. He develops a curious sensitivity about occurrences affecting himself. He is sensitive and easily hurt. He becomes apprehensive and readily develops anxiety regarding future events. He anticipates an unhappy future, even a presentiment of death. Conversely, the medorrhinum subject may experience on occasions a mental activity and a power of intuitive perception which appears to amount almost to foreknowledge. This approaches the cerebral activity of the lachesis patient who successfully completes at night, work which during the day he has been unable to complete.†

The medorrhinum patient shows a marked restlessness, both mentally and physically. This is not an unusual symptom in the sick and the peculiar modalities must be noted in order that

---

* This may be compared with the compulsion of the lueticum patient who does not object to being touched, but flinches when he touches anyone or anything which arouses in him a sense of contamination.

† This is another example of the inevitable rhythm of life activity. If as with medorrhinum there is excessive stress usually on the stage of preparation for activity in metabolism there will be occasional excessive energy shown in the performance of the cell function.

the physician can consider the remedy applicable to the condition. Here there is a definite physical restlessness in that he cannot keep still ; even in the consulting room he will constantly fidget and move things about, but there is not to be seen the physical agitation of zinc, or the restlessness which relieves painful symptoms as in rhus. tox.

The headache is often frontal, with a sensation as if a tight band were drawn round the forehead. Vertigo is aggravated on stooping and by motion, whereas relief is experienced when the patient lies down. (Conium has the opposite modality. Vertigo commonly occurs when the patient is in bed and is always aggravated when lying down.) Inflammation of the conjunctivæ may occur with a gluey discharge ; the patient experiences difficulty in separating the lids in the morning. It has proved of value in disturbances of vision : diplopia, or the patient sees objects smaller than normal (cf. platinum).

The rheumatic symptoms are important. Medorrhinum should always be considered in cases of arthritis, especially where there is a history of gonorrhœa, but the drug is of value, too, in any rheumatic condition when the symptoms agree, even when there is no venereal antecedence. The vertebral column is often sensitive to touch. There is stiffness in the lumbar region, and the drug has been used with success in cases of lumbago, following the strain of lifting. The joints are stiff and feeble, with a sensation of heaviness or want of power to move the limbs when walking. Sensitivity of the heel and tenderness of the ball of the foot is sometimes experienced. Damp weather relieves the pain in the limbs : an exacerbation of the pain is experienced at the approach of, and especially during, a storm, but cold weather, with or without damp, often intensifies the pain. The neuralgic pains of medorrhinum, too, are ameliorated by humid weather, and are aggravated by sudden sharp movements. The pains tend to change from place to place and appear and disappear suddenly.

The medorrhinum patient may show profound dental changes. The teeth are friable and dental caries develops (cf. thuja). Pharyngitis is helped by this drug, especially when the condition is relieved by gargling with salt water. This modality is of interest when it is recalled that the medorrhinum patient is generally relieved by sea air.

Burnett regarded gonorrhœa " as the mother of pus and catarrhs." The suitable remedy, frequently one of the sycotic drugs, has cured obstinate cases of nasal catarrh, with thick, greenish, yellow discharge : it should be especially considered in obstinate nasal discharges following a suppressed gonorrhœa and has a real value in sinusitis.

As a rule, the appetite is good, often increased, with a craving for sweets and stimulating foods such as salt, sour foods, pickles and beer. The abdominal pains may be severe, relieved by lying on the belly and aggravated by drawing up the knees (cf. colocynth). The patient is very constipated and finds that he can only open his bowels if he leans backwards. Medorrhinum is one of the most valued remedies for the treatment of asthma in both adults and children, especially where there is an hereditary sycosis. There is increased bronchial secretion. Dyspnœa is worse on the slightest exertion ; expiration is difficult. The sufferer finds relief by lying on the abdomen (cf. sambucus—where the patient must sit up). He kneels on the bed or bends himself over.* Attacks of bronchitis are benefited by medorrhinum when the characteristic modalities present themselves. The patient is relieved during damp weather and at the seaside. These two modalities distinguish this remedy from another most valuable drug for asthma conditions—natrum sulph.

In the latter drug, the patient's symptoms are aggravated both by damp weather and in the sea air. The skin of the medorrhinum patients (as with all sycotics), is cold and damp. An interesting circumstance found occasionally in the subjects is the presence of yellow spots on the backs of the hands.

Before the administration of medorrhinum, its outstanding modalities must be present (as with any remedy), if one hopes for a beneficial result. Generally, the patient's symptoms are relieved in damp weather. Rest helps most troubles and constipation is overcome by leaning backwards. Symptoms are aggravated when thinking about them ; during heat ; movement ; and thundery weather. The time aggravation of

* The child, and occasionally the adult, needing medorrhinum is often found to sleep in the knee-elbow position, with head bent down into the pillow. It has been pointed out that this is the only posture in which a human being can get the aid of gravity in draining his nasal sinuses.

troubles is definite—during the day and most especially in the early morning (3 to 5 a.m.).

A nosode has been made by Dr. John Paterson from a culture cf strains of diplococcus isolated from the bowel. It is named Sycotic Compound ; its general action is similar to that of medorrhinum and it is frequently a valuable supplement to this remedy.

MERCURY

Mercurius Solubilis. An impure oxide prepared according to a formula of Hahnemann's own which dates from his pre-homœopathic days and is still used by non-homœopathists in Germany. Triturations for lower and tinctures for higher potencies are made of this. Mercurious Vivus, the metal, prepared by trituration and as tincture for high potencies. The symptoms of these two are virtually identical and either may be given on the indications which follow.

Mercury has long been used in medicine and overdosing with it at one time was far from uncommon ; therefore, its gross effects upon the human body are well known to all physicians. It is not certain in what way mercury is absorbed, but it may well be that with this, as with other metals, insoluble particles are taken up by the leucocytes (from alimentary canal or after deep or superficial injections) and so reach the tissues, where by processes unknown (at present) they enter more deeply into the cellular life.

Acute mercurial poisoning, particularly by corrosive sublimate,* has marked local effects as well as more distant ones. If swallowed in any quantity, the symptom of a harsh metallic taste is followed by severe burning pain in mouth, throat, and stomach ; nausea and vomiting set in and blood and mucous membrane shreds are found in the vomit. Presently the involvement of the bowel is shown by tenesmus and loose and bloody (dysenteric) stools. Collapse with all its usual symptoms soon appears. The urine is suppressed or diminished and albuminuria with casts, epithelium and (sometimes) blood is almost invariable. Sugar has been found in the urine. The temperature is generally lowered. The mental state is usually

* Corrosive sublimate, the perchloride of mercury, is known to homœopathists as mercurius corrosivus : its general symptomatology resembles that of merc. sol., or vivus, but in the course of this article those conditions will be noted which specially indicate it, for it has certain spheres of very marked action.

either one of somnolence with attacks of vertigo or of restlessness. Consciousness is little affected. Death ensues from collapse or gradually from exhaustion. Of these symptoms, those of mouth and stomach are largely local, though there are specific symptoms here also (after more chronic poisonings) which are noteworthy. But the kidney and bowel symptoms appear however the poison is introduced and are therefore more profound and characteristic of the metal.

More chronic poisoning has often arisen as a sequel to incautious medication. The condition is known as mercurialism and is of the profoundest interest to the homœopathist. First of symptoms to appear are a metallic taste in the mouth and numbness or soreness of the gums and tongue. The tongue is swollen and thickly coated, the gums swollen and soft and the breath foul. The saliva is notably increased. If the poisoning continues ulcers appear on tongue (opposite the teeth), cheeks and gums and the saliva is not only profuse but irritating. Larger doses still may cause the teeth to fall out and gangrene of soft parts and even necrosis of the jaw to follow. Any caries of the teeth markedly predisposes to local poisoning effects.

The stomach and bowel are affected, so that anorexia, gastric discomfort, nausea and vomiting appear and colicky pains. The stools are generally loose, but periods of constipation often alternate with periods of diarrhœa. The first effect of the drug on the bowel in provers is usually to cause constipation.

Mercury is excreted by salivary glands and glands of mouth and throat, and to this process (and not to local irritation) is to be attributed the stomatitis and salivation of chronic mercurialism. The excoriations and ulcers follow, and if through carious teeth the ulcerative process reaches the periosteum, then periostitis occurs. Mercury has no such action on bone as phosphorus has and any necrosis is a sequel to the periostitis. The bowel is affected more than the stomach, for mercury is excreted largely here, mainly by cæcum and colon. Thus all the appearances of chronic dysentery may be produced, with ulceration and necrosis of tissue and its symptoms naturally are observed. Contrary to the usual belief, mercury (even calomel) does not increase the secretion of bile.

Skin eruptions are common : especially vesicular and pustular. Itching is worse from the warmth of the bed.

Several forms may be seen in the same patient. Desquama-
tion follows. Albuminuria has been observed and rarely
glycosuria. Diuresis follows the administration of mercury,
seemingly by a direct action on the kidney cells. As already
noted, corrosive sublimate causes nephritis more certainly
than other preparations of mercury, though other compounds approximate to it in mode of action more or less. An
actual necrosis may occur with the perchloride and phosphate
of lime is then deposited in the tubules. The result of all these
tissue disturbances is a more or less profound cachexia with
anæmia, weakness, fainting fits and restlessness. The pulse is
small and quick. The red corpuscles and hæmoglobin of the
healthy subject are said to be at first increased by mercury and
later diminished, while in syphilis the drug induces at first a
sudden fall and then a rise in both respects. This is a significant
observation for the homœopathist.

Mercury given medicinally, even in excessive doses, rarely
affects the nervous system, but workers in mercury mines or in
such manufactories as expose them to inhalations of the fumes
for long periods are apt to pass into a state characterised by
great irritability, with timidity and dislike of company. Sleeplessness and delirium with hallucinations may follow. Muscular
weakness is considerable and a general tremor (beginning
in hands and arms) is very characteristic. Neuralgias, anæs-
thesias, or localised paralyses occur, and the special senses
suffer, so that amblyopia, amnesia and deafness have all been
met with. Both the tremor and the sensory and motor symptoms are probably to be regarded as central and not as peripheral in origin.

The blood pressure tends to fall from excessive doses of
mercury. Nutrition (metabolism) appears to be improved by
small doses and therefore the cachexia of poisoning may be
partly due to a reversal of this favourable effect by excessive
quantities, but the local effects of the poison and their consequences mask the metabolic changes. But experience leaves
little doubt in the mind of the homœopathist of the power of
the drug over general metabolism.

The intestine and kidney are the chief points of excretion of
mercury, but sweat, saliva, milk, gastric juice and bile have all
shown traces of it after poisoning. In fact, it penetrates into

every organ of the body in time and is a drug of most profound and universal power. Excretion is very slow.

Mercury is naturally very poisonous to elementary organisms and preparations of it are much used as antiseptics. Its undoubted effects in syphilis are attributed to its power to kill spirochætes. It is more deadly to them in the test tube than to organisms of malaria or trypanosomiasis and some specificity of reaction is clearly present, since a solution of 1 in 200,000 is lethal. But it is by no means certain that this simple explanation of its curative action is sufficient. Now that chronic mercurialism is relatively rare, it has passed out of general observation that this condition can (and often does) present the closest resemblance to the effects of syphilis. Inasmuch as the drug poisoning generally occurs in syphilitic subjects, its effects are naturally masked by those of the disease, but a century or so ago more than one famous physician recorded the resemblances between them—among others, Hahnemann himself in his pre-homœopathic days. When the homœopathist claims that mercury is frequently the *simillimum* for a case of syphilis, the essence of his contention—the resemblance of symptoms producible by syphilis to those producible by mercury—has been admitted by many celebrated men who had no interest in homœopathy. Indeed, this resemblance has led more than once to the attempt to formulate a rule of treatment, such rules in practice being virtually always reproductions more or less detailed of the Hahnemannian generalisation. Professor Schulz, for instance, in recent days is clear and definite on the resemblance between the symptoms of drug and disease as a guide to cure, and lays great stress on mercury as an instance of the value of the rule.

In the main, to a homœopathist, the indications for mercury are found in the secondary stage of syphilis, but there they are nearly always clear and while generally he uses the lower potencies, he does not find it necessary to have recourse to the larger quantities fashionable to-day. Not that homœopathists do not sometimes make use of them, for they rightly maintain that the principle of similars is independent of the size of the dose and they admit that good results appear often to follow the larger dosage. But they retain great scepticism as to whether the drug effect is a parasiticidal one and they are well aware of the dangers of excess of mercury in the system, so that they use the larger dose with even more caution than their colleagues who do not share their opinions. They are much more disposed to believe that, since there exists some bodily resistance to the parasite confessedly sufficient in mild cases to effect a cure without aid of any remedy, therefore the true line of treatment is to endeavour to heighten this resistance. Since mercury indubitably helps to cure, they conceive that it works rather through increasing the efficacy of the resistance than through killing the parasite,* and point with more than interest to the resemblance between effects of the drug and effects of the disease. When the homœopathist treats syphilis with mercury he does so as an exemplification of his rule of practice and if the patient presented no signs characteristic of this drug, he would be disposed to give rather the remedy that was indicated by the whole symptom-complex.

The use of mercury for syphilis is so outstanding a feature of medical practice that it has to be thus considered as a particular application of the drug, but the distinctive knowledge of the homœopathist (from provings even more than from poisonings) defines the sphere of mercury for many conditions. Whenever the characteristic symptoms appear, mercury is the remedy of choice, syphilis or no syphilis, and, once again, syphilis should only be treated (and is only treated) homœopathically by mercury when it presents symptoms corresponding to those of the drug.

There are certain general symptoms of mercury brought out by homœopathic experience which often give the clue to the right use of the remedy. Thus, there is a sensitiveness of reaction to temperature, so that any change either in the direction of heat or cold worsens the patient's condition. He is aggravated by all forms of heat, a warm atmosphere or the warmth of the bed and alternately by the cold and the open air, also by wet damp weather. Many drugs suit patients averse from cold and many others those averse from heat, but the candidate for mercury dislikes both. It is the change which is resented. Another very marked symptom is that

---

* No doubt some spirochætes are killed by direct action when large doses are given, but the homœopathist would take this as an accessory action of the drug, not as its most important one.

disease conditions are worse at night, from sunset to sunrise.
This is the division of the twenty-four hours when syphilitic
patients are usually worse, and all the remedies predominantly valuable in syphilis show a nocturnal aggravation of
symptoms. Mercury shows it notably, but it appears under
hepar, sulph., arsen., aurum, nitric acid, etc. Tremor (of head,
of hands, of tongue, etc.) is pronounced in many cases that need
mercury. It goes on to paresis and paralysis and is accompanied by great restlessness ; sometimes it is exaggerated into
spasms, cramps, convulsive movements. It is often accompanied by fainting fits and in any case there is great debility.
Mind and body are alike weak : questions are ill-understood
and memory and will power deficient. But, on the other hand,
there is a great feeling of hurry and anxiety in the patient. He
talks rapidly in delirium and time seems to pass slowly ; everything is done hastily, though usually ineffectively. The drug
is often suggested in paralysis agitans. Coming to more
objective symptoms, mercury causes and cures profuse sweatings, which characteristically do not give any relief. For any
disease in which there is profuse sweating without relief,
mercurius should be considered as a possible remedy. It helps
acute and sub-acute rheumatism frequently when the symptom
is prominent. The sweat is often offensive as are many of the
excretions of the body. The mouth is so definite a point of
attack of mercury that it is natural that mouth and tongue
symptoms should be of value in selecting the drug, and an
offensive, sweet, mawkish odour of the breath and taste to the
patient are very characteristic. The tongue is swollen, flabby,
heavily coated, indented by the teeth and moist. Mercury is
rarely indicated in conditions when the tongue is dry. The
gums are swollen and sore, the teeth may be loose (pyorrhœa
is a condition where mercury should be remembered), the
saliva is thick and profuse : toothache from caries of the teeth
is more controlled by mercury (pending the dentist's aid) than
by any drug except perhaps creosote. There is great thirst. A
slimy mucus predominates in secretions that suggest mercury
as a remedy, together with pus. The nasal and pharyngeal
catarrhs are of this kind, causing soreness of the nostrils and
ulceration. Many nasal catarrhs respond to mercury. The
coryza is acrid and watery, more troublesome at night and

increased both by heat and cold. There is especially a general
tendency to middle ear disease and infcctions with involvement
of the Eustachian tubes may be cured. Mercury rivals pulsatilla in measles and scarlet fever when otitis media appears.
The discharge is purulent and offensive and the pain is aggravated at night and by the warmth of the bed. There are pains
in the throat, swelling and inflammation of pharynx and
tonsils, with secretion of thick and tenacious mucus : the pains
shoot up into the ears. Quinsy will often be helped, but the
throats that respond best are those that are markedly " septic."
In diphtheria the cyanide of mercury is the preparation of
election, and perhaps a majority of all cases of this disease need
it. The biniodide is also used : it has value in tonsillitis
and pharyngitis, but is inferior to the cyanide in diphtheria.
Swallowing is naturally difficult, but thirst is considerable in
these circumstances. The sore throat of secondary syphilis is a
typical condition for the use of mercury. Inflammations and
affections of the salivary glands are well in the mercurial sphere.
The unpleasant, sweetish, metallic taste in the mouth, which is
characteristic, naturally affects the appetite. Stimulants are
often craved, and sometimes there is great desire for food.
More often, however, there is dislike of all solids (sweets especially) and only liquids will be taken, for the thirst remains,
however much the appetite be lost. Digestion, however, in
conditions that suggest mercury is very defective. Sharp and
heavy pains, anxiety and vertigo, nausea and vomiting and
violent eructations proclaim the trouble of the stomach.
Though mercury may not increase the flow of bile, homœopathists find many symptoms of its pathogenesis referable to
liver disturbance. Thus, the region of the liver becomes sensitive and resents pressure and there may be a degree of catarrhal
jaundice. There is marked dislike to lying on the right side.
It should be noted here that many complaints are aggravated
by lying on the right side. However, hepatic symptoms that
call for mercury are rather those due to secondary than primary
disturbance of that organ. In the bowel it is principally the end
of the small intestine and the cæcum and colon that are affected.
Here, as already observed in the discussion of mercurial poisoning, acute inflammation and ulceration are produced by the
drug and the homœopathist thinks of it for dysentery, acute

colitis, and, in fact, all severe inflammations of this tract. The stools are loose, bloody, mucoid, with shreds of tissue. Pain is severe and both pain and diarrhœa are worse at night. There is much tenesmus and straining and the anus becomes very sore and excoriated. The peculiar modality regarding this condition is that no relief is experienced from the stool. Mercury is indicated in conditions where the patient will sit and strain. This is the opposite state of affairs to dysenteric conditions calling for nux. vomica. Here the patient is relieved if a little stool be passed. Probably bacillary dysentery more often presents mercurial symptoms than amœbic, but the homœopathist would review each symptom-complex as it presented itself, without prejudice, and if the complex suggested mercury, whatever the pathology, would administer the drug. Of all mercurial preparations, mercurius corrosivus (corrosive sublimate) is best adapted to cases of dysentery.

In less acute conditions mercury is often valuable when constipation, with hard and knotty stools, is present. Efforts at evacuation are difficult and ineffectual ; mucus is nearly always present and mercury is seldom or never indicated when this secretion is not in excess.

The genito-urinary organs are profoundly affected. Mercury (preferably merc. corr.) is one of the best remedies for recent nephritis. The ureter, bladder and urethra may each one (or all) be inflamed, with characteristic secretion of muco-pus. The end of the penis is particularly irritated ; the smegma increases in quantity and the itching and irritation lead the patient to much handling and pulling of the organ. Painful (nocturnal) erections and increased desire are common, but sexual power is diminished. All kinds of inflammation and ulcers of the penis are suitable for mercury and the drug undoubtedly attacks this region with a special violence, so that as far as ordinary locality goes the syphilitic chancre suggests mercury. But although there is often a degree of induration about the mercurial ulcer, it is rather the " soft sore " than the Hunterian chancre that is most typical of the drug. It is the secondary stage with enlarged glands, sore throat and skin eruptions that is most likely to give a mercurial symptom-complex, and the modern method of using arsenic at once and following with mercury commends itself to the homœopathist, as far as any routine procedure can. If, however, the symptomatology as a whole pointed to mercury, the homœopathist would give the drug whatever the stage of the disease.

Sweating of the external genitals is a common mercurial symptom. In the female sex, the periods are usually times of general abdominal discomfort. As a rule the menses are excessive. Leucorrhœa is profuse, worse at night, excoriating, and the external parts are sore, swollen, inflamed. In poisonous doses, mercury inflames the kidneys and the perchloride is one of the best remedies for the earlier stages of chronic nephritis. In general the quantity of urine is increased when the drug is called for.

The respiratory organs are chiefly affected in the air passages. The nasal and pharyngeal catarrh has been described, but larynx, trachea and bronchi are all affected. The inflammation is usually accompanied by free secretion of muco-pus and there may be ulceration. Cough and pains are worse at night. Thoracic discomfort and oppression, marked emphysematous conditions and bronchiectasis require mercury fairly often, and in certain pneumonias, especially those that do not resolve well, the claim of the drug should not be forgotten. Here the characteristic symptoms of the drug present themselves. The patient is restless with muscular twitching, intensely thirsty and bathed in a profuse sweat which aggravates the whole condition. The mouth is offensive, but the tongue is moist with indented margins by the teeth. Active delirium may supervene. The clue to successful use of the drug will be found generally in the mental condition, and in tongue and throat symptoms accompanying those of the chest. Palpitation and fainting on slight exertion are to be noted.

Regarding the special sense organs, inflammatory conditions of nose and middle ear have been already described as often suitable for mercury. The eyes show a chronic, obstinate conjunctivitis, with great thickening of the edges of the lids and tendency to agglutinate (cf. graphites). Corneal ulceration is frequently well treated with mercury and for iritis it is one of the best remedies. Naturally for syphilitic iritis it is specially to be remembered, but also may be indicated for other forms of the disease. The perchloride, iodide and sulphide (cinnabar) are here preferred to the metal.

Mercury causes lymphatic glands to swell. Periostitis, synovitis and neuralgias of big nerve trunks may all be accompanied by general mercurial indications. Bone pains are deepseated, intense and worse at night. Joints are affected notably, and when the heavy sweats are present giving no relief, when every change of temperature seems to worsen the suffering, as do touch, pressure and movement, and when the nightly aggravation of pain is marked the drug can be given with confidence in both acute and sub-acute conditions and in exacerbations of more chronic ones.

The skin when mercury is indicated is often yellowish and rough and subject to heavy sweat. Almost any kind of eruption—papular, pustular, urticarial—may be present ; chronic ulcers, syphilitic or other, with hard edges and slow to heal. Discharges are excoriating.

Drowsiness is a marked symptom of mercury, as of arsenic, but the customary nocturnal aggravation of symptoms naturally disturbs the sleep at night. Dreams are vivid and generally horrible : sometimes lascivious. Patients are very apt to talk and groan while asleep.

The best antidote for over-dosing with mercury is hepar sulph., and kali iod. has value also in this regard. Silica and mercury are incompatible. All potencies are valuable.

NATRUM MURIATICUM

The ions of sodium and chlorine are always present in body fluids and are essential to life. Sodium chloride is a substance of great osmotic power, and upon this physical property depend many of the results of large doses of it. When, however, the drug is given in potencies, these osmotic effects in no way come into play and therefore at first sight symptoms in provings dependent on them would not seem good indications for the choice of the remedy. It is, nevertheless, a fact that these symptoms have real value as suggestions for the curative use of the drug, and it is probable that subjects who are sensitive to the physical effects of large doses are also sensitive to the subtler non-osmotic influence of it. It is true that orthodox opinion regards salt as inert as a remedy in itself. But Loeb and others have found in lowly organisms that the sodium ion can have very definite effects and higher organisms (if sensitised by disease) may conceivably be influenced by potencies when non-potentised doses would be without action. This at least would be the claim of the homœopathist, for to him natrum muriaticum is one of the most profound remedies for chronic diseases and the clinical evidence of its power is extensive and persistent. To admit the claim is to realise again the extraordinary change in drug-potentiality wrought by homœopathic pharmacy, for only those who habitually use high potencies value this drug greatly, although to them it is an agent employed with confident expectation of good whenever the symptoms call for it. Dr. Schulz has praised small material doses of it, especially for some complaints of infants, and salt is a traditional remedy for some diseases (e.g., malaria), for which homœopathic experience also finds it often effective.

Provings and clinical use have elaborated a symptom-picture for the choice of nat. mur. that is definite and distinctive and there is no need to distinguish for purposes of drug choice between effects due to the physical properties of salt and those possibly due to its chemical action. If disease has modified the body in a way that can be matched by the osmotic effects of large doses of salt, that disorder is likely to be helped by the use of potencies of the remedy : inexplicable as the fact may appear, it is based upon a very prolonged clinical experience and could only be refuted by negative experience equally careful and thorough.

Natrum muriaticum produces anæmia and is a remedy for certain cases of it. Anæmia of a chronic kind, where red corpuscles and hæmoglobin are deficient without profound blood changes, is the most suitable form of the disease for the drug : the blood pressure is low, and when there is reason to regard adrenal secretion as diminished the symptom-complex often suggests nat. mur. Exophthalmic goitre following emotional stress also finds it remedy frequently in this drug. Emaciation and weakness are common symptoms besides anæmia and there is a general tendency to free watery discharges from mucous membranes as though the fluids of the blood were out of proportion to its solids—flowing easily away. The patients suitable for nat. mur. are sensitive to external stimuli, light, heat, etc. The circulation being poor, they are chilly and lack vital warmth, but also they greatly need air. These patients feel extreme of heat and cold. Many conditions are aggravated at the seaside.

The temperament that suggests nat. mur. is a melancholic one. Patients weep readily and find it very difficult to take pleasure in anything. Tears may be induced by pity or admonition without cause or may alternate with laughter. " Unpleasant occurrences are recalled that she may grieve over them."*

With their depression, however, they are irritable and apt to quarrel with any attempted consolation : they are averse from company and better alone. The causes of depression are usually personal and emotional. Fear of thunder is a notable symptom. Unhappy emotional experiences (*e.g.*, disappointed affection) are apt to give rise to mental conditions that are helped by this remedy as may also be the effects of fright or anger. Candidates for it much dislike to be pitied and conceal the cause of their troubles, though the mental depression is obvious enough. There may, however, be outbursts of rather hysterical mirth and both hysteria and hypochondriasis may find a remedy in nat. mur. Dr. Clarke made the observation that the depression varies proportionately to the .degree of constipation and nat. mur. produces (and cures) a definite type of constipation. Many undersized, ill-developed children are helped by this drug. They show the characteristic nat. mur. mental condition and general modalities, and, in particular, an irritability which resents interference from those around them.

Nat. mur. is one of the most prominent of headache remedies and the symptom-complex that calls for it is seldom without this feature. Typically, the pain is very severe, throbbing and hammering, incapacitating from any mental work. It begins about 10 a.m. (the time of aggravation of nat. mur. is usually from 9 to 10 a.m. for all symptoms) and goes on into the afternoon : often vision is affected at the beginning and flashes of light ("fiery zig-zags ") are seen. It is made worse by heat and relieved by fresh air. Eye-strain headaches persisting after correct glasses have been given, or due to over-use of

---

* Then can I grieve o'er grievances foregone
And heavily from woe to woe tell o'er
The sad account of fore-bemoanèd moan
Which I now pay as if nor paid before.

normal vision, often indicate this drug. There is some periodicity about the times of recurrence of these headaches which
occur every day or every third or fourth day.

Eye symptoms are prominent. The subjective sensations
with the headache have just been mentioned, but Burnett's
attention was drawn to the statement that young horses
reared on certain salt marshes developed cataract, and on this
hint he employed nat. mur. in this disease and he and others
have claimed considerable success for it. The conjunctiva is
chronically inflamed and the lids thickened and ulcerated (cf.
graphites) in many nat. mur. cases and the lachrymal secretion
much increased.

The appearance of the face is often enough to suggest this
remedy. Characteristically it is yellowish, pale, earthy and
greasy looking, the latter condition being intensified while
eating. The lips are dry and cracked or ulcerated : in febrile
complaints or coryzas, labial herpes is common. Acneiform
eruptions are also frequent and there is a profuse watery coryza,
leaving the nostrils sore, chapped or ulcerated. The nose feels
obstructed; hot and uncomfortable. The mouth also is frequently subject to chronic inflammations and small ulcerations
and may be cracked or deeply fissured. Tingling and numbness
about lips and tongue should be noted. The tongue is stiff and
dry, with a patchy appearance (what is often called a
" mapped " tongue) : frothy saliva is frequently seen along
the sides of it. The numbness and stiffness of the tongue which
leads to heavy speech often corresponds to children who are
late in talking, but this condition arises more through difficulty
in articulation than in mental backwardness as in baryta carb.
In spite of the dryness of the tongue, saliva is usually copiously
secreted.

There is more or less continuous thirst, dependent somewhat
on the constant desire for salt, also oysters. Bread is either
much liked or entirely disliked : fats are loathed. The appetite is variable. After food there are empty risings, nausea and
waterbrash and a general sense of impaired digestion without
great or persistent pain. The splenic region is often the site of
symptoms and some splenic disorders have seemed to react to
nat. mur. There is some general flatulence and usually marked
constipation with hard, dry, crumbling fæces, evacuated with

much straining and effort. The hard, dry stool tends to cause a fissure of the anus. Occasionally there is a profuse watery diarrhœa, often painless and coming characteristically about 9 a.m., or constipation and diarrhœa may alternate ; patients who are better for fasting or taking very little food are good subjects for natrum muriaticum.

Nat. mur. is a frequently indicated remedy in enuresis. The urine is increased and the sphincter weak, so that in women a cough may lead (as with ferr. phos. and caust.) to involuntary passage of some of the bladder contents. There is a notable modality here to be found, in that the patient finds difficulty in passing urine *if anyone be present*. The general state of weariness and exhaustion is reflected in the sexual sphere, where lack of desire or ineffective desire is frequent. In women there is often sterility : the menses may be profuse or scanty, but are seldom normal, and the depression and headache are apt then to be especially severe. As a rule desire is lost. Leucorrhœa if present is watery and profuse : there is an absence of the normal vaginal secretion in many cases. The backache, which is characteristic and common, is severe, affecting mainly the sacrum and lumbar spine and much relieved by pressure, *e.g.*, lying on something hard. Other aches and pains in the limbs are very common. They are not often persistently localised and are of a weary, tiring character and made worse by any prolonged exertion. They amount to symptoms of a general neuromuscular fatigue. Corns and warts and skin thickenings are frequent, the nails are often unhealthy : wounds heal slowly, and urticarial, vesicular and miliary rashes are apt to appear, besides facial acne. The margins of the hair are a characteristic site for this as are the flexor surfaces. The skin is often dry, though in febrile conditions sour-smelling perspirations occur which temporarily relieve the patient.

This drug is a valuable heart remedy. It may be indicated in hypertrophy of the heart, especially when the attacks of palpitation are aggravated by lying on the left side. There are violent palpitations and throbbings of the heart which shake the whole body and cardiac pains in many patients who need this remedy. The palpitation and sensation of faintness is aggravated by lying down, a very important modality. A sense of coldness in the precordial region is characteristic. Clinically nat. mur. is frequently found indicated in chronic morbus cordis and has so often improved even very severe cases that the homœopathist is bound to credit it with a profound action on heart structures and disease conditions. The pulse is quickened, but of low tension. The use of natrum muriaticum in Graves' disease has been mentioned. Certain chronic catarrhs, particularly of the upper respiratory passages, are helped by it when other symptoms correspond.

This drug is usually (and best) prescribed in chronic diseases where the mental and general symptoms suggest it. When acute cases have reacted well to bryonia, nat. mur. very often can be given to ensure complete recovery, but otherwise it comes to be thought of mainly in anæmic, tired-out, enfeebled conditions, with the characteristic headache and constipation. Such states may be due to more than one chronic disease. Particularly in malaria that has not responded to ordinary treatment is this drug useful or when the condition has resulted from administration of quinine. The aggravation from 9 a.m. to 10 a.m. is then of importance, and in the paroxysm the cold stage is severe and long. There is thirst throughout and the sweat relieves considerably, though there is much debility between the attacks.

Natrum mur. is one of our most valued remedies for the treatment of troubles resulting from emotional stress or strain. Its value lies less in its influence upon this or that tissue than upon its profound effect upon the deeper metabolic processes. As yet we have not the knowledge requisite to state precisely the nature and limits of its action, for the threads of the complex web of interacting forces that make up in their totality the life of an organism are not easy to trace. But provings and clinical experiments convinced (and still convince) homœopathists that the drug has a profound, harmful influence on the healthy when given in large doses and a profound curative influence on certain sick persons in minute doses. Acting on the principle of the choice of remedy by similarity of symptoms, a drug can be selected for a case of chronic disease although the full details of the metabolic defects in the patient are not known any more than the full details of the effects of the drug on the healthy. Let it not be for a moment imagined that the homœopathist despises such knowledge. On the contrary, he welcomes every experiment, every hint, that can elucidate in the least degree the puzzling pictures of chronic disease. But when the (largely) unexplained symptom-complex of a drug pathogenesis matches the (largely) unexplained complex of a case of disease, he assumes that similar, if unknown, processes are at work in each instance and expects that the drug in a small dose will affect favourably the disease condition which so resembles the one which it itself can produce in large dosage. The assumption is justified in practice so often as to make the homœopathic rule a valued guide to the careful physician.

As already mentioned more than once, nat. mur. follows bryonia very well. It also continues good effects begun by ignatia and apis, if these drugs begin to lose their power. Nat. mur. antidotes the ill-effects of excessive use of nitrate of silver. Illnesses dating from the local application of the latter drug have frequently defied treatment until the condition of this causation has led to the administration of nat. mur. It is almost exclusively used in spaced-out doses of high potencies, though Dr. Burnett used the sixth centesimal with success, and Professor Schulz has praised the use of a dilute solution of the pure substance.

NUX VOMICA

Tincture of Trituration of the seeds of the Strychnos Nux Vomica plant.

Strychnine and its analogue brucine are the chief active principles of this drug, but for homœopathists nux vomica tincture possesses qualities and powers that are not all represented in its alkaloids and since our provings are of nux vomica homœopathists turn to that. They value precision of indication far beyond concentration of the drug power, especially when the concentration involves a certain limitation of range. There are other alkaloids that resemble strychnine, notably gelsemine, and gelsemium and nux vomica have certain interesting points of comparison, although to the homœopathist they have mainly different, even opposing, indications. It will be valuable first to consider strychnine as it appears to the sceptic in homœopathy, for it is a much used drug and there is no reason why the homœopathist should not, if he chooses, avail

himself of its possible virtues. It is held from experiment and
observation that the main action of the poison is upon the
spinal nervous system. The special senses are rendered more
acute by small doses ; for touch, taste and smell the cause of
these results is probably central, but an action on the retinal
cells may be, partly at least, responsible for the effect of the
drug on vision. Homœopathists, it is perhaps needless to say,
regard heightened sense perceptions as one of the indications for
nux vomica and night blindness has been successfully treated
with it. Small doses of strychnine delay the onset of fatigue
and increase the capacity for muscular work. The power of the
drug is made use of to tide patients over emergencies and as an
emergency measure has a certain value of which homœopathists
can on occasion avail themselves. But it is important to
remember that this action does not mean that the increased
energy is obtained miraculously, without paying for it, but
merely that payment is deferred. This is the universal comment to be made on all effective drug action (homœopathic or
other) : it can only be effective by the utilisation of natural
reserves of power. It is quite sound practice so to utilise them
to defeat disease, leaving them to be reconstituted in the peace
of convalescence, but the homœopathist who aims at meeting
the " totality " of a case is chary of regarding only one symptomatic need so long as he hopes to meet the whole. The action
of strychnine on muscular energy may be used to help, for
instance, respiratory distress, but unless something can be done
to remove the initial cause of the distress the effect of the
strychnine can be but a temporary palliation of a symptom. It
may, however, be essential to do this, and strychnine is an
agent for the purpose. In poisonous doses strychnine causes
convulsions of spinal origin. They are reflex, being only produced in response to a sensory stimulus, but as reflex sensibility
is much heightened, the ·lightest stimulus avails to initiate
convulsions. It is the change in response to external stimuli
that is the essential effect of strychnine.

Probably all efferent nerve impulses from the spinal cord
are partly motor (to the appropriate muscles), partly inhibitory
(to opposing muscles) ; in strychnine poisoning the inhibitory
factor seems to be cut out so that all the muscles contract (the
contraction is always maximal, whether the stimulus be weak

or strong) and the resultant movement depends on the relative strength of the muscle groups. After some tremors or twitchings all the muscles in the body contract violently and remain so contracted for a time, with the subject cyanotic from cessation of respiration : prostration follows, then further spasms : ultimately death occurs in fatal cases from asphyxia, the respiration failing to return after a spasm for the state of prostration going on to respiratory failure. Before the general convulsions set in there is, as a rule, preliminary spasm of certain muscle groups, usually about the jaw and the neck. The general effects may be thus explained : An impulse reaching the cord may there take a number of paths, arousing different motor cells to activity or inhibition ; the influences that cause " spreading " of an impulse may be figured as varieties of resistance and the result of their interference is normally a co-ordinated movement. Under strychnine these resistances are greatly reduced, the impulse passes along all the motor paths more strongly and calls for a stronger reaction from the motor cells. It is also possible, though not certain, that strychnine affects motor cells directly. The resulting violent contractions are not co-ordinated. Medullary centres are affected as are spinal centres.

Depression and paralysis follow the violent stimulation of strychnine. Indeed, depression is mixed with stimulation very soon and greater fatigue is in evidence under strychnine than normally, though its appearance is delayed. This is a very important point to remember in using strychnine as an emergency agent. To spur the tired horse is proverbially an apparent remedy that often leads sooner to disaster.

When the effects on the respiratory nerve mechanism are alone considered, it is found that respiration is quickened by small doses, but if persisted in, the drug finally paralyses the centre. The heart is little affected directly. Small doses stimulate the vaso-motor centres, but larger doses soon produce opposite effects. In the alimentary canal, strychnine, like most bitters, stimulates the flow of saliva. The increased muscular activity resulting from the use of the drug causes increased body heat : glycosuria appears in small mammals and glycogen disappears from liver and muscles. Both these effects are no doubt secondary to the effect on muscles and respiration, and no homœopathist would from this expect the drug to be of any special value in diabetes, where the causation of the glycosuria is so much more profound.

This in outline is the action of strychnine as it appears to non-homœopathic physicians. One disease would seem obviously to call for it homœopathically, and that is tetanus.

It is of considerable interest that occasionally this drug has been used for this disease by non-homœopathists, though its symptomatic similarity is unmistakable ; certainly it would appear well indicated to any follower of Hahnemann. Good results have been reported from it, but it is difficult to collect enough cases for certainty, especially as at different times and places the virulence of tetanus seems to vary considerably. It is not the only remedy that homœopathy might find suggested. Hydrocyanic acid has claims from its provings and gelsemium (it is interesting to recall that the alkaloid of this drug is an analogue of strychnine), and in general homœopathists would not feel helpless in face of the disease for want of implements to test their therapeutic method. But the extensive experience in the Great War with anti-tetanic serum brought out some points in the disease which are worth a comment. The great value of the serum has been as a prophylactic ; as a remedy for the established disorder it has been in most cases a failure. In other words, once the toxin has become fixed in the spinal cord it is all but impossible to detach it or neutralise it. But the symptoms that resemble those of strychnine poisoning are the signs of the toxin fixation in the cord : that is to say, they are "ultimate" symptoms, and by the time they appear, the curable stage is for most cases past. The homœopathist should deduce the conclusion that the value of strychnine ought to be greatest before the characteristic spasms appear, the drug, as it were, occupying or fortifying the susceptible parts of the cord and so preventing the toxin from making good its attack. If the anti-toxin were not available, such a prophylactic use of strychnine would be at least worth a trial, but seeing that the value of the serum has been well established it would hardly be wise to neglect its certain claims for the more or less proble- matical ones of strychnine, and if strychnine treatment were combined with the use of serum in prophylaxis, a very long comparative series of cases would be needed before any valid judgment as to the value of the drug factor could be made. However, the convinced homœopathist, working on the basis of his method, would do well to combine nux vomica or strychnine with anti-tetanus serum (withholding for a time any dogmatic assertion as to its value, but using it as a possible help) and in the event of a definitely established case to treat, then strychnine would rank high among the drugs to consider.*

Nux vomica has been well proved and much used, and the moment the field of homœopathic therapeutics is entered the crude outline of poisoning and animal experiment takes on colour and shading and with precision in its application the remedy becomes a very valuable one. The two great characteristics of the remedy are spasm and exaggerated sensitiveness both emotional and physical. For example, there is sensitivity to cold atmosphere : chilliness is experienced on the slightest exposure to the open air or draught : the patient cannot get warm. The spasm and the increased sensitiveness which are so clear in the pathogenesis are naturally most important features from the homœopathist's point of view and unless both are present in some degree nux vomica is not likely to be indicated. The spasm may be of voluntary or involuntary muscle ; indeed, therapeutically, spasm of bowel, bladder, or rectum is a very common symptom calling for the drug, while irritability and sensitiveness combine to heighten the effect and frequency of the muscular contractions.

If aconite may be truly described as the drug of " anxious tension," nux vomica is pre-eminently the drug of " irritable tension." The irritability appears in the mental sphere ; subjects suitable for the drug are apt to be zealous and precise, prone to anger (especially to fits of excited temper), over-bearing and ardent. They are often actually spiteful and malicious ; this, at least, is the direction into which their temperament tends to degenerate. Nux vomica is a drug for the highly civilised races, for town dwellers, and those who

---

* If the work of Speransky and his group of workers be accepted (and it is supported by a large volume of experimental evidence), the sentences above would need to be reconstructed. But whether the damage to the nerve centres comes directly from the tetanus toxin or indirectly *viâ* the central nervous system it remains a possibility that a previous stimulation of those centres by the similar drug would have a protective effect.

under the stress of modern life develop both physical and mental symptoms. They are often sedentary brain workers, more inclined to the waste of nervous tissue than of muscular persons who get through their work largely on stimulants, addicted to the use of tea, coffee, alcohol, or are drugged subjects. Nux vomica is one of the best antidotes for drug or alcohol-taking (including medicine-taking, purgatives and patent preparations). Its subjects are more often thin and choleric than fat, nervous and melancholy in times of reaction from anger or excitement. The loss of nervous energy for which nux is suitable is the result of excessive waste and without a history of past excitement the remedy will seldom benefit. Candidates for it are apt to call themselves " bilious " ; they suffer from indigestion of a type to be described presently, they are addicted to condiments as well as stimulants and are often debauchees.   " Nux suits the old dyspeptic, lean withered, premature old age, always selecting his food, digesting none." But the nux vomica type is rather the Renaissance tyrant (Eccelino or Malatesta) than the heavy-jowled Nero type. The irritability may carry the patient to the verge of homicidal or suicidal impulses, but in its characteristic quality of suddenness and intensity, there is a certain " spasmodic quality " about even those mental symptoms. Thus the nux vomica patient is emotionally irrritable and over-sensitive. But this characteristic can be observed also in his over-sensitivity to external conditions. He is over-sensitive to stimuli of the special senses, e.g., to noise, light. He is extremely touchy as regards food, may display great care over its choice, but finds difficulty in digesting it. Through all these types tension and spasm may be traced.

Spasm plays a notable part in the symptomatology of nux in other bodily spheres. Nux can produce spasm of all voluntary and involuntary muscles. In the alimentary canal, for instance, appears one of the most distinct of all nux symptoms, a constipation characterised by frequent desire for stool which is nevertheless ineffectual. That is to say, the normal peristaltic rhythmic contraction is replaced by spasmodic contractions which cause pain but are not effective in forwarding the passage of the bowel contents along the tract. There are two modalities to be noted with regard to the nux constipation. Firstly, when the bowels are moved, there is temporary relief and the urging ceases for a time. Secondly, constipation where there is an absence of desire for stool is a contra-indication for nux. Sometimes a patient will require nux in whom there is diarrhœa, but then it will be found to be sudden, perhaps involuntary, and to represent a more violent degree of spasmodic contraction sufficient to cause untimely evacuation. These contractions are very painful and the pains are generally worse from pressure but relieved for a time after evacuation : the stool is often hard and large, but even when small there is the same difficulty in getting an effective clearance and a tenesmus after stool which suggests to the patient that the bowel is only partially emptied. Another peculiarity of the action of the drug in this sphere is that any pain may cause an ineffectual urging to stool. For example, a pain in the stomach after eating or a menstrual colic may induce an ineffectual urging to stool.

Another result of this spasmodic peristalsis is an interference with the circulation in the bowel and consequent hæmorrhoids. In nux patients these generally bleed freely ; indeed, as will be seen presently, hæmorrhage characterises the pathogenesis of nux vomica in other ways. These spasms of the bowel are very likely to occur in cases where a hernia has suddenly been forced through inguinal or femoral ring, the irritation of the pressure causing spasms which tend to aggravate the condition and so induce strangulation. Now, it need hardly be said that it would not be sufficient treatment for a strangulated hernia merely to administer nux vomica, but the administration of the remedy before strangulation frequently makes much easier the task of reduction.

In the upper part of the alimentary canal it is to be noted that the tongue in nux vomica cases is usually heavily coated and often dry and uncomfortable. There is a " scraping " sensation in the throat, worse from swallowing and accompanied by a salt or sour taste in the mouth, or a bitter and unpleasant taste. Often all food is insipid and a dislike is taken to meat, bread, coffee, or to tobacco, though as a rule before the disease has begun, the subject likely to need the drug is fond of meat and stimulants of all kinds and of tobacco. This is one of the few drugs wherewith appears a liking for fat food. In this, as in so many features, nux vomica and pulsatilla are diametrically opposed.

Heartburn and pyrosis are common symptoms in nux vomica cases, nausea and empty straining or periodical vomiting. Hæmatemesis may appear, but it rather suggests the bleeding of cases of gastrostaxis than of gastric ulcer, the " hæmorrhagic " powers of the drug being exemplified here. Pain in the stomach begins characteristically some time after the meal : it is a sensation of pressure experienced two to three hours after eating (cf. kali bic.—sensation of pressure immediately p.c.) and colicky pain with considerable flatulence and great desire to loosen clothing ; it arises in fact from the characteristic spasmodic peristalsis, which accounts also for the constipation. Hiccough (again a spasm) is common.

Redness and burning of the face (especially of the nose) after meals is a nux symptom and frontal headache after meals. Indeed, a flushed face is rather characteristic of the drug. There is often hunger and yet aversion from food. Gastric complaints that are relieved by it are not so much inflammatory as states of dyspepsia and irritation, especially such as follow the immoderate use of condiments or of alcohol, and it is the spirit-drinkers rather than the beer-drinkers whom nux helps. The latter are more likely to require kali bichrom.

The sensitiveness of nux subjects is shown by a tendency to faint easily from strong odours, from sudden pain, from straining at stool, from vomiting.

In the sexual sphere, desire is increased and very slight stimulus excites it. Labour pains are violent and ineffectual. The period in women is too profuse and too early and accompanied by cramping pains generally relieved by heat and tendency to faint. It may be followed by thick yellow acrid leucorrhœa.

In the respiratory sphere nux vomica produces little catarrh, although it reproduces well the features of a " stuffy " cold in the head, with congestion and obstruction and cures such cases readily. The coryza to which nux is applicable is stuffy indoors and fluent out of doors. The patient finds his condition aggravated in a warm room and better in the open air. This is a contradictory modality because nux, in general, is better from warmth. It is also responsible for a kind of asthmatic condition and is of great value in asthma. A dry, persistent, fatiguing cough, causing a splitting headache, is characteristic. In asthma cases the paroxysms will probably be worst about 3 a.m., for this is a marked time of aggravation of the drug. This marks, too, its value in sleeplessness which is considerable whenever the patient complains that he or she falls asleep quickly but wakes at 3 a.m., tosses about for hours and at last falls asleep again just before it is time to get up. The result of unbroken sleep (day or night) in a case that indicates nux is always favourable and it may be said of the drug that its subjects are worse when sleep is disturbed, better after undisturbed sleep.

Nux vomica does not produce any characteristic skin eruption, but violent and uncontrollable itching is a marked symptom of it.

Patients who benefit by this remedy are generally chilly, cannot get warm and desire heat. They are over-sensitive to cold, to the open air, draughts and to windy weather, especially dry winds. They are worse in winter, subject to chilblains and to cold, blue extremities. Damp troubles them much less than cold ; indeed, they may often be better in wet south-west weather.

The spasmodic quality of the drug suggests its use in all varieties of violent muscular contractions, e.g., strangury, biliary or renal colic, or in bladder conditions where there is painful ineffectual urging to urinate. The urine is passed in drops with burning pains, and when the general symptoms also agree in calling for it, it will speedily help, but as a rule there is considerable prominence of alimentary canal symptoms in the cases that need nux vomica. It is particularly suited to those who are meat-eaters and stimulant or drug-takers. The following general symptoms must be emphasised. The nux vomica patient feels generally worse in the morning soon after waking : his symptoms are aggravated after mental exertion, after eating, and usually in the cold air. Zinc is inimical to its action. It follows sulphur well and aconite : sepia may be regarded as its nearest analogue among drugs of a very profound and long-lasting action. Nux vomica may be of considerable value in chronic diseases, but requires some supplementing as a rule before a cure is obtained.

PHOSPHORUS

Saturated solution in absolute alcohol and potencies therefrom. Triturations of red amorphous Phosphorus.

This element, being exceedingly poisonous to the human body, has correspondingly been a valued remedy to homœopathists ever since their guiding principle was recognised, but for non-homœopathic medicine its worth is comparatively small. A century or so ago, however, it was credited with extraordinary remedial properties (without any clear realisation of the only method by which they can be fully utilised) and it has retained for the laity ever since an almost magical reputation. It is an essential element in the body structure, both in bone and in the nerve tissue, but it is its presence in the latter that is responsible for its popular reputation and there is a market for any preparation that can plausibly suggest that it will supply the system with extra stores of phosphorus. It will be seen presently that on the homœopathic principle it is often indicated in conditions which may accompany nerve strain and nerve diseases, so that no follower of Hahnemann would doubt that these preparations may have a high degree of usefulness at times, though their indiscriminate employment is to be deprecated and their dosage is unnecessarily large.

Phosphorus poisoning is not uncommon, and there is much knowledge available concerning its gross effects on body tissues. These may well be considered before proceeding to the study of the provings.

Phosphorus is not readily absorbed and unless finely divided quite large quantities may fail to have a fatal effect, but 1 to 2 grains may prove a lethal dose if absorption is achieved. Phosphorus vapour is absorbed by the lungs and phosphorus is readily taken up from oily vehicles. Water will only dissolve the merest traces. The red amorphous phorphorus being less volatile and soluble is much less poisonous than the common form of the element which is now (after a delay scandalously long) forbidden for the manufacture of matches. The chronic poisonings that used to result from match making were due to lung-absorption of the vapour and the local necrotic effect of the fumes upon the lower jaw was also frequent. Applied to the skin, phosphorus causes severe burns, but no systemic poisoning follows.

It is to the effect of the element (which has been detected unchanged in the blood after poisoning) that tissue changes must be attributed and not to the power of oxygen or hydrogen compounds of it. It does not coagulate albumen in solution when swallowed, but some hours after being taken into the stomach, pain and discomfort begin, followed by nausea and vomiting. Diarrhœa is less common, but occurs sometimes. These gastric symptoms may persist, but often disappear, especially if measures are taken to wash out the stomach ; but already enough of the poison has been taken to affect the liver (upon which the main action is exerted) and after an interval of quiescence of a few days, pain recurs and extends to the liver, which is enlarged, vomiting returns, generally containing blood, other hæmorrhages occur from nose, bowel and uterus ; extravasation of blood under'the skin, collapse and coma close the scene.

Albuminuria may appear early with fatty casts and fat globules : hæmaturia is common. Near death the secretion of urine may cease. Very noteworthy is an increase in the nitrogen elimination, in spite of the diminished food absorption. It appears mainly as ammonium lactate and would therefore seem to indicate excess formation of lactic acid in the tissues, but other nitrogenous constituents of urine are also increased (e.g., leucin and tyrosin). Phosphates are increased not from the poison taken so much as from increased tissue waste, and sulphates also rise. Homœopathists find that those who do well on phosphorus frequently have a great craving for salt, as though possibly in need of extra chlorides. No stress has been laid hitherto by investigators on increase or decrease of chlorides in the urine of cases of phosphorus poisoning, but the clinical symptom of craving for salt is a good indication for the remedial use of the drug. Retention of chlorides is seen in pneumonia, and phosphorus is one of the remedies most frequently indicated in cases of that disease.

Fatty infiltration and degeneration of cells, especially of liver, kidney and stomach and intestinal glands and muscles of heart and arteries, are the essential effects of phosphorus poisoning. As the liver cells become full of fat they swell or press on the bile capillaries and from this obstruction some degree of jaundice occurs. The glycogen of the liver is broken

up with formation of lactic acid. The fatty degeneration of the
kidney may give rise to albuminuria. The fatty degeneration
of the heart muscle counts for something in bringing about the
fatal termination of cases of chronic poisoning. Other muscles
may be affected. The central and peripheral nerves are little
changed in poisoning cases. The fatty degeneration of the
arteries (and possibly also the loss of fibrinogen from changes
in intestine and liver which render the blood less coagulable)
accounts for the numerous hæmorrhages characteristic of
phosphorus poisoning (e.g., hæmatemesis, hæmaturia, sub-
cutaneous purpuric hæmorrhages, etc., etc.). The bone marrow
in chronic poisoning becomes more active at first and red
corpuscles of the blood increase after small doses of phosphorus. With larger doses the bone marrow degenerates
and both red and white corpuscles ultimately diminish in
numbers.

The simplest explanation of the fatty degeneration caused
by phosphorus is that it is an acceleration of a normal process
and an autolysis, but that the accelerated distinctive metabolism is not completely carried out, so that the products of
the incomplete combustion (leucin, tyrosin, lactic acid) appear
in the excretions. Similar effects are found from chloroform
poisoning and are attributed to a similar cause. In yellow fever
and acute atrophy of the liver these disease manifestations
reproduce even more vividly the pictures of drug intoxications.
The resemblance between the toxic effects of phosphorus and
chloroform would suggest to the homœopathist the use of small
doses of phosphorus as a remedy for chloroform poisoning.
Unfortunately, the latter illness, when it occurs as the result of
anæsthesia, is often so sudden and overwhelming that no
remedy has much opportunity or time to develop its action.
It would be wiser to give phosphorus as a prophylactic, if there
were any means of determining beforehand the subjects likely
to be poisoned by chloroform, and even though the cases of
poisoning are very rare, it would do no harm to make routine
practice of giving a dose or two of phosphorus as a preliminary
to chloroform anæsthesia, preferably twelve hours beforehand.
It is needless to state that only by pursuing this method for
hundreds of cases would it be possible to come to any valid
conclusion as to whether or no the number of cases of chloro-

form poisoning were thereby diminished, but to administer a dose or two of phosphorus would add nothing to the seriousness of any patient's condition and it might conceivably lessen the risk of a catastrophe from the anæsthetic. This procedure is followed regularly in some hospitals where homœopathy is practised.

There are two other noteworthy effects of phosphorus deserving of mention before turning to the provings. Repeated small doses cause proliferation of the interstitial connective tissue of liver (especially) and kidney and can produce typical cirrhosis of both organs. It is not certain if it be a sequel to the necrosis of the actual liver and kidney cells, or a specific irritant effect on the connective tissue, but the fact that commencing cirrhosis of both organs seems to be very favourably influenced in many cases by phosphorus in the hands of homœopathists would suggest rather the latter than the former explanation.

Some years ago Wegner described the effects of minute doses of phosphorus on the bones of young animals, as amounting to a stimulant to the osteoblasts and increased formation of dense bone. This process he maintained to be followed by gradual absorption of cancellous bone and further dense bone formation, not only from cartilage but from periosteum also. Kassowitz, however, took a different view of the process : using larger doses, he produced appearances closely resembling those of rickets, a significant observation in view of the use of small doses of the drug for this disease, which is a practice not only of avowed homœopathists. As yet, while all observers admit a specific action of phosphorus on bone, there is not entire agreement as to its interpretation. By this specific action, however, the familiar necrosis of the jaw is explained : it is not the local irritant action of the vapour that is responsible, but the effect on the bone of the drug absorbed, for other bones (femur, radius, etc.) become more fragile ; the jaw by this action has its resistance to infection lowered and then if tubercle germs obtain access through a diseased tooth or sinus, caries ensues.

There is a sequel of some interest to these observations. Experiments by Wheeler and Neatby (*Journal of the British Homœopathic Society*, 1907) pointed to a marked influence of phosphorus upon the opsonic index of the blood to tubercle germs in both these observers. In one case repeatedly the index was found to rise for a space of days after administration of 3x potency.*

In the other case a single larger dose produced a typical opsonic curve with a preliminary fall (negative phase of Sir Almroth Wright) and subsequent marked rise. In this case a parallel estimation of the index to *Micrococcus neoformans* showed no change, suggesting that the influence of phosphorus was specific for tubercle. Since these experiments were made, much doubt has arisen as to the accuracy of opsonic measurements, but at least the evidence seemed clear and precise in pointing to a drug effect and if the coincidence of all the index estimations is to be read as accidental, it is a very remarkable phenomenon.

Assuming that it does indicate a specific influence † upon the body resistance to tubercle, it must further be admitted that phagocytosis does not appear to be an important part of this. But phagocytosis is so intimately associated with body resistance in general that it is difficult to avoid regarding any heightening of it as significant, at any rate to some extent. When in addition there can be noted the suggestion that phosphorus in poisonous doses lowers the resistance to tubercle and prepares the way for caries, any evidence that the same drug in smaller quantity raises resistance is more credible. Finally, the homœopathist caps both suggestions with the result of clinical experience, showing how frequently the symptom-complex of tuberculosis indicates phosphorus and how frequently the drug appears in such cases to do good, so that as far as it goes the experimental evidence justifies the choice from the general symptom similarity.

---

* The estimations of the index in all instances were made, of course, by an assistant absolutely unaware of the times of administration of the drug, so that the element of anticipation in the results can be eliminated. The estimator never knew if the result he handed in would confirm or deny the influence of the drug.

† An influence that is upon these two particular investigators. One of them at least would seem to any homœopathist a likely subject to respond to phosphorus. It is not inconceivable that for different subjects different remedies would be required to encourage the mechanism that raises the index. Arsenic and phosphorus have close resemblances in their poisonous effect on the body and conceivably arsenic might affect the index in some individuals, though upon the one of these experimenters who tried its power it had no such effect. No homœopathy worthy the name can exist without the most minute individualisation.

Phosphorus is a well-proved drug and homœopathists have ample material upon which to base their selection of it.

Taking first a survey of the general characteristics of the drug, it is found to be particularly suitable to diseases at the time of adolescence. Subjects susceptible to it are often delicate looking and rapidly growing ("outgrowing their strength," as popular phraseology has it) : they may be tall, but are fragile in appearance, narrow-chested, inclined to stoop, anæmic in complexion. Such slender delicate adolescents, often suggestive of incipient tuberculosis, physically easily tired, frequently show a definitely intelligent, perceptive, sensitive nature, both emotional and mental.

Such a type does not, of course, occur only in adolescents. The tall, slender, narrow-chested, frail adult, too, is to be found who has the constitution and symptom-complex that calls for phosphorus. There is a particular pale, lemon-yellow tint that suggests phosphorus at once to a homœopathist. It is almost entirely due to anæmia, but if slight jaundice accentuates it, the claims of the drug are enhanced. In colour, phosphorus subjects are often fair or red-haired.

This sensitive, impressionable, responsive phosphorus patient is a type often found in women. The metabolism is vigorous, the fires of life intense. They are often people where the problems of life, especially the sexual problems of life, have been vividly felt but unresolved. Such as these often produce the symptoms of phosphorus.

In the nature of the phosphorus patient, the outstanding characteristic to record is that of hyper-sensitivity. He is hyper-sensitive to all impressions, both emotional and physical. Physically he is sensitive to all stimuli of the special senses ; to odours, noise and light. Both smell and hearing are often abnormally acute, though phosphorus patients sometimes have a peculiar deafness in that they find difficulty in hearing the human voice.

Emotionally they are impressionable to their surroundings. They are described as being quick, sensitive and with lively perceptions. Thus, they are frequently perceptive, intuitive individuals having an awareness and understanding of the attitude of those around them. They may be even hyper-sensitive to psychical impressions, nervously excitable, likely recruits for new causes. Nevertheless, while likely to be roused to excitement over some new idea or emotion, they are as a rule apathetic and even slow to life in general. It is rather a condition of indifference to surroundings and occupations broken by flashes of excitement and enthusiasm that is characteristic. One of the most prominent emotions is fear, which is another aspect of the hyper-sensitivity of the phosphorus patient—fear of being alone, fear of the dark, of thunder, fear of illness or death. Not only is he frightened of storms, but the patient is disturbed generally and his complaints are likely to be aggravated or brought on by electrical disturbances in the atmosphere. For example, an attack of diarrhœa or palpitation may come on during stormy weather. The patient may be haunted by all sorts of imaginary things (*e.g.*, horrible faces). These impressionable individuals are apt to take fire easily and show anger, though not persistent rancour. They are restless, easily made anxious, cannot sit or stand still for a moment. Twilight and darkness affect them unfavourably. They may fly into tempers with their friends for little cause, but cannot bear to be left alone. In many conditions anxiety is allayed by the touch of another—for example, if someone holds his hand. The outbursts of excitability and anger sometimes prostrate this delicate subject, so that the opposite state of affairs develops. The patient becomes mentally and physically weary : he feels depressed and exhausted. Generally speaking, prostration of mind will come on after some mental effort and prostration of body after some physical effort. The phosphorus patient tends to be mentally over-active and suffers from it.

Objective nerve symptoms abound, as is not surprising, in view of the profound effects of the drug. Spasms, twitchings and especially fibrillary twitchings, concern the motor nerve mechanism, while numbness, formication, pain, show sensory interferences. Co-ordination is often defective, and, with the numbness of the feet and pains resembling lightning pains, the drug is sometimes suggested in locomotor ataxy. But a phosphorus symptom-complex is more apt to appear in nervous conditions following excess, or overwork, or hæmorrhage, or prolonged suppuration, or, again, after apoplexy. The spine in patients that call for phosphorus is frequently the site of burning pain, a sense of heat which seems to travel up the back into the head to the vertex (picric acid shows the reverse direction for the symptom). Phosphorus is often indicated in severe nervous disease, cerebral softening, post-apoplectic conditions, myelitis, polio-myelitis, less often in pseudo-hypertrophic paralysis. In every case, however, the whole symptom-complex should be considered. Burning pains are nearly as characteristic of phosphorus as of arsenic or sulphur : the palms of the hands burn, or burning sensations occur in patches (*e.g.*, between the scapulæ or in the abdomen).

In spite of these burning pains, the subjects suitable for phosphorus feel the cold very much and external cold aggravates many symptoms. Thus, cough will be excited on going from a warm to a cold atmosphere. (The reverse is true of bryonia.) Nevertheless, there are two notable exceptions to this general amelioration from heat. The head pains are definitely aggravated by all forms of heat and this aggravation from warmth applies to stomach complaints. There occurs a burning pain in the stomach that makes the patient desire cold food and drink and very characteristic is the condition when food is vomited after it has been swallowed a little while and become warm.

Phosphorus subjects (as already noted) have a great desire for salt. Their metabolism appears to need excessive quantities of it.

The tendency of the drug to cause all kinds of hæmorrhages has been brought out in the description of poisoning cases. To the homœopathist it is a most useful indication : hæmorrhages from every and any surface, from lung, kidney, bowel, subcutaneous hæmorrhages and excessive periods—all of these are phosphorus symptoms and one or more of them may give the deciding voice for the remedial use of the drug.

Phosphorus is on the whole a right-sided remedy and more suitable to complaints (*e.g.*, pneumonia) of the right side. The patients are often unable to lie upon the left side and relieved by lying on the right, a curious symptom difficult to explain, but, when present, a good indication.

Movement generally worsens the sufferings, in spite of the restlessness. Lying down (except on the left side) relieves. But the chief time of aggravation is from twilight to midnight, so that early sleep is very disturbed. There is a general amelioration of complaints from sleep ; even a short sleep helps the patient. Moreover, the phosphorus patient often sleeps better if he has had something to eat.

Mental exertion, worry and sensory stimuli (noises, light, even music) are apt to bring on symptoms of distress in phosphorus patients. These may take the form of headaches, neuralgias, etc. Grief, anxiety, in fact any emotion, are all apt to be felt excessively.

The photophobia of phosphorus is often more than mere hyper-sensitiveness, for the drug has a deep action on retina, choroid and lens as well as cornea and conjunctiva. For early cataract, for retinitis and glaucoma it may have real value. Its action on the kidney would confirm its use for albuminuric retinitis.

In the genito-urinary tract, besides its power to cause nephritis, which makes it especially useful in early cirrhosis of the kidney and in lardaceous or fatty degeneration, it influences the sexual organs of both sexes. Desire is increased usually to a considerable extent (even to nymphomania), but sexual power is apt to be deficient. The menses are profuse and too early. Pains and inflammations, even abscesses in the breasts, are prominent among the local symptoms of phosphorus.

The effects of phosphorus on the bones have been already noticed under the description of phosphorus poisoning. The homœopathic provings are full of symptoms of joint and bone pains. Joints are notably stiff, more stiff than painful. Hip and knee are specially affected. Caries is naturally a condition suggesting the use of the drug and it has seemed to help exostosis and other bony tumours. Pains (burning), cramps, numbness, weakness and inco-ordination are phosphorus symptoms.

The skin is subject to subcutaneous hæmorrhages : phosphorus is the first drug suggested by purpura, though Crotalus affects the blood (and liver) very similarly. Obstinate ulcers and scaly and pustular eruptions are noted in the pathogenesis and excessive sweating (especially night sweating) is common.

The alimentary canal symptoms are of high importance. The lips are dry, parched and cracked or ulcerated. The gums bleed readily and pyorrhœa is very likely to be present. The mouth and throat are dry and perhaps ulcerated or bleeding : the saliva is viscid, the tongue dry, brown generally in the centre, less often white or yellow, so dry and stiff that speech is difficult. There is often a sweetish taste in the mouth and a craving for salt may be profound. Hunger is common, abnormal desire for food and feelings of faintness if food is delayed : hunger persists at night, and sinking, empty sensations, affecting chest and abdomen. Generally the patient feels better after eating. With the hunger great thirst, but cold (or even iced) water is longed for, as it seems to allay the burning in the stomach. Hot food or drinks worsen the condition at once. Cold water (and cold food) are well taken, though they may be vomited later. Vomiting is often a kind of regurgitation : food may be thrown up in mouthfuls. Acidity seems to be increased and sour eructations are the rule : nausea, burning pain, pressure, distension, hiccough and waterbrash all testify to the deep disorder of the stomach. Hæmatemesis (less from ulcer than from oozing of blood) may occur.

The abdomen is usually exceedingly sensitive when phosphorus is indicated, though tactile sensitiveness elsewhere is not specially marked. It is associated with pain in the liver region, enlargement of the liver and often of the spleen and some degree of jaundice. Early cirrhosis and other liver diseases may find an effective remedy in phosphorus. The morbid anatomy of poisoning by the drug gives the homœopathist good grounds for its use in yellow fever or acute yellow atrophy. Crotalus has similar effects and uses.

The bowel becomes distended and pains and colic are usual. The stools are often very characteristic. Frequently they are loose, profuse, watery, very exhausting, but painless ; they contain blood, mucus shreds, undigested food. These stools may be passed involuntarily and the anus remains open, the sphincter being more or less paralysed. Hæmorrhoids are large and protruding and bleed freely. In less acute conditions there is often constipation and the stool is only passed with great straining and is long, dry and narrow, not bulky.

Occasionally in dysentery or other forms of enteritis with free secretion of mucus the discharge has a semi-coagulated appearance like that of boiled sago. This is an excellent local symptom for phosphorus.

The heart symptoms are largely subjective and aggravated by the temperament and emotions. Palpitation, faintness, dyspnœa are observed. The pulse is small and of low tension. The anæmia produced by phosphorus is profound and the drug is not only curative when general symptoms correspond in anæmia, but often modifies favourably the anæmias of profound disease (cachexia, lardaceous disease, tuberculosis) and is one of the most hopeful suggestions for leukæmia, pernicious anæmia, etc., though unless in very early stages it must be owned that no remedies are very promising in these diseases. It may be repeated here that lowered coagulability and tendency to hæmorrhage are susceptible to the action of phosphorus whenever the general symptoms of the case match those of the drug pathogenesis.*

The respiratory tract presents many symptoms in the provings and phosphorus is one of the most valuable drugs for larynx and lungs. Hoarseness and aphonia, spasmodic, dry, tickling cough, great laryngeal pain and sensitiveness, aggravation of cough from cold air, from talking or from laughing, paroxysmal cough causing vomiting—these are the characteristic features to be looked for in laryngeal or tracheal disease. The effect on the lung is indicated by pain, dyspnœa, expectoration of blood and mucus or viscid muco-pus. Heaviness, fullness and tension of the chest are experienced. Spasmodic asthma has been helped and emphysema, but it is for pneumonia that phosphorus is especially valued, and is one of the most frequently indicated remedies. A case of pneumonia calling for phosphorus has certain resemblances to one requiring bryonia, but the phosphorus patient is more alert and mentally active. The face is brighter and flushed (bryonia, dusky), the lips are dry and tend to bleed. He does not like to be left alone and experiences comfort from the presence of others. Even touch and gentle rubbing soothes and brings him comfort. The cough, which is dry and hacking, is accompanied by burning pains, the sputum is small in quantity and contains bright red blood. The tongue is dry and coated and there is thirst for cold water.

The profound effects of phosphorus on the system make it a suitable remedy for deep-seated diseases, and its relation to

* A phosphorus sensitive, while in apparent health, succeeded by taking a dose or two of the drug in low potency in producing a definite change in his electro-cardiographic record. Extra-systoles were the main feature of the alteration.

tuberculosis (especially of lungs, larynx, or bone) is emphasised over and over again when the symptoms produced by drug and disease are compared. Early cases in adolescents most often present symptoms that suggest phosphorus. When tuberculosis is complicated by secondary organisms the characteristic signs become less common.

The type of fever that calls for phosphorus is one wherein there are frequent shiverings, followed by flushes of heat and free sweating. Hectic fever patients often suggest the use of it and may benefit from it, but while it is often invaluable in combating the effects of long suppuration on nervous system, heart, or kidney, it does not seem to have much direct power over ordinary germs of suppuration. It is for this reason that if chronic tuberculosis or pneumococcal disease becomes secondarily infected, other drugs are needed to supplement the action of phosphorus, which is nevertheless effective against tubercle or pneumococcus alone.

Causticum and phosphorus are incompatible and it does not follow or precede iodium well. These facts are important, for causticum and phosphorus have many points of similarity in their pathogenesis and a choice has sometimes to be made between them. It should be carefully made, for if the wrong one be given the effect of the other subsequently is diminished or rendered null. Iodium is a most important remedy in tuberculosis of the lungs, so that again the choice between it and phosphorus should be made with considerable care. The reaction of patients to outside temperature are here a great help, for while phosphorus subjects are chilly, iodine patients love the open air and dislike warmth and hot rooms. Iodine candidates are also much less nervous and emotional and hæmorrhages are not at all marked in the iodine pathogenesis.

PLATINUM
The Metal called Platinum and Platina

Triturations of the metal are used for the lower potencies.

This remedy was introduced into practice by Hahnemann is his " Chronic Diseases," and remains almost exclusively in the hands of his followers. Since the introduction of colloidal metals in France, colloidal solutions of platinum have been prepared and used there, but no definite indications have been assigned to them, nor any special sphere of usefulness allotted. Professor Schulz has a little to say of it and some independent observations of the action of the chloride of platinum on the healthy. In five weeks each prover absorbed about 2 centi-grammes of the drug in regular doses of a dilute solution. The nervous system was the principal seat of its action. Weariness and distaste for mental exertion and drowsiness were marked symptoms, with severe headaches, principally occipital. In the spine and lumbar region pains developed and more definite neuralgias of the left arm and leg with paræsthesia and sense of muscular weakness. Abdominal pains were apparently refer-able to the colon : obstinate constipation and diarrhœa with tenesmus were both observed. In some provers a quick irregu-lar pulse with pain in the cardiac region appeared. Sweating (often at night), especially of the hands and feet, was a common symptom : acne spots and boils appeared and general skin irritation. The urine was increased in quantity and passed more frequently.

Its provings and clinical experience based on them have led homœopathists to very definite conclusions with regard to this remedy and its value is considerable when characteristic symptoms indicate it.

Several metals produce (and their use is prompted by) mental conditions : Gold and lead are suited to varieties of depression and melancholia, zinc and platinum are suggested by more unstable mental states, but whenever well marked, the mental symptoms rank high as indications for metallic remedies and platinum in particular is seldom successful unless the patient presents at least an approximation to its charac-teristic mental features. On the other hand, when these symptoms are present, great confidence can be placed in the remedy. The emotional state requiring platinum frequently arises in women who have undergone fright, prolonged excite-ment or shock. The mental condition of platinum at first sight appears to be one of rather rapidly alternating extremes, hilarity and anger, wretchedness and excitement, following one another with little pause between. Such alternations remind the observer of Ignatia and Crocus, but closer inquiry will reveal an underlying characteristic which is almost distinctive for platinum, although a somewhat similar feature appears in the pathogenesis of chamomilla. This characteristic is arrogance, an overwhelming pride in self and a contempt for others. It is not always easy to detect, for the pride is often contemptuously silent, but care in observation will discover it. The combination of this arrogance with mental instability is highly significant. But there are other symptoms that form good additional indications. A characteristic symptom is a loss of sense of proportion.

This may be found on the emotional side and developed into an illusion wherein the individual's imagination is such that she (or he) overestimates herself and her station in life, at the same time tending to disdain her acquaintances. Or, on the physical side, everything around her appears small whereas she herself is physically large. There may be present a desire to injure, even to kill, persons previously cared for. This may be an extreme development of the selfish arrogance, but it is sometimes accompanied by the most intense suffering and attempts to conquer the impulse. Further, there is often a tendency for the mental symptoms to alternate with physical nerve symptoms. These are mainly subjective (e.g., pain) and referred to nerve trunks or to the spine or to the sexual organs. Dr. Nash has recorded an admirable case illustrating this point (Nash : " Leaders "). The point is that when the physical sensations are present, the mental condition approximates to the normal and the mental symptoms appear when the pains or whatever are in abeyance. The pains appearing in the pathogenesis of platinum have the characteristics of coming on gradually and dying away gradually, exactly the opposite to the pains of belladonna, but similar characteristics are to be noted in the pathogenesis of stannum. Frequently there is numbness of the regions where the pain is felt, that is to say, the responses to tactile sensations are delayed or lessened. This symptom also appears under chamomilla, but there is usually much more active anger and bad temper when this latter drug is indicated : the patient needing platinum is seldom very angry, the feeling of superiority replacing wrath or conquering it. In spite, however, of this arrogance, fear is a prominent symptom in the platinum complex, fear of death (aconite), fear that something will happen, etc. : the fears become noticeable when the

patient's mood becomes melancholy and are less in evidence as
the mood changes to a brighter tone

Headaches are frequent in patients needing platinum (cf.
Schulz's provings) : they often seem to arise from emotional
causes and especially from sexual excitement or at the catamenia. The region of the head pain is not characteristic, but
an accompanying numbness of the scalp and the fact that the
pain comes gradually and goes gradually would strongly indicate platinum. Similarly with pains elsewhere, the gradual
onset and departure of the pain and an accompanying numbness
are general symptoms of great value as indications.

Together with these mental and nervous symptoms, those
which are most characteristic of platinum are symptoms referred
to and affecting the sexual organs. Indeed, it is highly probable
that the effects of the drug on the gonads and probably the
adrenals are largely responsible for the mental symptoms. The
normal internal secretions of these glands play a very large
part in determining the self-confidence, sense of personality
and courage which are notably lacking, for instance, in the
castrated. It is not difficult to imagine that a slight perversion
of these secretions might carry self-confidence over into arrogance, or an alteration in the rhythm of secretion cause courage
to alternate with fear. Be this as it may, symptoms in the
sexual sphere are of great importance in leading to a choice of
the drug. Females seem on the whole more susceptible than
males, but it is a mistake to regard platinum as exclusively a
remedy for women. Sexual hyper-sensitiveness is a marked
symptom : not inflammation, but erethism and hyperæsthesia.
This is accompanied by increased sexual desire and may lead to
masturbation. Both for the condition that has led to it and for
the nervous results of it platinum can be a sovereign remedy.
Violent sexual desire, even nymphomania or satyriasis, can be
controlled by platinum when other symptoms confirm the
choice of the remedy. The hyper-sensitiveness may reach the
point of pain so that the external genitals are unable to bear the
lightest touch. With this sexual erethism are associated pains
in the ovarian region, especially the left (Schulz's provers
confirmed this left-handedness of platinum symptoms), and
uterine hæmorrhage. Increased flow at the catamenia of dark
clotted blood. Platinum seems to predispose to hæmorrhage,

generally venous and clotted. The period is too early, too profuse, but not usually prolonged. Between the periods leucorrhœa is common. Cramps and spasms, even hysterical convulsions, may occur in relation to sexual disturbances and the mental state reacts on and is reacted on by the pelvic symptoms. Cramping, ineffective labour pains may find their remedy in platinum if the pregnant woman is otherwise of the platinum type.

Symptoms that suggest platinum are not infrequently found in pelvic cases of gross organic disease, e.g., prolapse, ovarian cyst, fibroma, etc. Each case must be judged on its merits with regard to surgical interference, use of pessaries, and so forth, and, at any rate for cysts and large fibromas, the practitioner will probably feel the need for surgery. But if the symptoms indicate platinum (or any drug) clearly, the use of the remedy will do much both before and after operation to relieve the patient, and should on no account be withheld, and if the gross change is recent and not giving rise to anxiety the indicated remedy is quite capable, when skilfully handled, of clearing up conditions at first sight unpromising.

The bane of the art of medicine is the recourse to facile generalisations—to treat every case precisely on its own merits should be the physician's ideal.

Apart from the sexual organs, platinum has a considerable number of abdominal symptoms, more to be referred to the bowel than the stomach and largely to the colon. Flatulence, colic and constipation are prominent : the abdomen is retracted, peristalsis spasmodic and ineffective. Indeed, the complex is so much like that of plumbum that platinum has been used as an antidote to lead colic. The stool, however, is more often clay-like and adherent, passed after much ineffectual straining : the plumbum stool, like that of opium, is more often like small black marbles. The alumina stool is more like that characteristic of platinum. Fasting generally aggravates conditions that call for this remedy.

Platinum is a drug which may be required in the treatment of the " syphilitic type." The characteristic mental symptoms will be found, and, notably, eye troubles such as squint and myopia. To the platinum patient, " everyone looks small mentally and physically" (Vannier).

To sum up : when platinum is indicated, the symptom-complex willl be mainly made up of abdominal (chiefly pelvic), mental and nervous symptoms and indications referable to the sexual organs have a special importance. It will often help meurasthenias and paresis and hysterical conditions and its characteristic symptoms being largely of an " intimate " order, require much care and patience to elicit them.

PULSATILLA

Tincture of the entire fresh plant of the Pasque flower, Pulsatilla Nigricans. This is allied to the Anemone Pulsatilla, but not identical with it. An American species has been partially proved, with results comparable to those of P. Nigricans, but preparations of the latter should be preferred.

Although all but unknown to modern medicine, outside homœopathy, pulsatilla had a considerable reputation in earlier times. Hahnemann found it in use for eye diseases, especially for ophthalmia and for a variety of other disorders and the provings soon showed that some at least of its empirical success could be attributed to homœopathy. Hahnemann appears to have had a large personal share in the provings of this drug and it has always been a remedy valued by his followers. Clinical use has supplemented the tests of it on the healthy and it can be prescribed with a good deal of confidence according to definite indications.

Pulsatilla causes well-marked local symptoms, mainly on mucous and synovial membranes and very definitely on the generative organs of both sexes, but especially the female. Probably this action is responsible for its relation to a very definite type of character and temperament. Wherever this type comes under observation pulsatilla has claims to be considered for its treatment. The prevailing mood of these individuals is one of yielding, gentle melancholy, often showing peevishness but seldom temper : they are lachrymose and easily emotional, moved to tears by the mere thought of suffering, especially of their own pains and sorrows ; sometimes they cannot relate their symptoms without weeping and self-pity and lack of moral and physical " backbone " are characteristic. The pulsatilla patients are not very emotionally hyper-sensitive to things so long as they do not really hurt, though patients may be easily hurt or upset. They like and seek sympathy, while at the time they are shy and self-conscious, absorbed in their own affairs, yet anxious concerning the impression they make on others. Their shyness and self-consciousness may cause them to be nervous in the presence of strangers, but their desire to appear well in the eyes of others and their liking of sympathetic understanding and sympathy make them responsive and, on the whole, easy patients to handle. They go easily from one mood to another ; while their prevailing atmosphere is one of melancholy, they can quite readily for a time be moved to laughter, often at trivial, childish things : they have seldom much intellectual power or interest, are unbalanced and hysterical. The anemone, the wind flower, moves to every breath of air, and the pulsatilla subject is changeful, never the same for any long time, moving through grief to hilarious mirth and back to tears again, but never showing much anger or determination or obstinacy. Thus, variability of symptoms is a great characteristic. It is a drug applicable to cases in which the symptoms tend to be contradictory and in which the characters of the symptom are always changing. Every symptom, emotional or physical, tends to present some degree of unexpectedness. The local symptoms are just as changeable as is the mentality. From day to day, characters of cough and expectoration or of joint pain or of stool will change as swiftly as do the mental features of the case, and this instability is always a strong indication for the drug.

These persons lack energy, both mental and physical, and consequently tend to put on fat : they are soft, sedentary subjects, who can be roused to momentary interest and exertion but speedily relapse to inertia and self-pity. Mrs Gummidge is a good example of a pulsatilla patient in middle life, but the type can be found at any age. It may always be remembered, however, that the attempt to register typical characters in relation to drugs does not imply that only those who approximate closely thereto can be treated with the corresponding remedies. The descriptions are of those most likely to respond well to the particular drug action, and in so far as patients come nearer to the type, either by nature or as a result of disease, so the probability increases that the drug will be of value for them ; but in certain (probably temporary) emergencies the local need of a particular remedy might be considerable, even though the general temperamental characteristics were absent.

It is a great mistake to think of pulsatilla as exclusively a remedy for women and children. It is true, however, that the particular, gentle, yielding, emotional temperament, changeable and weak, is very often found among women and children who have led a sheltered life. Those who have had to face realities of stress and difficulty generally harden and develop different characters or else go under. But however disconcerting it may be to masculine vanity, the characteristics that suggest pulsatilla are by no means exclusively feminine and the remedy often is indicated and successful for men. It affects the generative organs of both sexes very markedly : the testicles are swollen and painful, and the prostatic gland secretes freely. Emissions may be frequent and sexual desire is usually increased. Pulsatilla has general influence on the tissues of veins and is appropriate to conditions of venous hyperæmia and varicosis. Consequently it has a special relation to varicocele and in early cases is of great benefit. In the female there is usually also increase of sexual desire.

The menses are characteristically irregular, the interval being generally lengthened. The flow as a rule is scanty. Inframammary pain is often present as well as dysmenorrhœa of a more or less severe kind. Amenorrhœa at puberty, irregular, delayed and painful periods and a variety of nervous symptoms associated with them, respond well to this remedy in many cases. Even for epileptic convulsions first appearing at puberty and associated with irregular menses, the drug can be hopefully prescribed, and minor troubles, headaches, neuralgias, etc., yield readily. Whenever, indeed, complaints are associated with scanty, painful, irregular periods, pulsatilla should be thought of and, if any of its general symptoms are present, prescribed ; for its action on the generative organs is an essential feature of its pathogenesis and should be given full weight in determining its choice. Leucorrhœa, bland and non-irritating, frequently accompanies other pulsatilla symptoms and the period of the puerperium may need it. In parotitis the " metastasis " of the disease to the generative glands strongly suggests pulsatilla for this complaint.

As regards the reaction of the patient requiring pulsatilla to heat and cold, she is described as being both chilly and worse from heat. This apparent contradiction can be made clear. It is applicable to conditions when the patient's complaints are aggravated by all forms of heat. The circulation is not active and they dislike exercise, but their condition as a rule is one of low oxygenation. The venous system is congested and the oxygen content relatively low. Consequently there is a great longing for air : patients are better out of doors and worse in warm rooms and from warmth in general. They prefer cold applications to relieve pain and headache and cold food and drink in dyspepsia. Cold water relieves many of their pains, for example, the toothache of the pulsatilla patient is relieved by drinking cold water. So generally they feel better in the open air and the cold air, especially the cold *dry* air. It may be noted that cold *wet* weather sometimes aggravates their symptoms. But there is a chilliness associated with pulsatilla and a peculiar aggravation from cold. The patient may be upset by eating ice-cream or drinking iced water on a hot day. Again, he tends to feel chilly in the warmth : in a warm room : on a warm day : a sudden change to cold during the warm weather may bring on a complaint. Thus, though the pulsatilla patient is generally aggravated by heat, he is inclined to suffer if suddenly chilled when in heat. Symptoms are generally relieved by slow gradual movement, but pains are aggravated on beginning to move, the longer he has been at rest the worse this initial aggravation on movement is. Another noteworthy symptom is thirstlessness—even in fever, typical pulsatilla patients are not thirsty and this feature will often determine the choice of the drug. It has been said that " the patient instinctively dreads increasing the body fluids because the vessels (venous) are already overfull " : the phrase may be a convenient way of associating in the memory the thirstlessness with the venous congestion. The headaches of pulsatilla suggest congestion : they are dull and heavy, worse on stooping forward and relieved by tight bandaging. From several well-known passages of Shakespeare it may be concluded that a headache relieved by tight binding was a familiar type in his day. It is not so common in these times, and interesting speculation as to possible causes of the change in type might be made in regard to dietary and mode of life now and in the sixteenth century : but whenever a headache of this kind appears, pulsatilla is one of its possible remedies. The pain in the head shows the characteristic improvement from slow motion in the open air, aggravation from a warm room and from lying down. The headaches are often worse from using the eyes and from looking upwards. Looking upwards often produces a marked degree of vertigo, so that the patient describes herself as feeling " as if she had been turning round in a circle."

Joints are notably influenced by pulsatilla to the extent of swelling and pain. The choice of it in acute and sub-acute synovitis is determined mainly by the general symptoms, but in a characteristic case there would be a shifting of the trouble from joint to joint. Slow, gradual motion generally relieves and so do cold applications—both features opposed to the choice of bryonia. It has less value in chronic synovitis, though exacerbations of an old disease at the menses, if these were scanty and delayed, would suggest it.

The sweat may be profuse and perhaps sour and musty in odour. Skin eruptions are mainly of a character like the rash of measles : chilblains are common and small pustules. For varicose veins the power of pulsatilla over the venous tissue may be used. Hamamelis and Clematis compete with it here.

The other great seat of action of pulsatilla is the mucous membranes in general. Respiratory, alimentary, genito-urinary, all respond in the same way. From the mucous surface pours a copious, bland, creamy muco-pus and the tissue is swollen and engorged. Ophthalmia of this character yields quickly, and even corneal ulcers, while styes are a marked indication : nasal and bronchial catarrhs also respond well. It should be noted that the lungs and larynx are not notably affected and that with a typical bronchitis that calls for pulsa-tilla there will usually be great variations in the character of the cough in any subject. The copious expectoration will stop for a time and the cough become dry and fatiguing, or it will be dry at night and loose in the day or *vice versâ* ; or the cough will be troublesome only by day and cease at night, which is unusual when coughs are frequent and obstinate.

The alimentary canal symptoms indicate a general catarrh.

The tongue is white as if thickly (arg. nit. thinly) whitewashed, there is nausea and vomiting of mucus and a changeable diarrhœa, often with mucus in the stools. The drug is of no great value in deep inflammatory conditions of these regions, but is excellent for the catarrh that follows indiscretions in diet, indulgence in rich food, in pork or pastry for instance : there is the characteristic thirstlessness to look for and an absolute hatred of fat of any kind. Antimony is another most valuable remedy for such dyspepsias, but the mental characteristics when it is indicated are much more those of crossness and violent ill-temper than those of the tearful self-pity and longing for consolation of pulsatilla.

Pulsatilla affects the middle ear very markedly, and ordinary otitis media generally yields to it satisfactorily, whether or no suppuration has occurred. This is a last feature confirming others that give a leading place to pulsatilla in measles and sometimes in scarlet fever. Other less defined catarrhal affections and sequelæ, e.g., to influenza, may call for it. The inner ear is not so much in the sphere of action of pulsatilla except as far as its symptoms may be secondary to those of the middle ear.

The daily life rhythm is not characteristically influenced by pulsatilla. The changefulness of the drug shows in this respect, but there is very apt to be an aggravation of symptoms at twilight which should readily be read as a mental symptom. The characteristic temperament of pulsatilla yields easily to the suggestion of melancholy, of the transitoriness of life, the incompleteness of human effort, that readily arise at the end of the daylight. Venus is the evening star and pulsatilla patients are apt to pay homage to her in this and in other respects.

On the whole, the remedy is most valuable for many acute and sub-acute catarrhal affections of mucous membranes and often for synovitis. In chronic cases there will be generally stress to be laid on symptoms connected with the generative organs, when pulsatilla is required. It may be that its constitutional effect will finally be attributable to some modification of the internal secretions of the generative glands. Its chronic counterpart is silica and in spite of the fact that silica patients desire warmth as keenly as pulsatilla patients dislike it, any case that has benefited by pulsatilla is likely to improve more fundamentally on silica and any chronic case that has responded to silica will frequently find in pulsatilla a remedy for incidental minor disorders like catarrhs and neuralgias.

Pulsatilla may be indicated in anæmia—the characteristic that calls for it is one of low blood pressure with diminished red cells and hæmoglobin and, if anything, excess of white cells. It is an antidote to iron and to quinine (as well as to many other drugs) and if anæmias have been dosed ineffectively with " tonics," pulsatilla has a special value. Like nux vomica and sulphur, the drug may often have usefulness when beginning the treatment of an overdosed case. It acts on good indications promptly in all potencies. Spaced-out doses of the mother tincture often succeed admirably.

Pulsatilla is the antithesis of nux vomica in nearly every particular and this is noticeable in its effects on sleep, for while the nux patient sleeps early and wakes early and cannot sleep again until it is time to get up, the pulsatilla patient is slow in sleeping, but once asleep continues late in slumber.

RHUS TOXICODENDRON

Rhus Radicans is probably virtually identical with Rhus Tox. This tincture is made from the fresh leaves gathered just before flowering, at sunset.

The poison of the shrub is very virulent to those who handle it : actual contact seems necessary, even in susceptible subjects, in spite of some opinions to the contrary, but a very small amount ($\frac{1}{1000}$th milligramme) of the essential principle can produce symptoms. It is more active during the night and when damp conditions predominate : full sunlight weakens its action. An action so marked seems to indicate more than a power to irritate the skin by local contact, and provings and clinical use endorse the claim that rhus can affect this tissue after internal absorption. The effects of poisoning may be summarised thus : Redness and swelling of affected part, with intolerable itching and burning : vertigo and weariness follow. Face and eyes become swollen and eyelids agglutinate : there is restlessness, pain and fever. Vesicular dermatitis sets in with formation of bullæ and even appearances as of erysipelas : this may spread to mucous membranes. The mouth and throat swell, nausea and vomiting appear and irritative cough. Pains develop about the joints, and great lumbar stiffness : arms and legs may become numb. The fever may be accompanied by delirium and mental confusion and ends often with copious sweating. Urinary secretion is increased and diarrhœa is usual. Great general soreness and prostration are prominent symptoms.

This picture of poisoning will at once suggest uses of the drug for acute skin, joint and fascia affections and it is noteworthy that before Hahnemann, Dufresnoy used it for skin eruptions and rheumatism. There is one outstanding symptom of the drug which Hahnemann noticed early, which remains so characteristic of it that its presence always suggests rhus and in its absence the remedy is seldom indicated. This symptom is that the pains and sufferings caused (and curable) by rhus are at their worst when the limb or body is at rest and are relatively relieved by movement. Frequently there is great pain on first attempting the movement of an affected joint or limb, but with continued movement the pain gets less and less till it almost disappears : then after a period of rest the same sequence of phenomena has to be repeated. Carrol Dunham makes the further point that the pain returns if movement is continued until fatigue comes on. This symptom is the precise opposite of the intense worsening of pain on even the slightest movement that characterises bryonia and colocynth : it is more marked in the case of rhus than in that of any other remedy. This modality appears in the pathogenesis of rhododendron and other drugs. There is, however, a distinguishing modality between rhus and rhododendron. In the latter drug, the pains are immediately relieved when the patient begins to move, in contradistinction to rhus where the patient experiences great pain on beginning to move, though eventually he obtains temporary relief. It suggests that the conditions that will be benefited by rhus are those of inflammation in the ligaments and fibrous tissues near but outside joints, or in fasciæ and muscle sheaths, rather than those that implicate the synovial membranes, while the sphere of action of bryonia is rather with the latter. But whatever the actual morbid anatomy, affections of joints, nerves, muscles or fasciæ that present the characteristic of relief to pain from continued movement are likely to be relieved or cured by rhus. Following as a sequel to this leading symptom and correlated to it, is a second, namely, that the pains are apt to be worse by night than by day, the night being the time when the patient tries to rest, whereas in the day the inevitable more or less constant movement keeps the pains in the background. Pains are worse after rest as well as during rest, when rhus is required. Consequently, restlessness, a constant shifting of position to find ease, becomes characteristic.

Although rhus and bryonia differ thus diametrically in their characteristic reaction to movement of the pain which they cause, they are, nevertheless, often complementary remedies in the sense that a case often requires the one after the other, the characteristic symptom changing so as to give the indication for the change of remedy. In acute infections, too, they may run side by side. In the great typhus epidemic of 1813 Hahnemann found rhus and bryonia his main remedies, and the reaction of pain to movement was the chief distinguishing feature that guided his choice of one or of the other.

Another great general characteristic of rhus is the relation that the pains which are caused or cured by it have to damp. Aggravation of suffering from damp is a very marked symptom indeed. Even certain degrees of loss of power which have ensued on exposure of limbs to damp conditions (e.g., lying on damp ground) have been cured by rhus. It is likely that in these cases the fibrous sheaths of the nerves have been involved, for the drug shows little influence on central or peripheral actual nerve structures. Cold winds are harmful to patients who call for rhus, and there is an aggravation of complaint from thunder. Rhododendron is a drug whose patients are very susceptible to cold wind.

The power of rhus over joints and fibrous tissues leads to its use in a variety of sub-acute and even chronic affections, but a reference back to the symptoms of poisoning by it will rightly suggest a value for it in acute febrile diseases. Always, however, this restlessness, following on the attempt to relieve pain by movement, should be present before rhus comes strongly to the physician's mind. It may occur in enteric, paratyphoid, influenza, scarlet fever and other fevers. The patient is anxious, fearful and restless, continually changing his position. His mental apprehension and other symptoms are worse by night. Other rhus indications are a stuporous state, with muttering delirium. In certain cases the patient develops the delusion that there is a desire to poison him and therefore he will not take food or medicine (Hyos. Lach.). There is a clouded intelligence when delirium subsides and the special senses are dulled but not perverted, and notably there is a dry brown, cracked tongue with a triangular red patch at the tip and the rest of it coated. In such febrile states, the patient is intensely chilly.

In many less acute conditions with the general symptomatology calling for rhus, a somewhat similiar mental state is found. The patient is restless, anxious and despondent, often unable to sustain any mental effort. His anxiety and restlessness is increased at night so that he cannot remain in bed. In general, however, the restlessness of rhus is more due to physical discomfort or pain rather than to mental anxiety (cf. Aconite, Arsenicum).

Rhus is particularly suitable to affections of joints, tendons and fibrous tissues that are the result of overstrain (overlifting, for instance), or the effects of over-exertion of a group of muscles. Over-use of an organ or part of the body may present symptoms calling for rhus. For example, hoarseness following unusual exercise of the voice, worse on beginning to speak and relief by continued use, or, again, sore nipples in a nursing woman which are worse on beginning to nurse but relieved by continued nursing are illustrations of this characteristic of the drug. Also, not only the strains of prolonged exertion, but sudden sprains of a joint will respond well to it as a rule.

Apart from its relation to fibrous tissues, rhus effects the skin very acutely and is one of the great remedies for recent and severe skin diseases. Its power is less marked in proportion as the disorder becomes chronic, but recent and acute eczema, for instance, is well met by its prescription in many cases. The skin diseases that call for it are vesicular or pustular, even erysipelatous. Shingles is often helped by it. Itching and pain and free discharge are usual symptoms. Œdema is less than when apis is called for. The mucous membrane of the eyes is much influenced by rhus. It meets particularly an acute conjunctivitis with profuse lachrymation and pain. The deeper structures are less affected. In orbital cellulitis, rhus is very frequently indicated.

The respiratory mucous membranes are irritated rather than inflamed, though it may be required in the later stages of pneumonia where the patient is progressing towards the typhoid state. There is the typical restlessness through general discomfort and pain in the limbs which are temporarily relieved by motion. The patient is prostrate and should delirium supervene it is of a mild type. Herpes develop on the lips, the tongue is coated white with a triangular red tip. There is thirst for cold water though this aggravates the cough which is incessant and irritating, with scanty reddish-brown sputum. There is a dry teasing cough with tickling in the larynx which rhus can relieve and particularly if the cough and the hoarseness that generally goes with it are at their worst on beginning to speak and relieved by further use of the vocal cords.

Rhus Tox is a valuable remedy for the treatment of nocturnal eneuresis in children.

In the alimentary canal the mouth is dry and may be inflamed and ulcerated. Saliva is viscid and may be copious. The tongue is dry, red or brownish, but characteristically (as noted above) presents a triangular red tip : it is often cracked, inflamed, even ulcerated. Nausea and vomiting, with loss of appetite, are common, but gastric pain is not considerable. There is a desire for cold milk, sweets and oysters and an aversion from meat. The intestine shows more definite signs of involvement, with colicky pains and loose, bloody frothy stools, often contaning mucus and shreds ; more rarely constipation alternates with diarrhœa and there is a chronic painless morning diarrhœa that finds its remedy in rhus tox.

The effects on joints, nerve sheaths and muscles have been sufficiently indicated. Whenever these structures present pains that are relieved by continued movement rhus comes to be considered : if there is aggravation from damp to note or history of special strain, the choice becomes the more suitable.

There are several peculiar symptoms associated with rhus. Though the patient is chilly, he craves cold drinks which aggravate his troubles. The loss of appetite, as mentioned above, may be associated with sensations of emptiness and hunger, or dryness of the mouth with thirst. Attacks of asthma may alternate with herpes.

Patients who require rhus generally sleep badly, but the sleeplessness is due to increase of pain as a rule and rhus removes the symptom by relieving the suffering.

Radium shows a parallel to many of the symptoms of rhus, especially those affecting skin and joints and fasciæ. Its action is more profound. Rhus will antidote some of the effects of radium, but in spite of this, if a case has responded a little to rhus and yet remains uncured, radium will often complete the recovery.

SEPIA

Sepia Officinalis. Trituration of the (dried) substance from the ink-bag of the cuttle-fish.

This remedy is unknown outside homœopathic ranks, and owes its presence in the Materia Medica to Hahnemann. It is said that some preparation of the cuttlefish was used by ancient physicians, and (interestingly enough, in the light of the provings) it is also said that it was held valuable for genito-urinary catarrhs and for baldness and freckles, but to-day only homœopathists employ sepia, although for them it is among the most important of remedies.

Like pulsatilla, which, however, it does not closely resemble, it is apt to be considered as almost exclusively a remedy for the female sex, but in each case this view is mistaken. Sepia will be indicated, it is true, four or five times as often for women as for men, but its effect on the male sex when rightly prescribed is marked and satisfactory. In both sexes the starting point of its action is the generative gland system, and it is the predominance of diseases of these organs among women that make them need sepia more often than men. It affects the body so profoundly that it is difficult to resist the thought that, besides its marked relation to the tissues of the genital organs, it modifies in some way the internal secretions of the main sexual glands and probably others (e.g., adrenal). But it must remain at present doubtful if its effects are to be attributed mainly to alteration of quality or quantity in this respect. Very possibly the latter, since interferences with the general balance of internal secretions can be pleaded as causes of some characteristic symptoms. Adrenal secretion, for instance, seems often diminished and thyroid actually or relatively increased. Sepia will now and then affect thyroid enlargements favourably in a remarkable way (the general symptoms being present). Natrum muriaticum, which has points of comparison with sepia, is perhaps more often called for in chronic disease of this gland. Among the mineral constituents of sepia, magnesium is prominent, and this fact has no doubt a bearing on some symptoms of the drug.

Sepia has an extensive action on the organs and tissues of the body and the following are some of its important effects. It produces general relaxation of the tissues with resulting fatigue, weariness and exhaustion. The characteristic mental type to be described often accompanies a definite physical appearance. The whole organism is slack in fibre and relaxed and the lines of the face are not firm ; the body droops, the tissues are lax, the patient is nearly always tired and weary and the physical joy of life is unknown. Similarly, unhealthy fat may have replaced muscle to some extent, the face looks flabby and puffy. The drug produces a tendency to discharges from mucous membranes which are thick, bland and copious. The skin symptoms of sepia are of great interest. The yellowish tinge and tendency to deposit pigment in small patches occur not only over the skin of the face, but all over the body. The skin is unhealthy, in that it cracks readily and small injuries fester. Papillomata readily appear and thickenings and indurations. There is much itching and tendency to sweat. The eruptions are usually of small vesicles of papules. The hair follicles are notably affected. It is doubtful if any drug controls the falling out of hair better than sepia. It may be used for this both locally and internally and seems to have a real power to encourage new growth over thin (defluvium caputis) patches. All structures depending for power on non-striated muscles ten to be affected and weak.

Sepia is said to act best on brunettes, and is especially suitable to tall, slim females with narrow pelvis and lax muscles. The general relaxation of the tissues is reflected in the emotional state of the candidate for the drug, thus apathy is a keynote. A condition of physical weariness is accompanied by indifference and absence of joy in life. Thus the affective life of the individual is modified. She becomes unresponsive to the affection given to her by others and shows indifference to friends, at the worst, positive dislike of them. The apathy of the sepia patient is extended to her sexual life so that she is indifferent to her husband, averse to coitus which actually is often painful. With this general apathy of the affections, there is associated a definite nervous hyper-sensitivity, thus sepia subjects react violently to sense impressions : the sense of smell is acute, and odours, even pleasant ones, are not liked. There is often a complaint of consciousness of foul odour persistently, which (seeing that sepia is responsible for considerable nasal catarrh) is probably due to the increased sensitiveness, making the patient aware of a secretion which ordinarily would not rouse a conscious reaction. Sepia subjects are sensitive to light, especially to artificial light : marked photophobia is a strong characteristic of phosphorus which compares closely in many respects with sepia. Particularly when sepia is indicated is there intolerance of noise, sudden noises are unbearable and even slight sounds become the sources of irritation. There is great sensitiveness to music : even those who normally love it find it more of an irritation than a solace, becoming very acutely conscious of even the smallest lapses from perfect renderings, while the sounds that too commonly pass for music drive these sufferers to the very verge of distraction. All this hyper-sensitiveness leads on to a general mood of irritability which, on the least excuse or on none, breaks into fits of anger and rage comparable to those characteristic to nux vomica, a drug which often stands in a close relation to sepia. The irritability is absolutely intolerant of any attempt at consolation, the depression and melancholy that go with it (for it is a melancholy irritability) resents the least expression of sympathy, so much so that the sufferer shuns company and seeks solitude and is often (very characteristically) filled with dislike of those who normally are the most loved. With this prevailing mood, however, there may be intense sadness, even to weeping, but the self-pity that inspires it is proud and solitary, poles asunder from the easy, soft, yielding tearfulness that suggests pulsatilla. Among other drugs that have melancholy and weeping prominent in their pathogenesis, nat. mur. resembles sepia in the quality of this symptom.

Irritability, then, and melancholy with apathy and indifference to friends, and fits of temper breaking out on inadequate grounds, these are the prominent features of the temperamental condition which suggests sepia. There is also a considerable element of fear in the mental-complex that suggests this drug—anxiety and fear about real or imaginary evils, so that, even as with pulsatilla, the patient may be moved to tears in relating her (or his) symptoms. The fear may even lead to a dread of being alone, which does not contradict the aversion from society described above, since it is not due to a desire for company for the sake of its amenities, but to a purely selfish wish to be relieved of a personal anxiety. A certain greediness and indolence also appear in the selfishness that is characteristic of sepia. This mental condition is frequently met with at the two extremes of sexual life. Thus, from puberty to about the age of twenty-five, the period when the effects of the sexual glands become established and the first sex experiences have to be undergone, is a time when sepia is often required. Though sexual apathy is a symptom, it may be indicated in the ardent and physically passionate, whose desires may lead them to excess (*cf.* again nux vomica) : the effects of excesses resulting in sexual apathy may call for sepia. The drug is particularly to be thought of when the lowered state of health consequent apparently on sexual over-indulgence proves the starting point of such a disease as tuberculosis (see below). When gonorrhœa has passed the acute stage and its chronic sequelæ are threatening, sepia competes with thuja in value.

At the end of sexual life, at the climacteric, sepia is often needed and the characteristic temperament shows itself.

The use of sepia is not confined to the complaints of adults, for it is a valuable remedy for a certain type of child who displays a similar irritable moodiness. Generally such children are low-spirited, sluggish, tiresome and tired.

Vaso-motor instability is a marked symptom of the drug and flushes of heat (and also sudden sensations of cold) readily appear. Most characteristically, with sepia they travel from below upwards and end in sweating. The hands may be hot and the feet cold, or *vice versâ*. In general, patients who need sepia are chilly and feel the cold ; their circulations are poor, so that extremities become blue and chilblains readily appear ;

the arterial tension is low and venous congestion easy. But, even as with pulsatilla and carbo vegetabilis, the " venous " chilliness shows great desire for oxygen and the sepia subject demands air and resents stuffy rooms, so that even in winter windows may have to be widely open.

The skin appearances are often (not always) characteristic : freckles and excess of pigment are common on a sallow complexion and there is a yellowish streak across the nose spreading on to the cheeks (in the region characteristic for lupus erythematosus), which, as the " sepia saddle," has become a classical symptom. It is quite often seen in patients who indicate sepia otherwise, but, of course, it is neither invariably present nor, when present, an infallible indication : it is but one symptom, though a characteristic one. The skin sweats easily, particularly in the axillæ and about the genitals and the back, and the sweat has often an unpleasant smell, of which the patient is very conscious. The sweats may be drenching night sweats. Further, those who require sepia are very subject to invasions of the fungoid parasites, that manifest in such diseases as pityriasis versicolor and ringworm. There is no doubt that resistance to these invaders varies very much in different cases : sepia patients have a resistance notably low to them. Now it was long ago observed by Burnett that pulmonary tuberculosis or tendency thereto was often accompanied by just such a lowered resistance and this sepia symptom points to a real value that the drug has especially in early or threatening phthisis. Acute pulmonary symptoms need as a rule other remedies, but in the very early stages, or in chronic intervals, sepia has a definite place and should be thought of whenever the general temperament suggests it and especially if there are any noteworthy pelvic symptoms.

With the sallow freckled complexion and slack body goes a general air of intense weariness. Backache is almost a permanent condition and standing is an affliction to the patient. Hard pressure relieves the backache for a time, and though the pain is especially troublesome when she begins to move, violent exercise gives some relief, as often does the vibration of movement in a carriage or car. The circulatory deficiencies cause congestion of internal organs, so that there is a constant sense of dragging and bearing down. On pelvic examination, these symptoms in women will be at least partly explained by a general slackness of the pelvic structures and some greater or less degree of prolapse. Sepia has been called " the washerwoman's remedy," and, indeed, women who have to stand long hours at the wash-tub in a hot, steamy atmosphere with intervals of hanging out clothes, in weather possibly cold and wet, are very likely to develop physical conditions which result in a symptom-complex suggesting sepia, and if to their work is added over-much child-bearing and any degree of stimulant taking, the likelihood of the development of such disorders is increased. But whatever the cause, pelvic congestion and prolapse, with backache and bearing-down sensations, inevitably suggest sepia, and when the other symptoms correspond it can be given with considerable confidence. This is not to be taken to imply that there is any magic in the drug, for while it may not cure the condition while the causes that produced it still obtain, if they can be modified sepia will have great effect in removing their consequences, the drug acting (as drugs all but invariably act) by encouraging the natural tendency to recovery. Also, if the conditions cannot be modified, it is not beyond the power of the remedy to enable a better bodily resistance to be maintained so that relief can be secured, if not complete cure. Thus the physical condition of prolapse will very likely demand artificial support for the patient's relief, but if treatment is persisted in, there is ample evidence that the pelvic slackness that originally helped to indicate sepia can be largely repaired and that every now and then recovery is complete enough to enable the use of pessaries to be discontinued, and short of this success the ability of the drug to aid mechanical or operative measures is indubitable.

Besides the chronic backache and sense of weariness, sepia shows marked symptoms of pain in its pathogenesis affecting chiefly the pelvic region (rectum, vagina, urethra, etc.) and the head. The headaches are severe, hemicrania is common (with ocular symptoms, flashes of light and disturbed vision) : the pains are violent and often throbbing, resembling in many respects those caused by natrum mur. A good sleep relieves it, but if the patient is awakened from a short sleep the headache is aggravated. Such headaches are intensified by moving about the house, but vigorous exercise in the open air helps to work off the headache. Thundery weather makes the headache worse and is disturbing to the sepia patient in most ways. Vertigo may be accompanied by the sensation as of something "rolling round" in the head and this curious sensation may be linked in memory to one characteristic of pains in rectum and vagina, where, besides stitches and shootings of pain, there is a feeling *as of a hard round substance* in the passage. It is undoubtedly a spasm of involuntary muscle, for sepia acts markedly on sphincters, causing both spasm of them and paresis, or even paralysis. The symptom in the rectum may accompany both diarrhœa and constipation (the latter more often), and is not relieved by stool. Apart from head and pelvis, the pains caused by sepia are not noteworthy. On motor nerves it acts in the direction of spasm and later, paresis, mainly of involuntary muscles, though occasionally deep-seated spinal diseases (*e.g.*, disseminated sclerosis) will show (generally in women) a sepia symptom-picture and benefit markedly by its administration. Knowledge is still far from complete of the deepest actions of many remedies and any chronic illness whose complex of features suggests any drug clearly should be treated with it, whether or no the limited knowledge of its ultimate morbid anatomy confirms the choice. *It is always to be remembered that similar gross morbid anatomy in two or more cases may arise from causes by no means identical;* thus, more than one germ can cause pneumonia. But if the actual or impending tissue change is due in two cases to two different causes, the symptom-complexes will probably differ and demand diverse remedies. Further, a deep-acting drug, whose power possibly is exerted on a fundamental mechanism such as the balance of internal secretions, might well be indicated by symptoms arising from a disturbance of this mechanism, and, being administered, correct it with benefit to tissue symptoms depending upon it, even though the drug had in itself little or no special relation to these tissues affected. Sir John Moore in 1809 relieved the pressure of Napoleon on the Spaniards for a time by striking, not directly at the French, but at their line of communications. Similarly, a patient with a chronic disease may well require not a tissue remedy, but a corrective to the disturbance which is affecting the tissues.

However, the mere local action of sepia upon various regions of the body is pronounced. Probably the sites of its most important action are the genito-urinary tract, the alimentary tract and the skin, although it has a value also in certain respiratory diseases.

On the genito-urinary tract the objective symptoms in the male are those of chronic catarrhs, principally of the urethra, with congestion of the prostate and of the bladder to some extent. Warts may appear at the urethral orifice, and ulcers. The external genitals sweat freely and the secretion is apt to be foul smelling. There is increased sexual desire, but sexual intercourse is followed by great lassitude and fatigue. (This is also characteristic of salts of potassium.) The characteristic prostration, weariness and slackness of sepia are prominent in relation to the disorders of the sexual organs. The use of the drug is hereby indicated for gonorrhœa after the acute stage and chronic affections of the lower genito-urinary tract. The descriptions of the urine in the older provings strongly suggest bacilluria and from clinical experience it is highly probable that large doses of sepia lower and medicinal raise the system resistance to infections of the coli type in the urinary tract. High-coloured, offensive urine, with heavy deposits of urates and frequent micturition are characteristic. Sepia tends to produce both spasm and paresis (especially the latter) of sphincters and thus comes to be a remedy for enuresis, especially if the urine is irritating in quality as well as the muscle of the sphincter weak. It has a value in the nocturnal enuresis of children. It is characteristic that the involuntary passage should occur in the first sleep.

Upon the female organs the effects of sepia are even more marked. The periods are usually scanty (murex, in many respects an analogue of sepia, produces the opposite effect in this regard), in spite of the fact that with sepia the uterus is congested ; but the congestion is of a chronic type and leads rather to degeneration of function : sterility is a frequent accompaniment of the conditions that call for the drug and also a tendency to abortion may be cured by it. There is a general slackness of the pelvic floor, so that uterine displacements are almost inevitable. The patient may complain that she feels as if the whole contents of the abdomen will escape from her through the vagina. Thus, a favourite position is to be seated with the legs crossed to give support to this sensation of imminent protrusion. Backache (in sacrum chiefly), with severe bearing-down pains extending into the thighs, are prominent and the whole pelvic condition is apt to be associated with sensations of sinking and emptiness, which are referred to the upper abdomen, but seem to be reflex symptoms from the pelvis. Leucorrhœa is a common symptom, generally containing pus and the external genitals are apt to be irritated and inflamed. They also sweat readily after labour when it has been exhausting, either through prolongation of it or through previous poor health of the patient. Sepia symptoms are frequently prominent and relieved by the drug during pregnancy.

The alimentary canal is considerably influenced. The sallowness of the complexion indicates dyspepsia and portal congestion. There is often a yellowish tinge to the conjunctivæ and anæmia in some degree is common. There is a special loathing of fat food like that found under pulsatilla and a craving for spicy, bitter and pungent foods such as vinegar and sweets. On the whole, appetite is apt to be increased and may be excessive : the tongue is generally coated and is often specially sore at the tip. After food there are sour, burning risings in the throat, hiccough, sweating, flatulence. The patient complains much of " acidity " and the dyspepsia is of the type that accompanies the sensation of excess of acid, though it is uncertain whether the drug can actually cause an increase in the total stomach acidity. Waterbrash and nausea and vomiting may occur. The nausea is worse in the morning and tends to pass off after breakfast. Hence sepia is sometimes indicated in the nausea occurring during the early months of pregnancy. Particularly prominent is the gnawing, empty feeling, even soon after a meal, which patients call " sinking." Food relieves it (and sometimes other sepia symptoms) for a time, but it soon recurs. On the whole, eating generally aggravates the condition. Abdominal pain with flatulence and generalised discomfort is common. The character of the symptoms as a whole suggest a (not very severe) catarrh of the mucous membrane and a more significant interference with the quality and quantity of digestive secretions. Constipation is the rule, with scanty evacuations and much straining and with difficult discharge of even a soft stool ; the rectum may become prolapsed and the portal congestion shows in protruding and bleeding hæmorrhoids. The tenesmus giving rise to the sensation of a " ball " in the passage has been already noted : it makes the patient feel, even after a motion, as if the rectum were not emptied. Excoriations and warts and condylomata are common in the anal region.

The flushes of heat and the chills which testify to the vaso-motor instability of the drug cause a good deal of intermittent palpitation, which is likely to accompany pelvic and abdominal troubles, but there is no evidence that sepia affects the heart directly.

Besides the pains in the back, joint and muscle pains, with stiffness and tension and neuralgic pains, affect the whole loco-motor system. Whenever chronic arthritis is associated with chronic pelvic disease, or seems to have arisen in connection with a former leucorrhœa, sepia is worth remembering and its constitutional symptoms should be looked for. Spasms, rest-lessness and lack of energy are frequent. There is relief from external heat and aggravation from cold and from electrical changes in the atmosphere—before and during a thunderstorm— and the sulphur symptom of dislike of bathing appears also under sepia. The legs and feet are specially apt to be cold, while the upper parts may be hot : these weary achings are worse in the early morning and from almost any external calls on the patient, physical or mental exertion. Quite frequently, however, after violent exercise there is a real amelioration, as though for a time the general systemic circulation was improved. The patient generally feels her complaints to be aggravated in the forenoon and again in the evening. Rest and repose, at any rate, seldom bring any relief and after sleep there will be no cessation of the patient's complaints, but often the reverse.

There is very often considerable drowsiness during the day and broken sleep at night. The early morning is a bad time for patients who need sepia and they prefer to lie late in bed if possible, not because they are free from pain there, but because their very weariness suggests that any exertion will be intoler-able.

In the respiratory sphere sepia causes a nasal coryza (gener-ally one side at a time) with dryness of the throat and hoarseness. The cough is usually accompanied by considerable expectoration in the morning, which may be of mucus or of muco-pus. The cough is often spasmodic and accompanied by pains in the chest. The early stages of tubercle, when this disease comes on in middle or later life, are very apt to suggest sepia and the drug is of real value when the symptom-picture of remedy and patient agree at all closely.

It has already been noted that under the influence of the drug also the general resistance is lowered to parasites of the type of pityriasis versicolor and ringworm. The local treatment of these infections is all-important, but the constitutional value of sepia should not be overlooked here as well. The observations of Burnett on the relation of this phenomenon to pulmonary tuberculosis have been quoted above.

Sepia and lachesis are generally incompatible. This is important as both come much to be considered at the climacteric. But their general symptoms are different enough to make the choice generally easy between them. It often takes up and completes the action of nux vomica well and follows salts of sodium well. Nitric acid often proves the complement to sepia. When sepia is being given in high potency and in infrequent doses (and this is the best use of it), acute intercurrent pelvic symptoms, if so prominent that a remedy seems desirable, will often find that remedy in murex.

SILICA

Silica Dioxide—Flint. Prepared by trituration from pure Precipitated Silica.

This remedy is virtually unknown to physicians who have not studied homœopathy, although Paracelus and Glauber used it, but, like other minerals ordinarily considered inert, it passes under trituration into a colloidal state and displays marked powers of affecting the human body.

The mineral is widely distributed over the earth and is an element in the supporting structure of many plants. In the normal body-tissues only small traces are found, but it is a constant compound of the dental enamel and of connective tissue.

One very interesting observation with regard to it has been

made by German observers, notably Schwarz, who, experimenting with the Glashager Spring water, which contains 1 part
in 25,000 of silica, was able to show that in twenty out of
twenty-three subjects a marked leucocytosis occurred ranging
from 40 per cent. to 216 per cent. This observation is of great
importance, as will be readily admitted when the uses of the
drug have been further discussed.

Professor Schulz of Greifswald had made provings of silica
which agree generally with those of homœopathic text-books.
Among other observations, he confirms obstinate constipation
as a symptom which the drug can produce. Having observed
that such constipation is very common among infants fed on
sterilised milk, he was led to test samples of this food and found
that the silica content of it, though, of course, very small, was
high compared to that of unsterilised milk and derived no
doubt from the glass sterilising vessels, since modern chemistry
has shown that insolubility is only a relative term. Dr. Schulz
suggests that this silica may account for the frequent presence
of constipation in infants artifically fed and even perhaps for
graver symptoms.

Professor Schulz points out that certain mineral waters
recommended for chronic urinary diseases possess a relative
high silica content. Thus Vichy water contains 8 centigrammes
to the litre and the Wernarz Spring at Bruchenau 50 centi-
grammes to the litre. Careful examinations by Schulz revealed
the presence of silica in all connective tissue and demonstrated
also that the silica content varies inversely with age.* He has
also found it in pus and in the contents of ovarian cysts. Schulz
conducted a series of provings of silica in the Hahnemannian
way. The symptoms which his provers developed were those of
increased nervous sensibility with great muscular weariness and
sense of fatigue. The hands developed tremor, the knees gave
out on exertion. Then developed pains in the limbs following
the main nerve trunks—bone pains and marked pains in joints
worse in rest and relieved by gradual movements. Headache

* The recent researches into silicosis, the effects of persistent silica dust
inhalations, have confirmed and extended these observations. It is now
clear that the effect of the drug is very notably on the lymphatic system with
subsequent formation of fibrous tissue and that to this effect the symptom
of silicosis can mostly be referred. The homœopathist has long thought of
silica in relation to scar tissue and lesions therein. Occasionally round-
celled sarcoma has been notably influenced by it.

was constant and severe ; attacks of giddiness common ; sleep much disturbed by dreams. The hearing was definitely impaired in more than one prover.

Meteorism and obstinate constipation, alternating with attacks of diarrhœa, were symptoms of all the provers.

The urine was either increased or diminished, and Schulz quotes Breitenstein in this connection, who found in one case that the quantity of urine increased 37 per cent. under the administration of *equisetum*, which contains a large quantity of silica.

Acne eruptions and furunculosis occurred in the provers. Dandruff was marked with falling of the hair. Itching of the skin became troublesome and the nails grew malformed and tended to split.

The sexual organs in both sexes appeared to be stimulated.

The lymph glands swelled, a symptom to be noted in view of the power of silica to cause leucocytosis.

Sour foot-sweat with soreness and tendency to inflammations of the skin of the feet was a symptom definitely produced.

Schulz uses the drug chiefly for furunculosis and enlarged lymphatic glands, but he deduces from the increased silica content of the connective tissues of the young that the mineral may have a definite bearing upon normal growth and development and is inclined to use it for chronic maladies of childhood and infancy.

The provings of Professor Schulz here, as always, confirm those of homœopathists, but lack the precision and extent of the latter. They are most valuable confirmations of homœopathic beliefs, but a century of clinical use since Hahnemann proved and introduced this remedy enables his followers to be more confident in their recommendations of it than the distinguished Professor of Greifswald.

Silica is principally a remedy for chronic diseases ; its action is persistent and when well indicated and given in high potency it needs but infrequent repetition. It is applicable to states resulting from defective nutrition : such states as are brought on not by want of food but from imperfect assimilation. Hence it is well suited to weakly persons with lax muscles, often of fine skin, pale face and light complexion. It is also especially suited to sickly children who do not thrive, when the head is large for the body, who are sensitive to cold and damp and suffer from offensive foot sweat. Baryta carb. produces similar symptoms, but there the profuse head sweat of silica is absent, and there is none of the mental weakness of baryta carb. in the silica child who is self-willed and touchy, resenting interference and usually intelligent. A convenient mnemonic for the type of patient likely to be benefited by it is " want of grit, moral and physical," flint (silica) being " grit " *par excellence*. There is a prostration of mind and body which results in emotional and physical weariness, so that the patient is listless and uninterested, avoiding effort and responsibility, finding difficulty in concentration. On the physical side there is a sense of debility and weariness. The state of yielding may progress to anticipation and dread so that he develops a peculiar dread of failure in work which he is about to undertake, though actually when the time comes he does it well. Though inclined to timidity, shyness and tending to shirk responsibility, the silica subject becomes irritable, touchy and difficult when roused, often obstinate, this state may degenerate into a " fixed idea." It is in this the chronic counterpart of pulsatilla and many important symptoms of the two drugs are identical. For instance, under silica is found lachrymation, loss of taste, tendency to purulent secretions (especially, however, with silica to the thin, scanty pus, generally due to streptococcal infection, while the pulsatilla secretions are freer, of a bland muco-pus and often associated with staphylococcal invasions) : relief of joint pains from gradual motion (*cf.* Schulz) : photophobia. Generally speaking, when a patient has derived temporary benefit from pulsatilla, silica is likely to produce more lasting effects. It is interesting to note, however, that the reaction to temperature characteristic of silica differs from that of pulsatilla, since silica patients are very chilly even in a warm bed, and even when taking exercise they must be wrapped up. They take cold easily and the general chilliness is extended to chilblains of local parts, *e.g.*, icy coldness of legs and feet. They find relief from warmth (especially from wrapping up, *e.g.*, wrapping up the head for headache), while pulsatilla patients prefer generally cool air and are averse from heat. Dr. Kent taught that many patients who have responded well for a time to pulsatilla may require silica to carry forward the case. For, in some instances, the patient who has been a "hot" subject presents opposite modalities, becomes chilly and shows other silica symptoms. Many such cases finally revert to their original modalities when kali. sulph. may be given with benefit. Apart from its relation to pulsatilla, silica is indicated more for the patients whose troubles are brought on or aggravated by cold than for the warmer blooded : worse in cold weather, worse from uncovering, worse from approach of winter, worse before and during a storm and relieved in summer, relieved by wrapping up warmly, are all conditions characteristic of silica.

The relation to connective tissue noted by Schulz is endorsed and extended by homœopathists and equally by Schussler and his school. It has power over suppurative processes, chronic suppurative skin diseases, acne and old furunculosis and also in helping suppurations and sinuses and fistulæ to heal (cf. fluoric acid) ; it also influences scars and the development of keloid and neuralgic pains in scars. It is reasonable to associate its power to cause leucocytosis, with its influence on inflammatory processes. Occasionally (e.g., in chronic pulmonary tuberculosis) its use may have danger from its liability to rouse a chronic dormant inflammation to activity and free suppuration : in this respect its action is sometimes analogous to that of an overdose of a specific vaccine. Its power seems more marked over streptococcal than over staphylococcal infections, but generally speaking, when there is chronic suppuration in almost any part of the body silica will probably have a value if the general symptoms of the patient correspond to the provings. Particularly should it be remembered for inflammations affecting the neighbourhood of the nails, crippling and deforming them.

Silica is valuable to check excessive sweating, especially of the feet and hands and head. The sweat which indicates it is often sour and offensive. It is often successful in rickets ; and the characteristic symptoms of that disease can be parallel in the pathogenesis or confirmed as indications by clinical experience. If lymph glands swell, become inflamed and indurated and suppurate, silica is to be carefully considered. The excessive foot-sweat is a noteworthy symptom. When it is present, patients often adopt violent measures to check it, and, as no doubt it is an excretory effort on the part of the body, grave general symptoms are often found to follow its forcible suppression by strong local applications. Whenever there is a history of foot-sweat thus checked, silica should be thought of. It will often temporarily restore the secretion, with relief to the general conditions and then finally cure both the sweat and the disease of which it was a symptom.

Over-susceptibility to nerve stimuli should be noted as one indication for silica, together with a state of melancholy, with easy weeping, though they are averse to consolation (opp. pulsatilla). When there is nervous fatigue and neurasthenia, these symptoms often appear. A characteristic indication for silica is a severe chronic headache beginning at the nape of the neck, coming over the vertex and settling behind one or other eye (more especially the right). The headache is worse from cold air and mental exertion, relieved by wrapping up warmly and relieved by profuse urination—an indication of its toxic origin. Vertigo is often associated with it.

In the digestive sphere, the symptoms are more intestinal than gastric. Distension of the abdomen is a common symptom and the patient who needs silica is nearly always constipated. There is inertia of the rectum, the stool being passed with great difficulty, receding when partly expelled. Silica marina (sea sand) has sometimes proved very valuable in chronic constipation and constipation of infants will often yield to silica or alumina or lycopodium (which, it is interesting to note, contains both silica and alumina), but Schulz's suggestion as to sterilised milk (see above) must be remembered. Although the silica patient is an intensely chilly subject, there is often a desire for cold food and drink, whereas there is a disgust for meat and warm food. There is an aggravation from milk and so silica is a drug to be considered when mother's milk causes the infant diarrhœa and vomiting. (Æthusa : nat. carb. sanicula.)

The drug will be useful in almost any chronic condition when the general symptoms correspond and comes to be considered often in chronic inflammatory diseases of the chest, of the joints, of the kidneys, of the nervous system. Indurations and scars and thickenings should always bring it to the mind of the physician ; it may be useful in cataract and has a place in the palliation of recurrent cancer, especially scirrhus. Its tissue relation to connective tissue should be constantly remembered and its great value for the malnutritions of the young and growing. Like its counterpart, pulsatilla, it has a special relation to the external and middle ear.

Equisetum contains as much as 16 per cent. of silica. It is chiefly valuable in the more superficial urinary and bladder diseases, and, bearing in mind Schulz's experience, its effects may be largely attributed to its silica.

Mercury is quite incompatible with silica and they must never be given near one another in point of time. Hepar. sulph. and fluoric acid follow it well, as do also lycopod. and sepia. In rickets silica is often useful after calcarea and it follows graphites and phosphorus well. Its relation to pulsatilla has been already discussed. The characteristic headache and wrapping up is found also under mag. mur., which also has somewhat similar constipation symptoms to those of silica and foot-sweat. Unhealthy skin, where very little injury suppurates (i.e., lowered resistance to ordinary germs of suppuration), is found also in the pathogenesis of hepar, graphites, petroleum and mercury and ant. crud. markedly affects nails. Fluoric acid has great power over sinuses and fistulæ.

SULPHUR

Trituration of Flowers of Sulphur. A saturated solution in absolute alcohol is also taken as the mother tincture and potencies made from this. The quantity of sulphur dissolved is 0·035 gram sulphur to every 100 grams of tincture.

Sulphur is one of the oldest remedies in medicine, but of late years, except for homœopathists, who rank it among the chief potent drugs, it is little used except as an external application and as a purgative.

A large dose of sulphur readily causes a laxative action, with a certain slight catarrh of the bowel and with the purgation thus achieved the whole mass administered generally passes away with little or no absorption. A local effect is obtained, but not a general one. But if the drug is taken in small repeated doses, insufficient to produce at once active purging, then it is readily absorbed and profound effects produced, especially in chronic diseases. This is tacitly admitted by any physicians who make use of sulphur springs for chronic joint cases, for chronic syphilis, or for lead or other metallic poisonings, because the amount of sulphur in most sulphur springs is not large. In the famous springs at Aix-la-Chapelle, for instance, there is only 1 gram of sulphur to 250 litres, yet the virtues of treatment with it are renowned and the power of small quantities is surely thereby confessed. Homœopathists, however, are almost the only physicians deliberately to aim at the profound effects of the drug by administering minute doses of it. It has to be remembered that a small but essential quantity of sulphur is contained in the albumen molecule, so that it is not to be wondered at that quite a small disturbance of sulphur equilibrium in metabolism should have a marked effect. It should be added that the virtue of the sulphur in sulphur springs in producing improvement has been denied and the value of the treatment attributed to the general hygienic measures of hydrotherapy, the heat of the bath, etc. But it is nevertheless true that physicians in general continue to choose sulphur waters for certain complaints and not other waters, although if the sulphur were inert other waters should do as well. So that the verdict of general experience would seem to be that the sulphur *has* a value and it is at least interesting that the verdict of general empirical experience so often confirms the uses to which the homœopathist is led by his provings.

Certain experiments show a considerable increase in the urea excreted under the influence of sulphur. This suggests a heightening of general metabolism, a " speeding up " of body machinery and might account for some of the value of the drug in hastening elimination of metallic poisons or even toxins. Clinical homœopathic experience would certainly encourage a belief in this power.

Professor Hugo Schulz, of Greifswald, almost alone among non-homœopathic physicians, has a clear conception of the powers of sulphur. In this as in other matters his researches have led him to conclusions largely accordant with those of homœopathy, as he freely acknowledges, but the independence of his investigations adds great value to his confirmations of homœopathic experience. He has had sulphur " proved " under his own direction and bases his clinical uses of it upon these findings. He emphasises the great difference in the value attached to the drug by the two schools and is not unfairly critical of the somewhat complacent lack of experimental curiosity on the part of physicians, who, with the experience of the sulphur springs to give them suggestions, yet make so little use of the remedy and decry, without any personal investigation, the conclusions of those (like himself and the homœopathists) who have at least grounds of experiment for their convictions.

He quotes effectively the well-known lines from " Faust " addressed to the old and prejudiced imperial counsellors, which may be paraphrased thus :

" All you can't grasp is wholly lost on you,
All you can't reckon is, you deem, untrue,
All you can't weigh for you no weight can hold,
All you can't coin, can't pass, you think, for gold."

Wherever the truth lies in the homœopathic controversy, these lines are a fair criticism on the attitude (so terribly common) of the expert in the old to the experimenter in the new, as not only Hahnemann, but Harvey, Semmelweiss and a hundred others could testify.

Schulz points out first that sulphur is an invariable constituent of albumen, and second that the sulphur content varies with different tissues. Particularly are epithelial tissues relatively rich in it, and the relation of sulphur to the skin is a close one.

As a result of " provings," Schulz states that one of the early effects of taking small repeated doses of sulphur is upon the higher nerve centres. The first sign is a sense of discomfort, combined with increased sensitiveness and " nervousness " ; inability to concentrate and to pursue mental work follow with ready fatigue after relatively slight exertion. Lack of interest in life deepens into apathy, almost into melancholia. Drowsiness often increases : the sleep at night becomes heavy but unrestful and presently the patient begins to drop off to sleep at any time in the day, but occasionally the reverse phenomenon is seen and sleeplessness or light sleep broken by terrifying dreams appears. Both these opposed effects can be seen as a consequence of sulphur poisoning and sometimes even the one state will pass over into the other. This is an instance of a phenomenon which is found with great frequency in homœopathic provings, the phenomenon of the appearance of so-called primary and secondary symptoms. Thus a primary diarrhœa appearing under the influence of a drug will be replaced by constipation, a primary spasm by a secondary paresis, a primary neuralgia by numbness. Both effects are drug effects and therefore on the strength of the homœopathic generalisation, either should be an indication for the use of the drug if it appears in disease with similar characteristic qualifications. Clinically an attempt has sometimes been made to use either symptom-group as an indication, and to modify the potency of the drug according as the indication followed is primary or secondary. But the attempt has not been conclusively translated into practice, though it has value in acute or sub-acute diseases. In chronic disease most observers agree that either a primary or a secondary drug symptom can be used as a drug indication, and that, given that it is well marked, there is no clear evidence that it carries any necessity of high or low potency. Both high and low, in other words, will affect both primary and secondary symptoms. If a case calls for sulphur in its " totality," then sulphur (both in high and low potencies) will relieve either sleeplessness or tendency to excessive sleep.

The paradox becomes less paradoxical on consideration of other well-known phenomena. All life energies in cells are compounded of what may be called a building-up factor and a breaking-down factor, a reaction and a preparation for reaction. A secretion is a breaking down of a previously built-up substance, a muscle contraction an " explosion " of a previously prepared substance, a nerve impulse involves a chemical change for which a previous preparation must be made, and so on. Now the effect of a " stimulus " may be more exerted on one life factor than on the other. Opium is a nerve stimulant for a brief space, and it is as a stimulant that opium eaters take it as often as for a sedative, but its more abiding, predominant action is as a hindrance to nerve action, as a paralyser of muscle contraction. The most prominent action of a drug is apt to mask its opposite effect, but the latter is nearly always to be found if looked for. Now, it can hardly be doubted that the regulation of life processes is carried out largely by agents analogous at least to enzymes, and enzyme action has one great characteristic in that it is reversible. Yeast will break down sugar into alcohol and CO_2, but will also synthesise it out of alcohol and CO_2. If, then, what have just been called the life factors of building up and breaking down in tissues are controlled by enzymes, it is highly probable that one and the same enzyme controls both factors in virtue of this quality of reversibility, and if a drug acts (as it very well may) by influencing enzyme action (if not by directly supplementing it), then while its effect will very likely preponderate upon one factor, it is almost certain to some extent to affect both. But in this case its remedial effect in disease will depend upon the direction in which enzyme action is modified by the illness. Normally there is, as it were, a pendulum swinging with a definite rhythm and producing opposite effects as it swings in opposed directions. In disease the pendulum tends to become fixed to one side or the other : there may be excessive breaking down or building up with no capacity to break down. The effect of a drug which *ex hypothesi* influences the pendulum directly may very well be to set it swinging again, on whichever side it may have been fixed. This clumsy image may serve also to illustrate the advisability of discontinuing a drug when the desired effect is produced ; once the pendulum is set swinging again, to go on interfering with it might well produce new disorder. When a drug is being " proved " it will influence enzyme action first probably in the direction of heightening normal function, because as a cell exists to fulfil a certain function, there should be a certain definite readiness to perform it in response to any stimulus. The function of a muscle is to contract and the first effect of opium is to stimulate contraction. But after the cells have been thus abnormally stimulated into action, they are apt to revenge themselves by an abnormal reaction in the opposite sense and the reaction after an opium-produced contraction is a much more obvious lethargy. Non-homœopathic medicine inclines to make use of the secondary reactions, and, *e.g.*, uses opium to check diarrhœa. Homœopathic medicine, at any rate in non-chronic cases, inclines to use primary action and uses opium to relieve constipation, giving to that end a small dose, for the depth of the reaction is largely proportionate to the amount of drug given and a dose small enough to produce a primary effect may have no *obvious* reaction at all. In chronic diseases the disturbance to life is more profound. Here in practice either primary or secondary drug symptoms can be used as indications.

Returning from this digression to the consideration of sulphur, it must be next noted that Schulz finds attacks of giddiness a prominent feature in provers. The attacks are slight at first, but become repeated and may go on even to fainting. Particularly do they appear on rising after sitting, or after long standing, and the use both of alcohol and tobacco predispose to them. These phenomena are probably vaso-motor in origin and are to be associated with the characteristic attacks of " flushing " of the skin, locally or generally, with sensations of heat and cold. The heart's action is quickened at first and afterwards slowed : irregularity of pulse and palpitation are common symptoms.

Schulz's provers constantly developed headache under sulphur : the early morning on waking was a usual time for its appearance and it affected principally the forehead and brows. Sensations of congestion were common. Homœopathic provings find the vertex of the head a most characteristic site of sulphur action, but Schulz does not seem specially to have noted this and speaks of the frontal regions as chiefly affected. Conjunctivitis appeared, with swelling of the mucous membrane and increased secretion. Vision was considerably affected in some subjects, who complained of their sight flickering and of objects seeming veiled and indistinct. Peripheral nerve disturbances took the form of formication and discomfort rising to neuralgic pain, sometimes following the course of large nerves (e.g., sciatic), sometimes more generally diffused. The motor nerve involvement caused tremor of extremities and a general sense of muscular weakness. Also whole groups of muscles and definite joints suffered from pain and discomfort which recalled lumbago and rheumatism. In the respiratory sphere, catarrh of nasal, tracheal and bronchial mucous membranes appeared, with cough and increased secretion. The alimentary canal was even more definitely attacked. Herpes on the lips was seen several times ; the saliva increased, with swelling of the glands, the gums bled easily and were swollen. Anorexia, heart-burn, gastric distension with sense of pressure and fullness testified to the presence of catarrh of gastric mucous membrane. All the provers (taking small repeated doses) experienced at first constipation, with hard, dry stools : after a few days this passed over into diarrhœa. Distension from fermentation and gas formation and marked hæmorrhoids were usual sequels. The colour of the stools suggested a gradual increase in the output of bile under the influence of sulphur. Urine was generally increased : the genital organs in both sexes appeared to be stimulated.

Sulphur has an ancient reputation for affecting the skin, and the provers all showed marked effects of it on this tissue. Itching, crawling sensations and burning came first. Then the hair began to fall, the skin became dry and scaly and a tendency to local suppurations appeared, small boils and acne spots and inflammation round the nails. The skin under sulphur undoubtedly contains more blood and pigment is made and deposited more easily. Finally, Professor Schulz found good reason to think that the general level of body metabolism was heightened under sulphur and it is mainly in chronic diseases that he uses it to stir a system to better reactions by virtue of this general power. He notes (as homœopathists are interested to see) that the beginning of a course of sulphur treatment often leads to a temporary aggravation of symptoms, but regards such a phenomenon as hopeful and expects it to lead to final improvement. He also adds that old half-forgotten troubles may reappear under the influence of the drug and again regards this as of good augury for their ultimate complete disappearance. His whole point of view and practice with the remedy is of great interest and significance, and while homœopathists more often use high potencies and single doses of sulphur, Schulz's short courses of the tincture seem in his hands frequently to achieve admirable results.

From these confirmatory general provings it is time to turn to the more detailed indications of homœopathy. Sulphur to the homœopathist is inextricably associated with chronic disease (although there are many acute and sub-acute conditions for which it may be indicated), since Hahnemann formulated his famous doctrine of the " miasms " and their profound effects. The greatest of all race-poisons to him was the one he called " psora," and sulphur he indicated as one of the chief remedies for it.

Hahnemann's teaching, however modified in details, commends itself to the experimenting physician, in so far as chronic disease can be cleared up (with sufficient frequency at least to encourage the experimenter) by diligent application of the Hahnemannian method as worked out in detail by Allen, Kent and others. And since the practice is fruitful, the homœopathist can have no scorn for the doctrine upon which the practice is founded, however odd some of its expressions appear to-day. But there is no need here to spend words over the conception of " psora." Suffice it to make clear that Hahnemann probably did not mean by it ordinary scabies, as has been ignorantly asserted. He was aware of the parasitic nature of scabies and his psora was a very different affair, but it was one of the characteristics of it that skin symptoms (especially itching eruptions) should be prominent, and scabies was in his day often called psora and thus the confusion arose. The Hahnemannian doctrine of chronic disease does not mean any abandonment of homœopathy : the remedy is chosen by similarity and it is by its pathogenesis that sulphur becomes so frequently indicated. But an appreciation of the possibility of a poison underlying a chronic symptom-complex leads the homœopathist, when the remedies that seem obviously indicated fail or only relieve temporarily, to consider the drugs which may have a deeper action. Among these the choice must be made by general rather than local symptoms, by the general body reactions. Even when these are not very definite there is justification and value in the practice of administering a drug like sulphur, because of its well-established reputation of " clearing up " a case. Unquestionably it happens that the administration of sulphur often brings into prominence new or half-hidden symptoms which point the way to the real remedy, or else it speeds up a recovery that seems to hang fire and enhances the action of a drug which, though well indicated, has till then shown little power. The explanation may lie, as Schulz suggests, in its influence on general metabolism ; at any rate, from the days of Hahnemann it has been held good practice when a case does not respond well, to try if a dose of sulphur will not avail to help, and clinical experience justifies its use even when indications are few. Nevertheless, the symptoms of sulphur are many and definite and the better they are marked the more confidently can the prescription be made.

Most valuable of the indications for sulphur are the general ones, those that concern the patient as a whole rather than any one tissue. The drug is found to be particularly suitable to persons who approximate more or less to a type that may be defined as sensitive, even delicate, but slack, lazy, shiftless, lacking energy and will power, living on the wits rather than by hard work. It is sometimes difficult to decide whether their indolence is really laziness or due to an actual lack of physical stamina. There is an aversion to undertaking steady work and such people would rather undergo actual physical hardship than follow up work in a systematic manner. It must be understood here and whenever a drug is thus associated with a well-marked type of individual, first that the type described is only a guide to the physician and does not exclude exceptions, and second that it is a guide in two ways. Persons who conform to the type are to be regarded as having a constitution which will readily respond to the drug. If, indeed, they conform closely to (say) the sulphur type, then sulphur may be for them a general remedy capable of relieving most diverse complaints. Hahnemann would have said that they were "psoric" by inheritance, and, indeed, they may quite conceivably be persons starting life with a certain lack of balance of life forces (internal secretions or whatever), and sulphur may have the power of amending the ordinary deficiencies of their particular balance. Or, again, a person not notably of the sulphur type may approximate to it under stress of illness. The hard worker may overwork and develop the slack and lazy condition of mind and body that so often goes with this drug. Then clearly his life balance is disturbed in a definite direction, and again it is in the hope that sulphur will correct it that the prescription is made.

A characteristic (though not invariable) appearance of a typical case for sulphur is that of a spare, stooping, delicate-looking subject, very disinclined to stand, always ready to sit or lie down, but if compelled to stand, then constantly shifting about restlessly. It should be noted that this is not the only and invariable sulphur type. The drug is often applicable to the well-fed, well-nourished person.

In the sphere of mental activity the symptoms produced (and therefore curable) by sulphur are largely those compatible with a good average intelligence working under a cloud, as it were, and functioning therefore badly. Thus characteristic is a weak memory for names, for recent events, while affairs of the past are perfectly recalled. A condition somewhat similar is caused by lycopodium, but with this drug it approaches nearer to mild degrees of aphasia and allied states, the using of wrong words, omitting of syllables in writing, and so forth. The pathological mechanism may be partly toxic and partly circulatory. Candidates for sulphur are indisposed to any exertion, even to amuse themselves is too much trouble and work of any kind is a burden ; there is indolence of mind and body. Men and women who are born " tramps," who will endure a good deal of physical hardship rather than work steadily at anything, yet often possessing excellent abilities, these frequently suggest sulphur as their constitutional remedy. The " ragged philosopher " is a description that has a certain aptness. That is not to say that a general administration of sulphur would empty the casual wards of the workhouse, but does mean that many of the people who inevitably drift there are of a physical constitution which would find in sulphur a remedy for many troubles to which they are liable.

Patients who need sulphur often seem stupid and dull. They avoid conversation, take no trouble to answer questions or show any interest even in their own symptoms (though, in fact, they do note these carefully), but the stupidity is much more apparent than real, it is mental indolence and not lack of intelligence that produces the impression. Calcarea subjects, on the other hand, are often earnest and well-meaning, but really mentally slow and inactive. A sulphur subject would always rather dream or brood (it is flattery to call their broodings meditation, they are too lazy to think) than do anything else. It is not wonderful, therefore, that they are often melancholy, inclined to self-pity and hypochondriasis, but it is an inert condition, with little anger or pride or impulse in it. The tendency to brooding may become extreme so that the individual becomes absorbed in abstract, aimless philosophical or religious meditation. Sometimes the day dreams go on to illusions, Alnaschar visions that produce a foolish kind of happiness. Children who tend to day-dreaming are frequently much helped by sulphur. The complexion and hair in these cases are often fair and the eyes blue or light coloured.

There are several important general symptoms to be found in this drug. Very noteworthy is the skin condition : it often looks (and is) dirty, for the typical sulphur patient finds that washing irritates his skin and he avoids it : symptoms worse after bathing is a sulphur " keynote," as it is called. This is associated with a variety of skin eruptions to be described later, and with the presence of more blood in the tissue than normal (as Schulz notes), for wherever the covering layer is thin (lips, eyelids, orifices generally) there is a notable redness of the parts. The orifices are not only red and congested, they are often sore and hyper-sensitive, so that the passage of discharges and excretions over them is painful.

Corresponding to this permanent extra blood supply in the skin are the characteristic sulphur " flushes " of heat. The blood suddenly " rushes to the head," or to the chest ; heat and burning sensations of parts of the body occur, followed by sweating. These vaso-motor disturbances have a counterpart in the " sinking," " empty " sensations of which sulphur subjects complain. These no doubt depend on vaso-motor phenomena affecting the abdominal circulation. They are of great importance as sulphur symptoms. Several of the great remedies for chronic disease present them more or less, but with sulphur they are unusually prominent, particularly about 11 a.m. (also with sepia). That is a characteristic aggravation time for this drug for this particular symptom. It is of more than a little importance. The sinking sensations at this time of day are common in women of middle age, and are one of the most potent causes of the habit of spirit drinking, which temporarily relieves them. This, it need hardly be said, is a very undesirable practice and sulphur becomes a valuable weapon wherewith to fight it. The sinking often translates itself into hunger, and hunger in the forenoon or about noon may be equally read as a sulphur symptom.

The flushes are often associated with palpitation and sweating and sulphur patients always feel too hot. They want windows open and all the air they can get. Though they are worse from heat, they dislike the cold, especially the cold, wet weather. Dry, warm weather suits these persons very well. When troubled with breathing they want the windows and doors open. As regards the body, they tend to feel hot when covered and chilly when uncovered. Particularly at night (another great time of aggravation for sulphur symptoms) they are apt to find the bedclothes a burden. To toss the clothes off or put the feet out into the air is a habit that children (and others) often acquire when they thus feel the heat and it is a good broad hint to the homœopathist for sulphur. Heat and burning are sensations that come out again and again with this drug, both generally and locally. In the skin, itching goes with the burning and is markedly worse for the warmth of the bed. Indeed, the aggravation from the warmth of the bed is perhaps the most characteristic way in which sulphur patients show aversion to heat and it is true for joint pains, neuralgias, etc. Sulphur seems to affect the general life rhythm in periods of about twelve hours and noon and midnight will be the points about which aggravations of symptoms turn. The nightly aggravation of complaints is as characteristic as the aggravation from the warmth of the bed. Many of the complaints of sulphur are worse after sleep. Periodicity of symptoms in any periods of twelve hours or multiples of twelve suggests the drug. It has had success in chronic malaria and workers in sulphur mines in malarial districts are said to be immune from that disease.

The burning sensations of sulphur are marked throughout its pathogenesis. They are also prominent under arsenicum and phosphorus, but the subjects who need these are nearly always chilly and not averse to heat as are sulphur patients. Moreover, the burning pains of the first two drugs are relieved by heat, but in sulphur heat produces an aggravation and relief is found from cold. Aggravation from bathing is a general sulphur symptom. This does not apply only to skin conditions for there is a general aversion to washing. The patient does not feel any benefit from bathing, indeed he may experience an aggravation of his symptoms or feel generally unwell after a bath. It has often been noted that such subjects definitely prefer to take a bath in the evening just before going to bed.

The excretions of the sulphur subject tend to be offensive. The body smells unpleasantly, the breath is offensive, as are discharges from mucous surfaces. In spite of this, the sulphur patient is over-sensitive to bad odours and is offended by those which emanate from his own body.

Sulphur affects the head in all regions—forehead, vertex and occiput, perhaps most characteristically the vertex. The headaches are associated with the flushes generally. They are often periodical, returning every week or month. In spite of the general desire of sulphur patients for fresh air, the headaches (especially if one-sided sick headaches) are often worse in fresh air and relieved in a warm room. The head is hot and flushed and probably the brain congestion is relieved by the warm atmosphere that draws more blood to the surface. Exactly the opposite phenomenon is characteristic of arsenicum where the headaches are relieved by fresh air, though the patient generally needs warmth and hates cold of any kind. With the pain goes the characteristic of burning : the tendency of sulphur to develop acne spots shows well in the face and the symptoms are worse from application of water and generally worse at noon and midnight. Sometimes with the head very hot, the feet are cold in spite of the general tendency of sulphur patients to have hot, burning feet and hands. The eyes—at any rate, the superficial structures of the eye—are much affected by sulphur. The usual burning and itching sensations are accompanied by marked conjunctival redness and catarrh. There are feelings of dryness and of grit in the eye and later increase in secretion, though sulphur is not one of the drugs that produces very profuse secretion, as, for instance, pulsatilla does. Vision becomes dim from the congestion of the surface rather than from affection of the deeper structures. Broadly speaking, sulphur finds its place particularly in recurrent conjunctivitis of unhealthy children under suspicion of tuberculosis or syphilitic infection. Cases that do well for a time and relapse are here, as elsewhere, frequently indebted to the drug for a fresh start towards recovery.

Much the same may be said for the value of sulphur in chronic ear and nose catarrhs. It is especially useful in deafness following chronic middle ear disease and in the nasal conditions where there is no polypus formation or much mechanical obstruction, but a constant infection with frequent exacerbations, no great amount of discharge, but considerable discomfort. Sensations of itching and burning will, as usual, be present, and the nostrils are characteristically red in the sulphur case. Apart from these cases, when flushes are accompanied by tinnitus, sulphur often relieves the second symptom as well as the first. More acute cases of otitis in characteristic sulphur subjects react well to it, but the choice is likely to be made more on the general than the local symptoms. It follows apis well here. With chronic nasal catarrhs, sense of smell and taste are often lost and simultaneously a subjective sensation of unpleasant odours may be prominent. Secretions and excretions of all kinds in sulphur cases are usually foul smelling ; this is also characteristic of guaiacum, a drug that has certain affinities to sulphur and very notably with psorinum.

The alimentary tract is affected in certain definite ways. The lips are red, the tongue generally white with a red tip and edges, the pharynx congested with sensations of burning and dryness. The faintness and great hunger and empty feeling at 11 a.m. has already been noted as a characteristic subjective symptom. Thirst more marked than hunger is usual. The patient may complain of feeling hungry, but when he comes to the table he does not want to eat. There is a desire for highly seasoned foods, fat and sweets, though the latter is less prominent than with lycopodium or argent. nit. Sulphur is unquestionably of value in combating the craving for alcohol, especially a craving for spirits, in middle-aged women, where, as already observed, it seems to arise from the attempt to check the empty, sinking sensation which is so marked in the sulphur pathogenesis. Objectively under sulphur there is great tendency to flatulence, both gastric and intestinal, with rumbling and gurgling and emission of gas. Evidence also there is of portal stasis, hæmorrhoids and constipation. Constipation with rather large, dry stool (somewhat like those of bryonia) is the usual condition when sulphur is indicated, but there is a characteristic painless diarrhœa, coming on about 5 a.m. and compelling the patient to hurry out of bed for relief, which will respond quickly to this remedy. A similar symptom will be found under aloes. Sulphur and aloes are antidotes, and probably one of the reasons why sulphur (like nux vomica) is often valuable in constipation when much purgative medicine has been taken, is that many purgative pills contain aloes. Children who are in need of sulphur, besides the general symptoms already so much insisted on, frequently have a big, distended belly and emaciated limbs. Natrum sulph. is also a remedy for abdominal flatulence and diarrhœa, but, as a rule, the diarrhœa is more persistent (though it begins only on rising) and the abdominal pains more marked. There are differences also in the general symptoms of the two remedies, though no doubt the presence of the sulphur element in nat. sulph. is a link of some consequence. Prolapsus ani, tenesmus, hæmorrhoids, excoriation and soreness of the anus all appear under sulphur and the invariable burning and itching sensations are found.

In the genito-urinary sphere there is found the same redness, itching, burning sensation at the urethral and vaginal orifices and similar chronic, not very profuse, but rather irritating discharges. When gonorrhœa in either sex improves up to a point and then delays, a few doses of sulphur will often give the process of recovery a fresh start, if there are any general symptoms in the case that suggest the drug, or even if there are merely the obstinate objective appearances and an absence of well-marked symptoms. Similarly sulphur may help chronic prostatitis, sub-involution, chronic pelvic inflammation, whenever the remedies that seem more immediately indicated fail or slacken in effect. Aggravations of symptoms at night or at 11 a.m. and any characteristic flushings and sinking sensations and general dislike of heat and of bathing affected parts, are strong indications for its use. Enuresis in sulphur objects is often cured by it. It need hardly be said that the climacteric in women is a time then sulphur is almost sure to be called for ; here it competes with sepia and lachesis. As usual with remedies that have special virtues in chronic diseases, high potencies and infrequent repetition form the best method of administration.

In the respiratory sphere the power of sulphur to take up and complete the process of recovery from acute diseases is very marked. Occasionally when the general symptoms calling for it are very clear it will control a case of pneumonia effectively from the beginning, but more often its sphere is after the crisis, if resolution is for any reason delayed. Perhaps it is more often needed in lobar than in broncho-pneumonia, but many cases of chronic bronchitis benefit by a course of it and similarly chronic pleurisy, or chronic laryngitis, will frequently be helped. Sulphur symptoms are particularly likely to appear when the physician has reason to fear that tuberculosis is threatening and

even when the disease is unmistakably present the drug will
sometimes seem to arrest the progress of it. But in tuberculosis
a word of caution is required. The arrest of pulmonary tubercle
requires the effective mobilisation of forces of resistance at a
reasonably early stage. If for any reason this is not achieved
naturally or artificially, the disease often becomes chronic and
thereafter smoulders away with occasional exacerbations that
permit, in favourable cases, of great palliation and of the
leading of quite useful lives, but the trouble is rarely properly
arrested. Sulphur is invaluable in helping to mobilise the
resistance forces, and in early or threatening tuberculosis will
often clear up a case admirably, but sometimes the disease has a
stronger hold of longer duration than physical signs suggest.
Sulphur administered to cases wherein resistance has been
attempted without much success often leads to a violent
reaction, such as used to be seen after big doses of tuberculin,
and as, in some of those cases, the final result is to weaken the
patient and leave the situation worse, not better. Unless the
physician is convinced that the powers of resistance are good
and the disease early, sulphur in any potency above the thirtieth
should be given with some caution. When there is any doubt,
it is well to test the case with lower potencies, 3, 6, or 12, or the
tincture and only give higher potencies as the success of the
lower warrants. Characteristic symptoms that suggest it in
chest disorders are : great desire for air, especially at night ;
sense of suffocation ; oppression and burning sensations in the
chest ; stitching pains shooting through to the back, worse
when lying on the back or breathing deeply ; flushes of heat in
the chest rising to the head and face. Paroxysm of coughing
may terminate in sneezing.

In all chronic affections of joints, fasciæ and fibrous tissues,
sulphur springs have a reputation which homœopathy confirms
and extends. The choice, again, is largely dependent on the
presence of the general symptoms so often quoted, but especially notable are burning in feet and hands, aggravation from
bathing, stiffness, and cracking of joints, pain in back (felt
especially on rising after sitting) and cramps generally. The
drug will help osteo-arthritis, old tuberculous, syphilitic or
gonorrhœal joints or chronic rheumatism, when the symptoms
correspond.

The skin is greatly influenced by sulphur. The hair falls and fingers and toes and the surface generally tend to be dry, though local and partial sweatings (armpits, genitals, etc.) are frequent and generally offensive and after a flushing there is often sweating. The condition is rather one of irregular sweating, the skin too dry generally, but with excessive local or temporary perspiration. Burning and itching are prominent, relieved by scratching ; vesicles and pustules readily form and the skin grows rough, scaly and sore, made worse as to sensation by washing. There may be great itching with little to show for it but erythema ; pigment is deposited readily. Sulphur appears to lower the resistance to staphylococcal infection (this has been experimentally proved for calc. sulphide (hepar. sulph. which *cf.*), so that pustules and boils appear in the provers and correspondingly medicinal doses raise resistance and sulphur is admirable for pustular acne and furunculosis. Black gunpowder has been successfully used for suppurations and septicæmias, both streptococcal and staphylococcal, and no doubt owes much to the sulphur it contains.

Finally, sulphur is often a remedy for sleeplessness, when the patient tosses unrestfully, with constant and disquieting sense of heat and burning. Patients often wake at 3 a.m., as with nux vomica, and cannot sleep again. There is a general aggravation of symptoms at night with sulphur.

Sulphur on the whole is most successfully used in high potencies infrequently repeated. But *short* courses of the drug in tincture or low potency sometimes act very well. It is preeminently the chronic counterpart of aconite and whenever a case has done well up to a point sulphur will take up the torch and carry it on. It follows bryonia excellently, and mercury and calcarea follow sulphur well, but the reverse is not true. Sulphur seems sometimes to act in a complementary way to both pulsatilla and nux vomica, and, as a matter of fact, there are few remedies whose action it disturbs and many whose power it will seem to enhance.

THUJA

Thuja occidentalis. Arbor vitæ. Tincture of the fresh green twigs.

Thuja not only owes its place in the homœopathic Materia Medica to Hahnemann, but before him was used little if at all.

Nor, except for homœopathists, who prize it highly, has its fame increased since Hahnemann's day. Lewin has a word or two to say of the effects of large doses of it (taken as an abortifacient) : he notes that it does seem to affect the genital organs profoundly and that it has a relation to papillomata. Both these statements are more than confirmed by homœopathic provings and clinical results, but in addition the investigations of the homœopathic school have made precise the indications for this drug in a variety of chronic disease conditions.

It has been elsewhere stated that Hahnemann considered the foundation of any case of chronic disease to consist in poisoning by one or more of three " miasms." Of these he distinguished one under the name of sycosis and it was as the main remedy for sycosis that he valued thuja. The field of the sycosis of Hahnemann is covered to-day strikingly by the disease gonorrhœa,* and it is no small proof of Hahnemann's clinical insight that he recognised long before it became common knowledge the deep action of this deadly poison. Inasmuch as Hahnemann lived before bacteriology, the boundaries of his " miasms " are less precise than they might have been if he could have drawn them some decades later and no doubt he may have included under sycosis cases not obviously gonorrhœal ; but, on the other hand, homœopathy, always concerned at the bedside rather with body reactions than with body enemies, finds the same remedy frequently indicated in symptom-complexes, arising from diverse causes, but arousing the system to similar reactions. Thuja, therefore, while very frequently required in gonorrhœa, can also be a remedy for other conditions, and the homœopathist chooses it by its indications among the symptoms rather than by the presence of one specific germ of disease.

One of the features by which Hahnemann distinguished sycosis was a tendency to the development of warty growths and especially of soft cockscomb-like papillomata, bleeding readily and moist with an unpleasant secretion. It has been already noted that Professor Lewin finds evidence of a specific power of thuja over papillomata and the provings well confirm this belief. Whenever papillomata are present, and most of all

---

* Other disorders associated with coccal infections often come into the thuja sphere of action.

when they show characteristics outlined above, thuja comes swiftly to mind, not that it is the only remedy for such new growths by any means, but because it is a very prominent one. It has a further relationship to more serious new growths, and even malignant tumours have seemed to yield to it, as in the once famous case of Marshal Radetzky. Particularly, however, polypi or fibromata (*e.g.*, epulis) or papillomata that are the result of chronic irritation by discharges will find a remedy in thuja. Even nasal polypi can often be helped, obstinate as they are. Thuja will influence the catarrh that accompanies them, and if it does not cause the growths to dwindle (occasionally it does even this, though slowly), it will often do something after their removal to prevent recurrence.

Thuja is one of the remedies that suits those whose complaints are much aggravated by damp and cold, but especially by damp. The unfavourable reaction readily takes the form of catarrh of mucous membranes through the lowering of systemic resistance to germs of catarrh and for infections of the upper respiratory passages and genito-urinary tract, and for certain chronic gastric conditions, when damp and cold aggravate the symptoms, thuja comes well forward as a likely remedy. A kindred drug is sulphate of soda, but the discharges that fit this medicine are more profuse and purulent. The discharges that suggest thuja are free, but not excessive, of muco-pus and generally foul smelling.

Chronic catarrh, sensitiveness to damp cold and tendency to new growths are, then, leading indications for thuja, but there is another, even more important. Thuja has a marked action upon the skin, producing either scaly patches suggesting psoriasis (often pigmented), warts, or condylomata, or a definitely pustular eruption, not as a rule covering very wide areas, but suggesting in the individual pustule the characteristic pock of small-pox. For this reason thuja has been used for small-pox considerably and there is reason to believe that it has real value in the disease ; but the eruption is even more like that of vaccination and it is the relation of thuja to vaccinosis (as Burnett called it) that has become significant. In so far as it is generally used to decry the value of vaccination (a question not here at issue), the fact is generally denied or made light of that various chronic disease symptoms not infrequently seem to start from vaccination, successful or even unsuccessful. But all physicians are familiar with chronic skin troubles that appear thus to begin, and Burnett collected many cases of chronic neuralgia, chronic dyspepsia and constipation, etc., besides a tendency to papillomatous growths, all seeming to date from the time of vaccination, especially when the operation had been repeated at intervals in the way generally recommended as a prophylactic against small-pox. He therefore classified these conditions together as varieties of vaccinosis, related them to Hahnemann's sycosis,* and, from the similarity of symptoms, treated them largely with thuja, and, as he claimed, with marked success. His work has been followed up and it may at once be said that there are few homœopathists who do not consider thuja whenever a case gives a clear history of vaccination as the starting point of chronic disease symptoms (particularly skin symptoms).

The question deserves further consideration, however. Apart from vaccination, chronic skin troubles, neuralgias, dyspepsias, etc., may present thuja symptoms and respond to thuja. But clinical observation finds that a starting point of disease in vaccination is an additional indication for the drug, and even when other thuja symptoms are not prominent this relationship may hold good for the relief of the patient. More difficult for many physicians is the whole conception of " vaccinosis " as an entity of disease. However, there is no question, first, that vaccine lymph contains a powerful toxic agent, and, second, that the body reacts to it sometimes violently. Further, several germ poisons (e.g., influenza) produce effects which continue long after the acute stage is past. There is nothing, therefore, inconceivable in the conception that vaccine lymph should (in susceptible subjects, and these alone are in question here) produce remote and lasting effects. Clinical observers who look for evidence of this will find it, and Burnett's views can be taken at least as a working hypothesis. Even if the risk of " vaccinosis " be conceded, it is not a very frequent or often a severe sequel of one vaccination. Repeated vaccinations are more likely to give rise to it and the element of risk should be

---

* Burnett, of course, did not mean that vaccinosis and gonorrhœa were identical, but that both affected the system similarly (though gonorrhœa more virulently) and were therefore not to be regarded as falling under Hahnemann's heading of sycosis.

weighed against the prophylactic power for which the operation is undertaken.

Another general antidotal effect of thuja has been clinically discovered and emphasised by the late Dr. Clarke, and that is its power to relieve chronic symptoms brought on by abuse of tea. The headaches and subjective heart symptoms, sleeplessness and dyspepsia of tea drinkers to excess are frequently relieved promptly by thuja when the mere cessation of the poison has brought no early relief.

The thuja patient is frequently an individual with dark complexion, black hair and unhealthy skin, though children are often light haired. It is pre-eminently the remedy to be considered in the treatment of illnesses following vaccination and maltreated gonorrhœa and where there is a history of snake bite or small-pox. It has been found to be both preventative and curative in an epidemic of small-pox. It aborted the disease and prevented the pitting when the disease had developed.

To these general features that characterise the drug can now be added regional symptoms in detail. The thuja patient is a sick person, of soft fibre, easily exhausted and easily prostrated. His appearance is characteristic, he is sickly looking with a waxy shiny face that looks as if it has been smeared over with grease. Mentally he is anxious, indisposed to do anything and with a disposition to weep ; he is especially so affected by music. This mental condition of dejection and depression may even approach melancholia and is then apt to be characterised by fixed ideas. These are usually fantastic (*e.g.*, a delusion of fragility, as if the body were brittle and would easily break ; or he imagines there is a living animal in the abdomen ; feels as if he were under the influence of some superior power). He is apt to be ill-humoured and peevish ; a characteristic symptom is that he will act hurriedly and talk hastily and he is extremely scrupulous about small things. Slight degrees of aphasia or allied conditions (*e.g.*, use of wrong words in writing or speaking) are not uncommon.

There is a definite influence on sleep and thuja is suited to patients who wake early and cannot sleep afterwards (*cf.* nux vomica). The dreams are often of falling from a height.

The headaches which indicate the drug cause much mental

confusion ; they are often dull and stupefying, but relieved by the open air. Sharper pains are not uncommon in small spots and feelings as of a tight band round the head. Vertigo usually accompanies the headache. The morning on waking is a common time of aggravation of chronic headache, or the evening at bed-time. In this latter case it frequently prevents or disturbs sleep. The skin of the scalp often sweats and eczematous eruptions or warty growths often appear in cases that are helped by thuja.

The special sense organs show the effects of thuja in chronic catarrhs and tendency to develop overgrowths of tissue. Thus, not only papillomata, but granulations (e.g., anal), polypi and fibromata can be benefited. Conjunctivitis with lachrymation is marked, and, remembering the deadly effect of the gonococcus on this structure, any local measures adopted for the cure of gonorrhœal conjunctivitis should be supplemented with thuja as an internal remedy. Burnett had a saying that " Gonorrhœa is the mother of catarrh," meaning thereby that uncured gonorrhœa, even if latent, predisposed to all kinds of secondary infections of nearly all mucous surfaces. Thuja certainly affects all mucous membranes, tending to cause mucopurulent, copious, foul-smelling discharges, and therefore, on grounds of similarity, its curative relation to gonorrhœal cases becomes emphasised.

The alimentary canal is a site of marked action of thuja. It affects the teeth profoundly ; the roots become carious, while the crown remains sound, or relatively sound. The gums are swollen and inflamed. Pyorrhœa alveolaris is certainly often helped by the administration of the remedy. Ranula and epulis are both conditions for which thuja has been given with success. The tongue is usually clean or only thinly coated and often is red and painful. The power of thuja to antidote excess in tea-drinking has been already mentioned and great tea-drinkers often present a tongue of this character, even when (as often they are) constipated. There is a chronic post-nasal catarrh characteristic of thuja and a chronic pharyngitis with swollen veins and unhealthy mucous membrane.

The appetite is capricious. There is often a mawkish or sweetish taste in the mouth, to relieve which the patient craves salt. Cold food is preferred and a very little as a rule

satisfies the appetite. Burnett thought that inability to take
food in the morning at breakfast was an indication for thuja.
In many ways the beginning of the day is a time of special
suffering for thuja subjects. It is a noteworthy clinical observation that in the twenty-four hours, the twelve hours that include
the time from sunrise to sunset are usually the worst for
gonorrhœal subjects, while those who are syphilitic suffer most
during the twelve hours that include the time from sunset to
sunrise.

Every sign of chronic catarrh of the stomach is present :
eructations, vomiting (mucus and food), nausea, discomfort,
pressure and flatulence. Acute pain is not so common and
signs of actual ulceration rare. The sensations are rather those
of weight and pressure. Abies nigra, a plant allied to thuja, has
a deserved reputation for similar gastric conditions, when the
sensation of a lump in the stomach after food is very clear and
definite. The catarrhal condition appears to extend throughout
the greater part of the bowel, with flatulence and discomfort
and soreness as accompanying symptoms. There is marked
constipation and tenesmus and the anus shows hæmorrhoids or
condylomata, cracks or fissures with great frequency. Offensive perspirations are usual in groin and round buttocks and
genitals. Occasionally there is an early morning sudden
explosive diarrhœa.

In the respiratory sphere there are again signs of catarrh.
The larynx is affected and trachea and polypus of the vocal
cord has disappeared under the drug. There is not much
evidence of effects of thuja on the lungs, but the whole bronchial tract is influenced. Sputum is of muco-pus and cough
irritating and explosive. Asthma is a disease wherein at times
thuja has great power. It is to be chosen largely, however, from
general symptoms, such as aggravation from damp weather
and association with a history of gonorrhœa or of repeated
vaccinations. With regard to the latter, the asthma of sycosis
frequently produces symptoms during the attack which call for
arsenicum. In such cases, in order to clear up the condition
it becomes necessary to follow the palliative drug with an anti-
sycotic remedy such as thuja (or natrum sulph.).

The genito-urinary sphere is one of the utmost importance
for the action of thuja. In the female are to be noted as indica-

tions for it gonorrhœal symptoms of all kinds, discharges, condylomata, ulcers and swellings. The periods are *too early* but scanty, with severe pains often centred in the left ovarian region. Tendency to abortion, especially with a gonorrhœal history, calls for thuja. But the drug also meets the late effects of gonorrhœa, chronic inflammations of uterus, tubes and ovaries and all the aches and pains and weariness that accompany these. The implication of the joints (especially of the sacro-iliac) is a further indication, and whenever osteo-arthritis is or has been accompanied by leucorrhœa or pelvic symptoms, even with no clear history of gonorrhœa, thuja should be remembered.

In the male the effects of both acute and chronic gonorrhœa are similarly countered. Urethritis, prostatitis, varicocele, ulcers, condylomata and balanitis—any of these local conditions suggest thuja, and if the general constitution of the patient is not definitely opposed to that which indicates the drug, this is the remedy of choice. The more chronic effects of gonorrhœa are signally helped—persistent urethritis and prostatitis and arthritis. There is some evidence of the effect of the drug on the kidney tissue. Sharp pains in the kidney region may be experienced, and in the urinary passages a continuous urging to urinate and often severe cutting pains after urination. In this connection a keynote of thuja may be mentioned. A pain experienced in any part of the body may be accompanied with frequent micturition. But it is rather the passages from ureters to bladder and then the urethra that feel the influence of thuja most, and for any recent inflammations in those regions it has definite claims for consideration. Sugar, blood, mucus and albumen have all been found in the urine of subjects under the influence of thuja, but the mere presence of any one of them would not be sufficient indication for its use without some further symptoms from the general pathogenesis.

It may be appropriate here to consider the question of local applications (irrigations, etc.) in gonorrhœa. Comfort and cleanliness demand some irrigation, but the homœopathist is, as a rule, inclined to doubt the value of the very powerful antiseptics that are fashionable. It is clear that their use does not avail to prevent a greater or less degree of generalised infection. Urethral discharges may quickly cease under their use and the patient apparently recovers more quickly than if they are not used, but bitter experience most frequently shows that the disease is latent, not eradicated. The local inflammations are body reactions to the disease and any cure must rather proceed from within outwards (by increase of the natural, phagocytic and other defences) than from without inwards, for the strongest antiseptics will not penetrate very deeply into the tissues. Thuja acts by encouraging the general resistance, and when it is well chosen it is generally enough to use simple saline solutions for cleanliness and avoid the powerful antiseptics. By this means speedy relief to the pain and discomfort is usual, and though sometimes the discharge is slower to disappear, subsequent relapses are less common and the hope greater that the disease has been eradicated. Each case must be treated on its own merits, but as a general rule this treatment is the best in final results.

Subjects in whom gonorrhœa is uncured are often sufferers from subjective cardiac symptoms. Those that indicate thuja are palpitation (worse morning), cardiac anxiety and stitching pain and a slow, weak pulse, with occasional bursts of tachycardia.

The joint conditions have already been discussed. Gonorrhœal arthritis, acute or chronic, may be helped by thuja, and even when there is no clear history of this disease it is worth a trial if there is much worsening of symptoms from damp and if local foul-smelling sweats are present. Movement generally relieves pains to some extent and heat (oddly enough) is not often grateful when locally applied, rather the reverse. Pyorrhœa as a cause of arthritis is another possible indication for thuja.

Muscle sheaths and fasciæ may be effected in cases that respond to thuja, and a few years ago a most extraordinary improvement was effected by this drug in two cases of the rare disease myositis ossificans, treated at the London Homœopathic Hospital. Both were advanced cases of the disease and one was well known to most of the hospitals in London. The improvement made under thuja was well-nigh miraculous and sustained. In both these cases the drug was chosen on the whole symptom-complex, not on the local muscle symptoms, but it is interesting that each case, considered quite independently, worked out to the same remedy and justified the choice of it by its response.

Finally, the skin in thuja subjects may show a variety of eruptions, papular or pustular, eczematous or like psoriasis. The nails suffer, chilblains are common, the sweat glands are active (sweating is generally more on parts uncovered), and extra pigment is deposited. The tendency to warty growths is marked.

The general modalities of thuja are : an early morning aggravation of symptoms from 3 a.m. onwards, also at 3 p.m. the patient is chilly ; worse cold damp air : worse bright light : worse sun : worse during the waxing moon : the left side of the body is predominantly affected. Pains are worse at night and worse from the heat of the bed. Pains are frequently found in localised small spots and often accompanied by frequent micturition.

TUBERCULINUM

Introduction to the Study of the Nosodes

In this section of the Materia Medica there have to be considered a number of different remedies, but all alike in that they take their origin from actual diseased tissues or (latterly) from bacterial cultures. Long before bacteriology was established as a subject for scientific enquiry it occurred to one or two homœopathists (notably Dr. Swan) that the obvious manifestations of toxic conditions such as skin eruptions and discharges should contain poisons which could be turned to account as remedies on the basis of symptom similarity. Several such preparations were made and proved so successful that their number has been constantly augmented. The material of the discharge or fluid from an eruption or actual diseased tissue (e.g., in the cancer nosodes) was mixed with lactose, triturated for a starting point and potencies prepared therefrom in the usual way. As they were never used below the 6th centesimal and usually in the 30th and upwards, any question of there remaining any repugnant morbid material did not arise. They were (and are) called nosodes, a name implying their origin from actual diseases.

Later, when bacteriology became a flourishing branch of

medicine, cultures of specific germs were used as the basis for potentised remedies and the modern Staphylococcin, Streptococcin, etc., are so prepared and also the whole range of bowel organisms.

It is held that influenza virus (and others) can be grown on certain tissues. As the virus cannot be isolated from its medium as a germ culture can, a vaccine of the virus has to include the tissue on which it is grown and this again is analogous to the procedure of the homœopathists.

This, then, is the mode of origin of the nosodes and the group includes a number of remedies and is extensively used in homœopathic therapeutics. Although they include the prime agents of the corresponding diseases, the method of preparation and potentisation makes them closely similar to rather than identical with the sickness from which they are derived, just as culture on a culture medium and killing the culture makes a vaccine something less than the actual poison of the disease. It can be regarded in our phraseology as *simillimum* rather than as *idem*, so that vaccine therapy has always interested homœopathists who see in it a procedure analogous to their own. The resemblance has often been admitted by eminent men from Von Behring onwards. It was, of course, developed without any thought of the homœopathic heresy but that fact makes it all the more deeply significant to the followers of Hahnemann.

Some of the nosodes (*e.g.*, Psorinum, Medorrhinum, Leuticum, Tuberculinum) have had some testing on the healthy, but it must be admitted that their symptomatology (in some instances quite extensive) has been mainly worked out clinically on the reactions of patients. Since, however, the clinical evidence has had in the best instances many years to accumulate and has been checked by the experience of many practitioners, it can be relied on to give trustworthy indications for the use of these remedies.

The less well proved ones are associated with their corresponding diseases and characteristic disease symptoms can (with due care) be taken as indications for the use of the nosode in any disease. To the homœopathist a nosode is a poison to the body just as any vegetable or mineral may be, and the rule of similars should therefore apply to it and make it available as a remedy. For instance, a severe backache might find its remedy in variolinum, backache being a characteristic symptom of smallpox,* if other symptoms fitted into the picture.

It is true that this use of the nosodes of acute disease is not common ; usually there are many other drugs with a more extensive symptomatology to be considered and a more exact choice can be made from among them. It is probable that the acute sickness elicits so specific a reaction that the uses of its nosode, apart from its own disease, are bound to be few. Experience appears to point to that conclusion. One interesting fact emerges from experience in acute diseases. If a case is severe and remedies either poorly indicated from lack of effective vital reaction or failing to produce results from the same reason, then a dose of the nosode may prove to be just the stimulus required and either suffice for cure or carry the patient to a state wherein another remedy will be well indicated and successful. This is particularly true of certain types of pneumonia that were terribly in evidence just after the last great war. The septicæmia was severe, far too often fatal and, although homœopathists succeeded in achieving a lower mortality than the average, it was far higher than that which they usually see in pneumonia, at least in hospital cases. In private patients the results were good, but the onset of the disease was often insidious and far too many of the poorer cases delayed applying to the hospital until there was little chance for them. In these circumstances it was more difficult than is customary with pneumonia to find the *simillimum*. Much the best results that were personally known to us were achieved by Drs. Teale and Bach with a polyvalent intestinal vaccine prepared from a number of severe infections. At the time of the worst epidemic we did not know of it, but it was used in sporadic similar cases later, and these without exception cleared up quickly and conclusively. It was given hypodermically in small isolated doses, the effect of each being observed before repetition was considered. After

* It would be rash to assume that any, even well marked, symptom of a disease can be read as an indication when it occurs in a case of sickness independent of that disease. The nosode is not identical with the disease toxin in the way, for example, a massive dose taken by a prover of arsenic is identical with the potentised arsenic given to a patient who reproduces the prover's symptoms. If or when the nosodes are symptomatically proved, uses may be found for them.

These statements apply particularly to nosodes of acute diseases, and their use in acute disease conditions to which they do not pathologically correspond.

injections there would be a brief rise of temperature of half a degree to a degree or more, and then within a couple of hours a fall like that of a crisis. Often no further rise of temperature would occur, and no further dose be given. Sometimes fever would return and a second dose be given. Occasionally a third was required, if the fever yet did not finally end. But three doses were rarely used and more than three never, for if so many failed no further ones availed. Naturally, the earlier the first dose was given the less often was more than one dose needed. The success of this vaccine was typical of the way in which the well-indicated remedy acts.

One country hospital obtained great success with a nosode potentised direct from the sputum of several cases, but this procedure was relatively unsuccessful in London. Probably such a nosode would need more strains of organism than were actually used in order to be generally effective.*

To sum up the matter so far, nosodes of the acute diseases do not appear to be of great curative value in the course of the actual diseases to which they are related, with the important exception of the polyvalent vaccine (or nosode) in acute septic pneumonia. It is, however, just possible that in other acute diseases they might find a place in very severe and overwhelming cases and if other remedies fail they should then be remembered.

The great usefulness of the acute disease nosodes lies elsewhere in two spheres. First, that of prophylaxis. In any epidemic the corresponding nosode can be given for this purpose, and will be found valuable. Generally speaking, a dose of the 30th potency will protect for at least a fortnight. For more persistent and recurrent infections like influenza, in our judgment the nosode influenzinum is best mixed with one of the T.B. nosodes, either tub. bov. or bacillinum (Burnett). All the tuberculins suit that type of patient who seems to pick up nasal catarrh on the least provocation and the mixture suggested is effective against the common cold as well as against influenza.

* In these terrible epidemics the modern sulphonamide preparations were unknown. But as far as pneumonia is concerned Hahnemann's followers have never felt themselves to be ill equipped for cure. On the contrary, they expect success, so that they do not hasten to leave their well-tried and effective weapons for others till the latter have been very well tested, though naturally they do not, and will not, neglect any weapon of proved efficacy.

A monthly dose of the 30th potency is usually sufficient to confer protection. Generally there is a slight reaction (mild pharyngitis probably) for twelve to twenty-four hours after a dose.

The other sphere of usefulness has two divisions. If a case of an acute disease is slow in convalescence, apt to relapse, a dose or two of its nosode will work wonders : e.g., Pneumococcin for a lobar pneumonia that is slow to resolve, or Morbillinum for a case of measles where chest catarrhal symptoms are persistent. In all such cases the nosode seems to give a fresh impetus to powers of recovery. It is true that great polycrests like sulphur or lycopodium will often work effectively in such emergencies and if any one of them were well indicated by symptoms it should be given. But so often in these cases there is a fundamental deficiency in recuperative power, and that generally means few and uncertain symptoms, since characteristic symptoms are as much (or more) the expression of body reaction as of disease attack. It is precisely where there are no very clear indications for a remedy that the nosode can help.

The other value of these nosodes is one of particular interest. It has been realised by several physicians (notably by Dr. Clarke and Dr. Burnett), but Dr. Tyler of recent years has done great service in insisting on it. In treating chronic cases it frequently happens that enquiry into past history reveals that the patient dates the beginning of trouble to an acute illness, saying, " I have never been really well since I had measles (or diphtheria or whatever)." In such a case it is remarkable how often a dose of the corresponding nosode (preferably in high potency) starts the case on the road to recovery or at least to marked improvement. The indications for supplementary remedies become clearer and the response to them more marked.

It is true that certain remedies have long been regarded with favour for some conditions dating from previous disease poisonings, as e.g., thuja for ill effects of vaccination, but without forgetting or underrating these, the nosodes of acute disease are most valuable. Even when the association of the acute attack and the chronic condition has not been observed by the patient, the history of a severe experience of this or the other acute disease would warrant an experimental use of the corresponding nosode in a case refractory to obvious remedies.

Many of our French colleagues distinguish a group of patients as "Tuberculiniques," meaning by this term that they are specially likely to develop tuberculosis, and that dangerously.*

One of their indications for the "tuberculinique" is a history of a severe attack of measles or whooping-cough, both of them diseases not infrequently followed by tubercular manifestations. In such cases these physicians employ one or other of the tuberculins, but it might be well to remember also the disease nosodes such as morbillinum and perhaps give them the first chance to stimulate effective reactions.

These two preparations have recently been protentised by Messrs. Nelson and are now available.

TUBERCULINUM

In this study of tuberculinum we propose to approach the subject in the following manner. We shall first enumerate the various tuberculins more generally employed by homœopathists. Then we shall consider the type and general reactions of the individual who usually benefits from the administration of tuberculin in potency (the "tuberculinique" of the French).

Finally, having taken note of the gross effects on the body of tuberculin injections, we shall give the detailed symptoms of this remedy as known to homœopathists and refer briefly to the shades of difference in symptomatology between the various potentised tuberculins.

Sources of the Tuberculins

Bacillinum. Dr. Burnett was the first to employ this nosode. His preparation was made from typical nummular sputum and tubercle bacilli were demonstrated in it, but it must have contained as well secondary pus organisms, streptococci, staphylococci of possibly various kinds. Bacteriology was not an advanced study in those days, and we have no details recorded beyond the presence of tub. bac. It may, however, safely be regarded as polyvalent, and this may make it specially valuable in certain cases.

Tuberculinum. Preparations have been made from tubercular

---

* Calmette held that a "tubercular" state preceded the appearance of the bacillus; it is on this state that the physicians in question concentrate attention.

abscesses derived from the human body, though the infection was probably a bovine strain.

Tuberculinum bovinum. This is the preparation of which Dr. Kent principally writes, though he has not detailed a definite symptomatology that would lead the prescriber to choose this remedy in preference to any of the other potentised tuberculins. Tuberculinum bovinum is made by triturating with sugar of milk the tubercular glands of infected cattle.

Aviaire is prepared from chicken tuberculosis and appears to act most markedly on the apices of the lungs.

Bacillinum testium is a nosode prepared from a tubercular testicle and was considered by Clarke and Burnett as having a more direct relationship to the lower part of the body than the pulmonary bacillinum.

*Tuberculin of Koch. This preparation is made from cultures of the human bacillus of tubercle which are triturated with lactose and potentised.

Tuberculin of Denys. Our French colleagues have potentised a filtered broth in which cultures of tubercle bacilli have been grown.

*Residual Tuberculin of Koch. A culture of Koch's bacilli in broth is filtered and the residual emulsion from which the potency is made contains the different substances which enter into the constitution of the microbe.

The Serum of Marmorek is obtained from animals injected with successive doses of tuberculin.

Tuberculin of Rosenbach is made, we understand, from tub. grown symbiotically with tricophyton and has on occasion been employed, though not in potency.

Comments on the Relationship between Tubercular and Bowel Infections

The indications for tuberculinum are perhaps more circumscribed in Britain and U.S.A. than in France. For our colleagues there to all intents and purposes identify tuberculosis and the state they call " tuberculinique " with Hahnemann's psora. It must be emphasised that the " tuberculinique " has not necessarily any obvious recognisable signs of active tubercle ; the patient is one in whom tubercle will find a

---

* These two preparations have recently been potentised by Messrs. Nelson and are now available.

favourable soil so that a manifestation of it is inevitable sooner or later unless fortune is favourable. All homœopathists accept and work on the conception that a nosode can be valuable independently of its corresponding disease, often indeed more valuable in such circumstances. But in thinking of tuberculosis and pre-tubercular states as psora, our French colleagues extend the range of tuberculin to cases wherein many of us would look to the other nosodes.

Those who use the bowel nosodes believe that there is a very close relationship between this group and the tuberculins. We have only to remember the frequency with which dyspepsia precedes pulmonary developments to realise that the ground favourable to one also favours the other. It may well be that either group may act as effective aids in these conditions and both sides can claim results to bear out their contention. Possibly, too (for we have much to learn about the bowel flora and its possible mutations and their causes), differences of climate and natural dietary may play a part. The French homœopathists (and to some extent those in U.S.A.) maintain that they find the non-lactose fermenting organisms less persistently than we do. But before accepting this experience as final we have to be certain that the technique employed in the search for them is identical in all countries. Our most expert investigators of these organisms find that even apparently negligible differences in the preparation of the medium may affect certainty in determining the presence of this group of organisms.

The practical conclusion at this stage, in view of the good results obtained by both contestants, is to regard the tuberculin group and the non-lactose fermenting group as both to be considered seriously in obstinate chronic disease. Particularly if one group fails should we be ready to consider the other, since only by very extended and careful observations of both can any valid conclusions be drawn.

General Indications for Tuberculinum

In studying the application of the nosode to tubercular constitutions and tendencies, it is convenient to recognise two states in which tuberculinum is especially likely to be indicated.

The first is the pre-tubercular state, the " tuberculinique " of the French, a term first employed by Dr. Vannier to imply the type of individual who has a predisposition to tubercular infection. The tendency is manifested particularly by nervous and circulatory disturbances which will be described later in detail. To this Dr. Vannier would add that such individuals show characteristic signs of what he describes as "intermittent elimination," by which he means repeated exacerbations of local symptoms, e.g., periodic migraine, attacks of diarrhœa, intermittent fever, etc.

The tuberculinique is known or at least suspected first and foremost from the family history. If tubercle has taken toll of near relatives, the patient may be unduly susceptible to it. Next the personal history of previous illnesses, special stress being laid on severe attacks of measles or whooping-cough, both of which infections, if badly met, are significant. Otherwise the general type is one which our ancestors called " scrofulous " and recognised as closely related to tuberculosis.

The other condition where the nosode can so often be looked to for help is one wherein the patient has suffered from a tubercular lesion, has apparently recovered but still retains the toxin in the system to which the body reacts, giving rise to symptoms calling for tuberculinum.

The skin of the tuberculinique is often delicate and complexion attractive, with long eyelashes and fine hair. The appetite is capricious and there is difficulty in putting on weight. They are seldom fat, and bodily exertion easily fatigues them. But they may grow rapidly, shoot up in height without corresponding muscular development. There is an extreme variability in all their symptoms. The emotional state varies and is often unbalanced : for example, there is a tendency to fits of irrational bad temper and a restless changefulness in their approach to life. There is a similar variability in the physical symptoms ; for example, the stools may be constipated and hard on some occasions, soft on others.

Superficial disturbances of the circulation are seen ; there is a bluish pallor of the skin, a purple condition of the extremities and chilblains are usual. Circulatory derangements are characteristic. Hypotension is usual, though arterial tension is often raised temporarily by taking coffee. Palpitation often occurs on waking, but the cardiac symptoms in general are usually relieved by the taking of gentle exercise. The tuberculinique has difficulty in going to sleep and difficulty in awakening, but when he does fall asleep he is likely to sleep well. He is easily fatigued and is not generally energetic and this lack of vitality shows itself in the readiness with which he takes colds. Dr. Vannier records an interesting objective sign where a lesion of the lung has existed. The tuberculinique tends to develop an erythema on the chest wall following friction. Should friction be applied to both sides of the anterior chest wall, a marked redness will appear and will persist for several minutes on the area overlying the affected part of the lung. The susceptibility of pulmonary cases to fungoid skin eruptions is described later in this study. The tuberculinique is mentally alert, though later on this vivid responsiveness may burn itself out and thus the individual becomes intellectually sluggish, though emotionally agitated. From adolescence onwards (or even before) there is often seen a rapid ripening of brain power and any noteworthy creative gifts come speedily to fruition. The outstanding example of this is the poet Keats, but in lesser degrees and in other arts the same development is seen as though there were a sort of prescience that life will be short so that there is a hurry to complete expression of experience. The patient may be aware of the feeling. There is a famous sonnet of Keats which illustrates this point. With this mental acuteness often goes a keen interest, almost an obsession, with sexual matters that is, however, not accompanied with any special sexual potency, and the clash between desire and power may produce an emotional conflict. The small dose of any poison may be a stimulus where the large dose is destructive, and it is probable that a disease toxin may often encourage (or seem to) ideas, and images. It may even lower the barrier that shuts off the unconscious and play a part in "inspiration" which is so intimately related to this part of the mind, as F. W. H. Myers argued convincingly long ago in the chapter on Genius in "Human Personality." The converse evidence appears now and then ; we know of at least one case where successful treatment of a chronic intestinal infection markedly lessened the inventiveness and flow of ideas which had earned as an author a living for the patient.

The Gross Effects on the Body of Tuberculin Injections

Lewin, writing after the first enthusiasm for tuberculin injections had waned through the manifold disasters which followed the first use of them, but before there was great experience of smaller doses, made his symptomatology therefore as the result of massive doses and (mainly) from their effect on cases already suffering from tuberculosis. But he speaks of the effects also in the non-tubercular, and has no hesitation in attributing *all* the results that he chronicles to the preparation and not to the original disease that was pre-existent. Thus rise of temperature following rigor is usual with the non-tubercular, and as high a point as 106·7° has been noted. More rarely it becomes persistently subnormal. A marked leucocytosis and jaundice followed in at least one such case. As the tuberculin was given hypodermically, a distinction should be drawn from effects at the point of injection and others more remote. Redness and œdema locally were frequent, but swelling of lymph glands, healthy as well as those already tubercular, was common and noted in the mediastinal region more than once. Swelling of the joints with effusion, again of healthy as well as diseased ones, occurred, and considerable pain which increased at night. Skin eruptions were usual : erythema, urticaria, papular and vesicular eruptions were frequently observed.

In the alimentary canal, glossitis with abscesses of the tongue or suppuration of the gums, acute parotitis, splenic enlargement, persistent vomiting and diarrhœa were objective symptoms observed, and subjective ones included loss of appetite, nausea, gastric and intestinal pain. One case developed acute inflammation round the navel and in some lupus cases the mucous membrane of ileum and lower bowel was found to be attacked. Presumably there was no previous disease in these regions in these cases, but perforation in existing tuberculosis of the bowel also occurred. The kidney was severely affected on many occasions. Polyuria, often with fever, appeared ; sometimes oliguria and often death. Acute nephritis was demonstrated in certain cases. Naturally albuminuria with the passage of casts was often observed, and sugar and acetone were noted more than once in the urine.

The effects of material doses of tuberculin on the urinary

system is of especial interest to the homœopathist, for certain physicians have remarked on the value of the potentised tuberculin in renal affections, though they advocate caution in its administration where the skin, intestines and other eliminatory functions do not act adequately. In chronic cystitis good results have been observed from the exhibition of tuberculinum.

In a woman suffering from lupus the period was delayed after tuberculin injections and pregnant women have been known to miscarry after its use.

Nerve and brain symptoms include somnolence, even deep, and its obverse sleeplessness. Violent headache was frequently observed, and neuralgic pain in limbs and intercostal regions. Œdema and hyperæmia of the brain were noted *post mortem*, and serious mental symptoms, delirium with fever and confusion of mind, hallucinations and illusions followed injections on several occasions. In lung cases tubercular meningitis developed more than once after tuberculin. Conjunctivitis was observed, and also disturbances of vision with the subjective experience of seeing colours. This did not disappear for a considerable time after ceasing the drug. The heart was notably disturbed, and not only in tubercular cases. Palpitation, rapid pulse and pain with anxiety were the symptoms. Death followed in some cases with every sign of an acute cardiac crisis. Blood pressure was usually lowered and the hæmoglobin content diminished. The lung and larynx symptoms are mainly to be read as aggravations of existing disease in those suffering from tuberculosis of these regions. Lewin makes no mention of these symptoms affecting non-tubercular cases, and latent T.B. is so widespread that it would be difficult in any case to be certain that symptoms that might occur in the apparently healthy were not actually due to the lighting up of a quiescent focus. But of the power of tuberculin to aggravate, even disastrously, pre-existent T.B. there can be no doubt, and from a homœopathic standpoint that would make the drug suitable for help to similar cases provided the right dosage could be found. When much more cautious administration was adopted, many men in many places believed that favourable results were obtained, but we think to-day that the general judgment would be that the evidence is suggestive rather than conclusive on this point even when small doses are used. The followers of Hahnemann using almost entirely potencies and much less frequent repetition are still of the opinion that the drug can be useful, but pulmonary and laryngeal cases demand the utmost care in the use of it.*

With the possible exception of miliary tuberculosis, the tuberculins are mainly used in this group of patients for such as are becoming chronic, fibrosing rather than cavitating, going downhill but slowly. Here an occasional dose of tuberculin does seem to give a fresh start and enable the other remedies to become effective.

The foregoing is ample evidence of the gross effects of tuberculin. Morbid anatomy when a " similar " drug can be found to it is often a great help to the prescriber, particularly in palliating incurable chronic cases and relieving symptoms. In acute illness a " similar " morbid anatomy, e.g., bryonia in pleurisy and pneumonia, can often prove a good guide to cure, though every homœopathist prefers a wider symptom resemblance. Therefore this tuberculin symptomatology is here recorded. It will form a good starting point for the finer indications to which we now turn.

General Considerations of the Homœopathic Use of Tuberculinum

There are a number of preparations of tuberculinum employed by homœopathists. The indications for any one of them are similar, not unnaturally, and it will be most convenient to group the characteristic symptoms in one description and then give such hints as we can for preference of one preparation over another in special cases. Kent's account of tuberculinum bovinum contains few outstanding diversities in symptomatology that would lead the prescriber to the choice of the bovine tuberculinum in preference to any other, and in his study of tub. bov., he has grouped together symptoms from the provings and clinical observations obtained from the records of various other tuberculinum preparations. Our experience

---

* A markedly increased frequency of laryngeal T.B. is recorded by Lewin as having followed the early reckless use of tuberculin, and if the drug has the power in excess to encourage such development, then in sufficiently smaller dosage it should tend to check it.

over the past ten years is that we prefer the potency of
Koch's Tuberculinum. He holds tuberculinum to be closely
associated to psorinum and uses it in cases where well-
selected remedies " hold the case " for shorter periods than
usual through vital weakness and deep-seated disease.* Thus
intermittent attacks of fever in debilitated subjects, each
of which may respond to treatment reasonably well, but
where they recur on the least provocation and on every
occasion call for a new remedy, such a condition would
indicate tuberculinum. This changefulness in symptomatology is, of course, a general characteristic of tuberculinum.
Kent makes use of the conception of the tubercular background
which Burnett first developed and claims that children with
actual or suspected tubercular parentage can often be cured of
T.B. glands with it and, he adds, of adenoids.† Most homœopathists have found tuberculinum of help in cases of enlarged
tonsils and adenoids and tub. bov. is generally preferred,
though the other preparations have claims to consideration.
Probably in general very high potencies are best here.

Tuberculinum should always be considered in the treatment
of mentally deficient children. Where there is arrested development, mental or physical, for example, delayed dentition, it is a
particularly valuable remedy. Many cases are recorded wherein
a backward child has been stimulated to normal development
following the administration of tuberculinum.

Mental and Emotional Symptoms

The predominant characteristics in this sphere are those of
mental weakness and depression. This is mirrored on the
physical side by a corresponding state of relaxation and debility.
The " Spes Phthisica " is rarely present in cases that need
tuberculinum. On the contrary, hopelessness and weariness of
life are common. The patient seems crushed emotionally and is
depressed ; he is melancholy and complains on the slightest

---

* Kent never knew nor used the bowel nosodes.
† In the course of the last two generations medical opinion has changed
more than once on the matter of operations for the removal of tonsils and
adenoids. It has swung from advocacy of wholesale removal of any enlarged
tonsils with a few (mostly homœopathically-minded) physicians refusing
any and every surgical interference, to the present attempt to select only the
persistently septic ones for removal.

provocation. He becomes hyper-sensitive and nervous and is especially sensitive to music.*

Particularly in children there is peevishness and fretfulness and a tendency to outbursts of bad temper. Indeed, sudden fits of fury in a child from little or no apparent cause would turn the thoughts of most homœopathists to this remedy.

The variability of the symptoms of tuberculinum has already been mentioned, and this characteristic changefulness is to be found in the emotional state of the patient who becomes irritable and agitated. He has a constant desire to change his place, and nowhere is he able to rest content. The restless condition of the mind of the tuberculinique may show itself in an abnormal urge to travel ; a desire to do something different ; to change his doctor, and so forth. Dr. Elizabeth Hubbard has described this feature very graphically : " The traveller, the great cosmopolite, ever in search of new people, new ideas ; the faddist, the consumer of cults."

As the patient is always frail and tired, exertion brings on intense fatigue, mental and physical, and so he has an aversion to mental work and any intellectual effort.

The tuberculinique when in health may be of a placid, cheerful nature but when a restless agitation develops in such persons this change of disposition naturally is very noticeable to his friends and a valuable indication for tuberculinum, for homœo-pathists consider that alterations in outlook and in emotional responses are of the highest importance in guiding the prescriber to a remedy.

Head Symptoms

Periodical sick headaches, even the most severe ones, respond to tuberculinum in suitable cases. Recurrence is usually every fortnight, sometimes weekly, and it is charac-teristic that changes in weather (particularly damp conditions), excitement, overwork, gastric disturbances, may precipitate an extra attack. Intense pain " as of an iron band round the head " is a modality noted by Hering. Burnett described an interesting confirmation of this when he found that tuber-

---

* In sanatoria there is always a proportion of patients who drift from one place to another, never carrying out treatment wholeheartedly anywhere and never doing well.

culinum had the power to set up pains that seemed to be
situated deep in the head. The pains may be severe and cutting,
movement aggravates them. The pains are often accompanied
by cold sweat on the head which recalls calc. carb., and this
drug and silica follow tuberculinum well.

Gastro-Intestinal Symptoms

The pre-tubercular type (the tuberculinique) may eat well,
but even while so doing there is loss of weight or even emaciation. Later the appetite is poor or absent; there is an aversion to
meat but sometimes a desire for cold milk and large quantities
of cold water. Now and then there is a sinking sensation in
the stomach that causes desire to eat, but there is always
loss of flesh with gradually increasing weakness and weariness.
Constipation alternates with diarrhœa. In the first case the
stools are large and hard, in the second there is a marked
morning aggravation so that an early morning diarrhœa may
drive the patient out of bed (sulphur ; aloes).

Menstrual Symptoms

The menses are apt to be too early, too profuse and long
lasting.

Respiratory Tract

Subjects for tuberculinum are generally martyrs to the
common cold and the temperature often rises in the evening,
the face becoming flushed, even purplish. Respiration tends to
be rapid, but should the attention of the patient be occupied,
respirations assume a slower and more normal rate. A hacking
cough coming in paroxysms follows and disturbs sleep. In
these conditions there is a longing for air, windows must be
open and there is an attempt to breathe deeply, for warm rooms
cause a feeling of suffocation. Expectoration is thick and
profuse, and comes away easily. The left lung is more usually
affected in pneumonic conditions, and tuberculinum should be
considered in cases of unresolved pneumonia (especially where
there is a history of T.B.). Should this remedy be called for
and given, a reaction following its administration can be
recognised by a transient rise of temperature which lasts a few

hours. A local and general improvement in the condition of the patient usually follows. Young girls who are feeble and tired and in whom the menses are suppressed may develop a hacking cough and a chest where the physical signs are suspicious of tuberculosis. Such cases often derive benefit from occasional doses of tub.

Pains in General

The whole body feels sore and aching and pain seems to be in the bones. Warmth and movement relieve the suffering which is intensified by rest and standing and rhus tox. will often be thought of, especially as the pains are aggravated by wet and stormy weather. If rhus has frequently helped attacks but has not prevented recurrence, tub. bov. should be remembered. Heat locally relieves these aches and pains. A more detailed account of the relationship between rhus tox. and tuberculinum will be given under the description of the special symptomatology of the potentised tuberculinum prepared from a residual emulsion of Koch's bacillus.

As with sulphur, the muscular exertion of standing is worse to endure than any other : the patient feels he must move about.

Skin

The skin is apt to itch, but scratching worsens the condition. Eruptions are mostly vague and indefinite but may resemble erythema nodosum. Burnett noted a marked susceptibility to parasitic affections like ringworm, tinea versicolor, etc., in patients that did well on tuberculinum. He generally prescribed and valued it as a remedy for ringworm, using his preparation bacillinum. Clarke stresses an eczematous thickening of the margins of the eyelids as an indication for bacillinum and notes a general time aggravation : worse at night and early morning, but when there is a tubercular background and in actual tuberculosis of the lungs, the sluggish rather than the acute cases, where free muco-purulent bronchial secretion complicates phthisis, he finds it particularly valuable. Tubercle bacilli have been found in old chronic bronchitic cases sometimes with, of course, other organisms. These would be suitable cases for bacillinum, but being a mixed nosode, it would not be contra-indicated by the absence of actual T.B. There is sweating on the slightest exertion and at night. The sweat stains the linen yellow.

Summary of Modalities

Tuberculinum is specially indicated in delicate narrow-chested individuals who are easily fatigued, nervous, and have poor power of recuperation. There is a characteristic changefulness in the symptoms both physical and mental, and symptoms tend to begin suddenly and cease suddenly.

The subject is very susceptible to changes in the weather, to cold dampness and draughts and particularly to every electrical change in the atmosphere. Though he is chilly he longs for fresh air and opens windows, he feels better for example when riding in a strong wind. Most tuberculiniques feel worse at the seaside and an aggravation from sea air is a feature of the drug.

Being physically slack and easily tired his complaints are worsened by exertion and standing, though there is a general aggravation after sleep. He is sensitive both physically and emotionally, an example of the former is seen in the readiness with which he takes cold on the slightest exposure, of the latter in his sensitiveness to music.

This is a powerful constitutional remedy, and when other polycrests act only for a short period and such remedies have to be changed frequently, tuberculinum is a drug to be considered and given if the symptoms agree.

Outstanding Indications for the Lesser-known Tuberculins

In the above outline of the symptomatology of tuberculinum, the characteristics of bacillinum, tuberculinum prepared from a tubercular abscess and tuberculinum bovinum have been grouped together. Other preparations have been used, however, and some knowledge of their individual indications have accumulated. We propose to outline these briefly.

Tuberculin of Koch. This was one of Clarke's favourite remedies for the after effects of influenza vying with psorinum. He thus endorses Kent's association of the two nosodes. Years ago, before the high temperature treatment of general paralysis of the insane was tried, Jauregg of Vienna gave tuberculin injections to insane patients. There appeared to be a steady

clearing up of mental confusion in a number of cases and Clarke
thought that potencies of tuberculinum should not be forgotten
in insanity if there were any other symptoms suggesting it.
Clarke records symptoms of weariness and aching in the limbs
and joints but is less insistent than Kent on the general relief
from movement. Much of his general symptomatology is
clearly taken from actual T.B. cases of glands, joints, lungs,
larynx, etc., and he would naturally give it in tuberculosis, not
as a rule in the acute manifestations but when a chronic case
seemed to need a stimulus.

Patients suggesting potencies of Koch's tuberculin do not
readily put on weight in spite of all efforts that are made with
suitable dietary. There is a tendency to digestive disturbances,
accompanied by a bad taste in the mouth and bad breath.

There is an aversion to food, especially sweets, and he
experiences nausea at the sight or smell of food, even cold milk,
which he desires, nauseates him.

Attacks of offensive diarrhœa are usual and the urine may be
offensive, the odour suggesting the presence of B.C.C.

Apart from these special symptoms, there are few other
indications which would lead the physician to give Koch's
preparation rather than the more familiar bacillinum or tub.
bov.

Residual Tuberculinum of Koch. We are indebted to Dr.
Vannier's observations for the record of the special indications
for this tuberculinum. He considers this preparation is of more
value than others in the subject who has recovered from an
attack of tuberculosis but who is still under the influence of the
tubercular toxin in the system. In these patients the reaction
of the body to the toxin is usually of an arthritic order and
results in the production of fibrous formation : for example,
induration round the joints or tendon contractions. In such
cases, Dr. Vannier believes, should a potency of the residual
tuberculinum be given, the body will be stimulated in such a
way that symptoms will appear indicating rhus tox., which can
then be given with great benefit. Again, he would think of this
remedy for old tubercular patients who later on develop a
periodic complaint such as migraine, and in general he appears
to regard the patient who requires the residual preparation as
very much more frail than the average candidate for tuber-

culinum. Patients look pale and ill, with pale bluish lips. They are incapable of leading any but the quietest of lives and any slight emotional or physical upset may precipitate some acute attack.

Aviaire. This is one of the least potent of the tuberculins and has come to be thought of for individuals who display a persistent tendency to "take cold." It has a real value as a prophylactic for this susceptibility to germs of catarrh. The same may be said of the serum of Marmorek which can be repeated with little danger of reaction more frequently than some of the other tuberculins. This may be of advantage when continuous infection is prevalent for people constantly exposed to it. Bacillinum is another excellent prophylactic against colds, and can be combined to advantage with influenzinum. Aviaire has also helped in advanced pulmonary cases where it would be dangerous to use a more active preparation for fear of producing a harmful reaction, but where the patient benefits from a milder stimulus. Its prophylactic virtue is less effective. It has also been regarded as a valuable remedy in influenzal bronchitis and in some cases of bronchitis following measles.

Serum of Marmorek. A potency of this serum may be given with benefit to patients who react badly to other remedies and at the same time show progressive wasting. Not only is it effective as a prophylactic for the common cold but also for the treatment of inexplicable febrile attacks where there are no obvious physical signs to account for them. We recall the case of a young women who suffered from intermittent fever and vague joint and bone pains for several months, but after receiving the apparently indicated remedies without result, a rapid improvement was experienced after the administration of this serum in potency. There is some resemblance to sulphur in its pathogenesis. The skin is rough expecially the skin of the back, the lips red and the tongue dry, red and furrowed.

Tuberculin of Denys. Of the serum of Denys we have little experience, but our French colleagues have a place for it in the type of individual who, though of tubercular tendency, has good reactions and often does not appear ill. Indeed he may be of a florid, large, even fat, appearance, though he is easily wearied on exertion which may induce pyrexia. Sudden attacks of weakness and great depression at irregular intervals develop or a sudden anorexia and gastric disturbances with nausea, vomiting and diarrhœa. Pulse tension is persistently low. Sudden illnesses with no obvious cause, whether coryza, headache, vomiting and diarrhœa, in subjects apparently in good health, are considered to be indications.

The Tuberculin of Rosenbach has never become well known to practitioners and has received less fame than perhaps it deserves. In lupus particularly it has helped considerably and under it we have seen a case recover from a condition which presented every symptom of acute pulmonary miliary tuberculosis. We hesitate to make the definite claim that it was a case of this disease, as recovery was complete and permanent, but no symptom was lacking in the picture to suggest that diagnosis. There was temporary amelioration from tuberculin in potency, itself a suggestive sign, and when the Rosenbach tuberculin was given (hypodermically, not in potency) response was immediate and recovery thereafter uninterrupted. It is put on record here for further observation and testing on similar cases. The preparation might be worth remembering in tubercular meningitis.

Dosage

Potencies from 30 upwards are most commonly used for all tuberculins. Burnett used bacillinum mostly in the 200th, many physicians prefer the 1m and upwards especially for the tuberculinique and apyretic cases of phthisis. In phthisical cases complicated with a mixed infection, Nebel advises the administration of a single dose of tuberculinum 1m which he claims will clear the case so that a syndrome will present which will permit the accurate choice of an antipsoric. Should a relapse occur after the antipsoric treatment, he prefers to follow up the treatment by the administration of a high potency of a nosode corresponding to the most virulent organism found in the sputum, staphylococcin, streptococcin, pneumococcin or whatever. He summarises the treatment of phthisis as follows : "Accurate bacteriological analysis of the sputum is essential ; the choice of the nosode (tuberculinum in the first place and later such nosodes as streptococcin if present in quantity in the sputum) clears up the picture, and so proceeding on the one side etiologically, on the other side symptomatically with antipsoric remedies, the disease is dominated." On the other hand, many physicians hold the view that the incautious use of the higher potencies may result in a severe and even dangerous aggravation of symptoms and consider any potency above the 30th to be deprecated for the initial dose when lung or larynx is affected, if indeed they employ the nosode in these cases at all.

The repetition of tuberculinum must always be most carefully watched and only infrequently repeated. Tuberculinum is called for to treat many conditions in childhood and here more frequent repetition may be made than on adults. Dr. Fergie Woods believes that tuberculinum needs more frequent repetition in children's complaints than almost any other " chronic " remedy. Dr. Borland recently recorded a mode of administration of tuberculinum to children adopted by some American physicians who recommend the giving of doses of increasing potencies of tuberculinum from the 1*m* to the *cm*—two of 1*m*, two of 10*m*, two of 50*m* and two of *cm*. These are given on successive days, two doses of the 1*m* on the first day and so onwards to the end.

VERATRUM ALBUM

The White Hellebore. Tincture made from the root-stocks (plants of Alps and Pyrenees) early in June, before flowering.

Hellebore was a drug largely used in the ancient world, and the Greek physicians appear to have used both the white (veratrum album) and the black (the Christmas rose, helleborus niger), but principally the white, the subject of this chapter. The two plants are classified in different natural orders and have different pathogeneses.

Hahnemann wrote a once-famous essay on the " Helleborism of the Ancients," and in it discussed the old use of the drug as an " evacuant." It used to be taken in large doses as a regular " cure " in spring and (less frequently) in autumn. Mental and nervous diseases were held to be specially suitable for its action, but many other disorders were treated by it. The dosage was large and the risks of the treatment considerable.

Lewin (" Die Nebenwirkungen der Arzneimittel) speaks of the local use of veratrin (alkaloid of v. album) as producing an occasional local redness and swelling, with pricking, burning sensation and neuralgia, not only locally but in parts of the body far removed from the actual application. A rash may appear erythematous, petechial, rarely vesicular or pustular. Taken internally, salivation may occur with subsequent dryness of the mouth ; loss of appetite, burning pain and vomiting are constant. Children are specially susceptible. Abdominal pain and diarrhœa (choleraic) are common symptoms. A slowing of the pulse rate is very characteristic and may lead on to collapse. Fainting is a prominent symptom. The heart muscle appears to be affected harmfully. The patient is pale with dilated pupils : cold sweats and cramps are frequent.

These are the cruder symptoms of the drug. The provings fully confirm them and lead to more precise indications. Veratrum album produces a picture of collapse with prostration, coldness, blueness, accompanied by profuse discharges and such symptoms call strongly for the use of this remedy.

A. Copiousness of Discharges

The former use of veratrum album as an evacuant provides the keynote to the general symptom that the discharges are copious. This applies to the vomit, the diarrhœa, the sweat, the urine. If there is salivation, it, too, will be profuse. So rapidly does the body lose water in these ways that symptoms of collapse appear, faintness, rapid exhaustion and prostration ; the skin becomes blue and cold, the face " hippocratic," and, as always when much fluid is lost, violent cramps are experienced. Needless to add, these symptoms make ver. alb. one of the great remedies for cholera and choleriac diarrhœas ; especially the cold sweat, the copious evacuations (vomiting *as well as* diarrhœa) and collapse call for it.

B. Coldness

Coldness of the whole body ; rigors and frequent shiverings ; *cold sweat on the forehead* or elsewhere ; skin cold and blue. In spite of the coldness, external heat does not relieve, but, if anything, aggravates the symptoms. This group of phenomena recalls camphor, but the copious discharges of ver. alb. serve to distinguish its pathogenesis from that of camphor.

C. Frequent Fainting

This is not only to be noted as a result of the collapse following the evacuations, but is characteristic of the drug when these violent symptoms are less marked. Thus veratrum album may be applicable to fainting following emotional stress or exertion. It is due probably (as Lewin suggests) to a direct effect on the heart muscle. Characteristically the pulse is slow and weak and the blood pressure is low and veratrum alb. has a definite place as a heart remedy for the cardiac effects of severe or prolonged illness. Cases where cratægus is valuable will often benefit by some doses of ver. alb. The patients show the characteristic coldness, but are worse from heat.

D. Mental Symptoms

These have a special interest in view of the ancient uses of ver. alb., and indeed Hippocrates noted that "Hellebore can cause madness and sometimes can cure it." The symptoms that suggest this drug are characteristically violent : Violent delirium, violent mania, destructive, lascivious and frequently accompanied by filthy habits (eating fæces and so forth). Religious excitement may be present and sexual symptoms are more common still. Nearly always the diagnosis of the remedy will be clinched by some of the symptoms from the foregoing groups and the choice would be confirmed by coldness : collapse and other general symptoms of the drug. Thus stramonium presents violent mental symptoms as does belladonna, but neither of these shows the characteristic pale, cold, sweating skin of ver. alb. On the contrary, the face is red and congested. The violent attacks characteristic of ver. alb. often alternate with sullen silences, but the silences do not mark cessations of the violent emotions, for if disturbed the patient may break out most furiously.

When these characteristic symptom groups are remembered, the indications for ver. alb. are not likely to be overlooked. There are a variety of subsidiary symptoms not likely to be found without some at least of the more important mentioned above, but leading to valuable uses of the drug. Thus, there is a form of constipation that ver. alb. will relieve where the stool is hard and large, perhaps in rounded black lumps, with frequent urging and colic somewhat as with nux vom., but distinguished by cold sweat, faintness and prostration and worsening from heat.

Further, ver. alb. is a marked cause of pain and will relieve all kinds of neuralgias (trigeminal, sciatic, etc.) and headaches : it will also help dysmenorrhœa, when prostration and perhaps vomiting and cold sweat are present. Heat worsens always ; the pain compels the patient to move about, but no relief follows. This sometimes is noted with pains referred to joints and fasciæ (so-called rheumatic) and worsening from damp is an additional indication. When dysmenorrhœa is violent and gives rise to emotional disturbances of a violent nature, the drug is particularly useful. Ver. viride frequently relieves dysmenorrhœal pains.

In the respiratory sphere there is a marked, irritable tickling, referred to the region behind the sternum and causing violent cough.

In many ways the drug is suited best to cases occurring at the extremes of life, childhood and old age. Thin, choleric subjects respond to it well and emotional persons generally.

The green hellebora (veratrum viride) has not been very extensively proved but has been found very useful in certain cases of pneumonia. Some American observers claim to have shown how the drug can raise the opsonic index to the pneumococcus. The cases that need it are acute, with a tendency to violent delirium, marked throbbing of arteries of which the patient is very conscious and a tongue heavily coated but with a red streak down the middle.

THERAPEUTIC INDEX
AND REPERTORY

It has been repeatedly stated that the homœopathic physician, in his approach to drug therapeutics, does not place emphasis on disease entities but rather on the reactions of the body to disease.

To these reactions and symptoms shown by the sick individual, he exhibits a remedy which is known to have produced similar reactions and symptoms in the healthy.

Nevertheless, as this approach is unfamiliar to the orthodox inquirer for whom this book is intended, the following index of disease reactions is appended.

But this is for the purpose of directing attention to the more usual remedies used for any specific illness and also with a view to *reorientating the outlook* of the inquirer to the homœopathic technique.

This index, we believe, will indicate the *method* by which the curative remedy is chosen to treat the sick.

Naturally, as the volume only includes thirty-eight remedies, the following list cannot be regarded as exhaustive.

Its value lies in the fact that the indications for a prescription are made easily available for some of the more usual drugs in a number of disease conditions.

THERAPEUTIC INDEX
AND REPERTORY

GENERAL SYMPTOMATOLOGY

Anæmia
secondary
(following
hœmorrhages) China, 152
Ferrum
Met., 171
Ferrum,
Phos., 174
Manganum, 227
Phosph., 270
Puls., 282
Nat. Mur, 246

Anæsthesia
to combat the
effects of Ant. Tart., 65
Phosph, 262, 263

Asthma
onset 2–4 a.m.
Must sit up
and bend for-
wards Kali Carb., 196
ameliorated by
mountain air Lueticum, 216
ameliorated by
sea air Medorrhinum, 235

Asymmetry
of various organs
of body Lueticum, 217
Ant. tart, 69

Backache
aggravates—
pressure Kali Carb, 196.
ameliorates—
pressure Nat. Mur, 249
Rhus,
Sepia,

Cancer
Arg. Met., 85
Cartilage
hypertrophy Arg. Met., 85

Chorea
Constipation Cimicifuga, 154
ameliorates Calc. Carb., 137
Bryonia, 127
Lycopodium, 224
alternating with
diarrhœa Mercury, 237, 238
Nat. Mur., 247
Nux vom., 256
with much strain-
ing Sepia, 296
with hard stools
frequent urg-
ing and pro-
stration Veratrum alb., 351

Diarrhœa
exhausting, pain-
less, profuse.
Dehydration Phosphorus, 269
cold drinks aggra-
vate Ars. Alb., 101
fœtid with ex-
haustion Baptisia, 107
from exposure to
cold Calc. Carb., 135
during dentition Chamomilla, 141
on beginning to
eat Ferrum. Met., 172
with exhaustion Ars. Alb., 101
no relief experi-
enced from
stools Mercury, 243

Ear Affections
Aconite, 50
Chamomilla, 142
China, 144
Manganum, 230
Pulsatilla, 281
Silica, 303
Sulphur, 315

Epilepsy
*post-menstrual
epileptic* Lueticum, 213
Eating
*aggravation of
abdominal
symptoms* Sepia, 295

Food Aggravations
Alcohol, Ignatia, 184
coffee, Ignatia, 184
milk, Ars. Alb., 100
Pulsatilla, 281
Silica, 302
*stimulants (beverages, spirits,
narcotics)* Chamomilla, 138
tea Thuja, 323
eggs Ferrum. Met., 172
food, rich, *aggravates* Pulsatilla, 281
Silica, 302
*fruits, watery,
aggravates* Ars. Alb., 100
oysters aggravate Lycopodium, 223
sweets aggravate Lycopodium, 223
Fevers
diphtheria Apis, 73
Baptisia, 105
Lachesis, 201
*diphtheria with
prostration* Manganum, 228
Mercury, 242
Exanthemata
*measles with
nerve symptoms* Gelsemium, 178
*with otitis
media* Pulsatilla, 281
scarlet fever Apis, 73
Baptisia, 105
Belladonna, 114
Pulsatilla, 281
Rhus, 284
*associated with
nerve symptoms* Gelsenium, 178
hectic Ars. Alb., 96
Phosphorus, 271
influenza Baptisia, 107
Bryonia, 123
Gelsemium, 178, 179
Rhus Tox, 285
intermittent China, 151
Natrum Mur, 250
malaria Rhus Tox, 285
Sulphur, 314

Exanthemata—*contd.*
rheumatic Aconite, 52
violent onset Aconite, 46
sudden exposure to cold Belladonna, 120
Bryonia, 125
Ferrum Phos., 176
enteric Baptisia, 105, 109
Bryonia, 123
Gelsmium, 180
Lachesis, 201
Rhus Tox, 285
of violent onset Aconite, 46

**Gastro-intestinal
Affections**
Baptisia, 107
*sensitive to light
touch but hard
pressure relieves* China, 151
Lycopodium, 223
*aggravations
from drinking
iced water* Aconite, 50
*nausea and
vomiting
with thirst-
lessness* Ant. Tart, 66
*relieved by
vomiting* Ant. Tart., 66
Exophthalmic
goitre Natrum Mur, 246
Gonorrhœa Medorrhinum, 231, 232, 235
Thuja, 320

Headache
*aggravations,
cold,* China, 149
Silica, 302
*cold dry winds
in the plethoric type,* Aconite, 49
Ameliorates,
cold, Ars. Alb., 99
Bryonia, 124
Cimicifuga, 153
Lycopodium, 221
Phosphorus, 267
Sepia, 293
worse lying, Belladonna, 116
Mercury,
Platinum,
Rhus Tox.,

Headache—*contd.*

movement aggra-	
vates	Bryonia, 124
pressure aggra-	
vates	China, 149
pressure amelio-	
rates	Apis, 170
	Arg. Met., 83
	Bryonia, 124
gradual pressure	
ameliorates	Belladonna, 116
worse thunder	Sepia, 293
associated with	
pelvic condi-	
tions	Cimicifuga, 153
with disturbances	
of vision	Gelsemium, 178
with aura of	
flashes of light	Natrum Mur, 247
periodic	Tuberculinum, 342
ameliorates ly-	
ing with	
head high	
in bed	Gelsemium, 178
lying on pain-	
ful side	Ignatia, 184
of copious	
urination	Gelsemium, 178
	Ignatia, 184
	Silica, 302
ameliorates	
warmth	Lueticum, 215
	Silica, 300

Larynx

affections	⎱ Aconite, 51
with sudden	⎰
onset	Belladonna, 119
from exposure to	
cold	Calc. Carb., 135
laryngeal spasm	Chamomilla, 142
	China, 150
	Ignatia, 184
Leucorrhœa	Calc. Carb., 134
	Chamomilla, 142
	Cimicifuga, 145
	Ipecac., 190
	Kali Carb., 197
	Nat. Mur., 249
	Nux Vom., 258
	Sepia, 295
bland	Pulsatilla, 278
excoriating	Mercury, 244

Menses

irregular and	
scanty	Apis, 74
	Cimicifuga, 154

Menses—*contd.*

scanty	Natrum. Mur, 249
	Pulsatilla, 278
dysmenorrhœa	Apis, 74
	Belladonna, 118
	Chamomilla, 142
	Cimicifuga, 154
	Gelsemium, 180
	Ignatia, 185
	Lachesis, 207
	Nux Vom., 238
	Platinum, 271
	Pulsatilla, 278
	Veratrum Alb., 352

Nausea

accompanies all	
complaints	Ipecac., 186
with desire to	
vomit but	
vomiting	
does not take	
place	Ipecec., 186
not relieved by	
vomiting	Ipecac., 186
relieved by	
vomiting	Ant. Tart., 66
with hœmorrhage	Ipecac., 187
morning—better	
after breakfast	Sepia, 295

Œdema

with burning	
pains, cold	
ameliorated	Apis, 70

Pains

in gastric affec-	
tions relieved	
by eating	Anacardium, 62
relieved by	
warmth	Anacardium, 62
aggravated	
cold food	Anacardium, 62
Paralysis	
with tremor	Gelsemium, 178
post-diphtheretic	Gelsemium, 177, 178
following damage	
to ant. horn	
cells	Manganum, 229
Pneumonia	
early stages with	
sudden onset	Aconite, 51
	Belladonna, 119
early stage	Ferrum. Phos., 175
	Ipecac., 189

Pneumonia—*contd.*
extremes of age
periods (chil-
dren and old)   Ant. Tart, 67, 68
later stage   Ars. Alb., 102
left-sided   Lachesis, 207
especially   Bryonia, 123
   Phosphorus, 261, 270
   Sulphur, 317
   Tuberculinum, 343
unresolved   Lycopodium, 225

Rheumatic Conditions
   Apis, 74
   Bryonia, 125
   Cimicifuga, 153
   Ferrum, 173
sensitivity of bone   Manganum, 229
   Medorrhinum, 234, 241
worse at night and worse on movement   Mercury, 245
backache
   lumbago   Ant. Tart., 69
   better hard pressure   Sepia, 291
   occipital
   nape of neck backache }   Baptisia, 107
   limbs   Baptisia, 107
chr. arthritis   Lueticum, 216
gonorrhœal arthritis (movement relieves, heat aggravates   Thuja, 327

Septicæmia
   Baptisia, 105
   Lachesis, 201, 208
Skins
acnœ   Natrum Mur., 248
acnœ and furunculosis   Silica, 299
alopœcia   Ars. Alb., 103
   Lueticum, 215
brittle nails   Natrum Mur., 248
callosities   Natrum Mur., 248
defluvium capitis and grey hair   Lycopodium, 222
defluvium capitis   Ars. Alb., 103
dyshidrosis   Ars. Alb., 103

Skins—*contd.*
eruptions
   infectious exanthemata, e.g., variola and vaccinea   Thuja, 321, 323
   bullous, e.g., impetigo   Ant. Tart., 69
   bullous and vesicular, e.g., pemphigus, herpetiform lesions, warty excrescences, e.g., lichen planus   Anacardium, 61
   macular, papular   Lueticum, 215
   never itch   Lueticum, 216
   itching worse for the warmth of bed   Mercury, 237
   pustular   Ant. Tart., 68
   eczema—burning itching worse at night   Ars. Alb., 103
   secondary infections ulceration
   erythmata   Belladonna, 114
   erysipelas and erysipeloid rashes   Apis, 72
      Belladonna, 114
      Rhus, 285
   erythema nodosum   Manganum, 229
   exaggerated formications   Coca, 163
   ulcers and gummata   Lueticum, 215, 216
   ulceration and itchy at night with vesicular, pustular eruptions   Mercury, 237, 245
   herpes labialis   Natrum Mur., 248
   urticaria   Apis, 74
      Calc. carb., 137
   warts   Nat. Mur., 248
Sprains   Arnica,
      Calc. Carb., 137
      Ferrum Phos., 173
      Rhus, 285

**Teeth and Tooth-
    ache**
*aggravation
    following ex-
    posure to cold
    dry winds*   Aconite, 50
hot drinks   Chamomilla, 140
dental caries   Medorrhinum, 234.
                        Mercury, 241
                        Thuja, 234, 324

Thirst
*large quantities
    at fairly long
    intervals*   Bryonia, 124, 128
*small quantities
    frequently,
    little   and
    often*   Ars. Alb., 124
*intense for cold
    water*   Aconite, 50
*accompanied by
    hunger*   Belladonna, 117
Thirstlessness   Apis, 73
                        Ant. Tart., 66
                        Gelsemium, 180
                        Pulsatilla, 279
Thirst   Mercury, 241
*excessive for cold
    drinks, even
    iced water*   Phosphorus, 269
*more   marked
    than hunger*   Sulphur, 316

Tongue
hot, fiery   Apis, 72
red, dry   Ars. Alb., 100
*dry, cracked or
    ulcerated*   Baptisia, 107
mapped   Natrum Mur., 248
*dry, furred, yel-
    low, red streak
    and brown in
    centre*   Phosphorus, 269
*triangular,   red
    at   the   tip,
    cracked*   Rhus Tox, 286
*tongue   coated,
    sore tip*   Sepia, 295

Urinary Affections
*constant urge to
    urinate*   Aconite, 51
enuresis   Nat. Mur., 249
*nocturnal
    enuresis   in
    children*   Calc. Carb., 132
                        Rhus Tox, 286
nephritis   Apis, 73
*retention   of
    urine in chil-
    dren resulting
    from shock*   Aconite, 51
*retention—spas-
    modic*   Belladonna, 118
urethritis   Arg. Met., 84

GENERAL MODALITIES

Altitudes
*aggravates (moun-
    tain sickness)*   Coca, 162, 165
**Appearance   and
    general physical
    indications**
pale and sickly   Ant. Tart., 66
besotted   Baptisia, 104
*dark hair and
    dark   com-
    plexion*   Bryonia, 123
Child
    *light   com-
    plexion, blue
    eyed, white
    skin,   head
    sweating*   Calc. Carb., 132
Adult
    *fat, flabby,
    lacks energy*   Calc. Carb., 132

Appearance—*contd.*
    Brought on
    by
1. *emotional
    excitement*
2. *fear*
3. *exposure to
    cold*   Aconite, 51
*sallow or dingy
    yellow*   China, 149
*pallor, delicate
    skin,   malar
    flush on exer-
    tion or excite-
    ment*   Ferr. Phosph., 174
*face   haggard,
    puffy, flushed
    cheeks*   Kali. Carb., 197
*thin, dark, sal-
    low skin*   Lycopodium, 219

Appearance—*contd.*
*yellow, pale,
greasy-looking* Nat. Mur., 248
*lean, premature-
ly old, nervous
and melan-
choly* Nux. Vom., 256
*slender, delicate,
adolescent,
suggestive of
incipient
tubercle* Phosph., 265
*fat, soft, seden-
tary, indulg-
ing in self pity* Pulsatilla, 277
*anxious, fearful,
restless, con-
stantly chang-
ing his posi-
tion* Rhus. Tox., 284
*face sagging, sal-
low " sepia
saddle,"
" lupus ery-
thematosus "* Sepia, 291
*brunette, tall,
slim with nar-
row pelvis and
lax muscles* Sepia, 288
*weak, with re-
laxed muscle,
light com-
plexion and
fine skin* Silica, 299
*head sweat in
children* Silica, 300
*sensitive, deli-
cate, slack,
restless, lack-
ing energy* Sulphur, 311
*sickly looking,
unhealthy
skin and of
dark com-
plexion* Thuja, 323
*delicate, com-
plexion attrac-
tive, long eye-
lashes, dark
hair* Tuberculinum, 336
*face red, con-
gested* Veratrum Alb., 351
Aversions—food
bread Nat. Mur., 248
butter China, 150
coffee Calc. Carb., 136
Nat. Mur., 248
fat Pulsatilla, 281
Sepia, 295
greasy food Nat. Mur., 248

Aversions—food—*contd.*
meat Calc. Carb., 136
Ferrum Phos., 175
Lueticum, 216
Rhus Tox., 286
milk Ant. Tart., 67
Ferrum Phos., 175
Chilled suddenly
in warm
weather,
brings on symp-
toms Pulsatilla, 279
Cold *in general
aggravates* Anacardium, 62
Arg. Met., 86
Ars. Alb., 94, 103
Baptisia, 107
Belladonna, 113
Calc. carb., 131,
135
China, 151
Cimicifuga, 156
Coca, 165
Ferrum Met., 171
Ignatia, 184
Kali Carb., 194
Lueticum, 215
Lycopodium, 222
Manganum, 230
Nat. Mur., 246, 247
Nux. Vom., 255
*except head and
stomach com-
plaints* Phosphorus, 261
Sepia, 291
*aggravates all
symptoms* Silica, 301
Sulphur, 313
Thuja, 321
Tuberculinum, 344
Cold and heat ex-
tremes
aggravate Ipecac., 191
Lueticum, 213
Mercury, 240
Nat. Mur., 247
Coldness with rigors
but external
heat does not
relieve Veratrum Alb., 350
Cold damp weather
aggravates Ant. Tart., 69
Thuja, 321
*aggravate rheu-
matic symp-
toms, especi-
ally lumbago* Ars. Alb., 103
Calc. Carb., 131,
135

Cold damp winds
and weather   Rhus. Tox., 284

C o l d   d a m p
weather   Manganum, 230

Cold drinks
aggravation   Ars. Alb., 100

Cold food
sweets   Mercury, 242
   Tuberculinum, 346
tobacco   Calc. Carb., 136
   Ignatia, 184

Bath aggravates
symptoms   Sepia, 296
   Sulphur, 314

Coitus aggravates
symptoms   Kali Carb., 197

Contradictory
symptoms   Ignatia, 181

Discharge, onset of,
ameliorates   Lachesis, 202

Desires
abnormal food
(children—
capricious
diet)   Calc. Carb., 136
acids   Ant. Tart., 67
alcohol   Coca, 164
bitter food   Sepia, 295
bread   Nat. Mur., 248
eggs   Calc. Carb., 136
fats   Arsenic, 100
   Nux Vom., 257
   Sulphur, 316
lemon   Belladonna, 117
milk   Apis, 73
   for cold milk Rhus Tox., 286
oysters   Apis, 73
   Calcarea, 136
   Lachesis, 206
   Lycopodium, 223
   Nat. Mur., 248
   Rhus. Tox., 286
pungent foods   Aconite, 50
   Sepia, 295
salt   Nat. Mur., 248
   Phosp., 261, 267
   Ferrum Phos., 175
   Medorrhinum, 235
   Thuja, 325
   Veratrum, 349
sour milk   Calc. Carb., 136
   Sepia, 295
seasoned a n d
spicy food   Sepia, 295
(vinegar)   Sulphur, 316
s p i r i t o u s
liquors   Lueticum, 216
   Sulphur, 308, 316

Desires—*contd.*
stimulants of all
kinds   Nux Vom., 357
sweets   Kali Carb., 136
   Lycopodium, 223
   Medorrhinum, 235
   Rhus Tox., 286
   Sepia, 295
   Sulphur, 316

Aversion from
meat   Rhus Tox., 286

Electrical atmo-
spheric disturb-
ances   Medorrhinum, 235
   Phosphorus, 266
   Rhus Tox., 284
   Sepia, 293
   Tuberculinum, 345

Fatigue
after slight exer-
tion   Ferr. Met., 171

Heat
aggravates   Aconite, 53
   Ant. Tart., 69
   Apis., 70, 72
   Lachesis, 203
   Nat. Mur., 247
   Pulsatilla, 279
all forms of heat
but sometimes
w a r m d r y
weather suits
them   Sulphur, 314
humid heat
aggravates   Baptisia, 109
   Gelsemium, 181
   Lachesis, 203
heat and heat in
bed aggravate   Thuja, 328

Motion
movement aggra-
vates   Ant. Tart., 69
   Baptisia, 107
even slightest   Bryonia, 122, 123
in heart con-
ditions   Gels., 180
   Ignatia, 184
   Manganum, 230
   Tuberculinum, 344
m o v e m e n t
ameliorates   Arg. Met., 86
   Chamomilla, 142
   Lycopodium, 222
   Rhus Tox., 283
   Thuja, 327
gentle movement   Ferrum Met., 173
   Ferrum Phos., 176
   Pulsatilla, 280

Motion—*contd.*

mo v e m e n t — *gradual*	Silica, 298
m o v e m e n t — *vigorous*	Sepia, 291
m o v e m e n t — *rapid in* open-air, *walking or riding*	Coca, 165
Worse beginning to move	Anacardium, 55
	Rhus Tox., 283
	Sepia, 291
Worse—movement but restless	Phosphorus, 267
Night. *Symptoms worse in bed*	Aconite, 53
Open-air—*better*	Apis, 74
	Lycopodium, 221, 222
	Pulsatilla, 279
	Sulphur, 313

Pains

ameliorated by cold	Apis, 70
	Chamomilla, 138
	Sulphur, 314
heat ameliorates	Ars. Alb., 94
	Phosph., 267
	Belladonna, 113
pressure amelio-rated	Bryonia, 128
hard pressure ameliorated	Ignatia, 184
come and go sud-denly	Belladonna, 114
worse at night— worse with heat of bed	Sulphur, 314
	Thuja, 328
small spots — pains	Thuja, 324
stitching and cutting	Kali Carb., 194
unaffected by rest or move-ment	Kali Carb., 194
aggravated — ly-ing on affected side	Kali Carb., 194
Periodicity of com-plaints	Ars. Alb., 94
	China, 149
	Ipecac., 191
	Nat. Mur., 248
aggravation of symptoms — twelve hourly, e.g., noon and midnight	Sulphur, 314

Posture

worse lying down	Ant. Tart., 69
worse—standing	Calc. Carb., 137
worse—lying on the affected side	Kali Carb., 194
ameliorates—ly-ing on the abdomen	Medorrhinum, 235
ameliorates—ly-ing unaffected side	Belladonna, 122
ameliorates—ly-ing affected side	Bryonia, 122
with head up-lying	Gelsemium, 178
better sitting up	Ant. Tart., 69

Pressure

aggravates, ex-cept head symptoms	Apis., 70
	Lachesis, 203
	Kali Carb., 194
ameliorates	Bryonia, 122
	China, 152
hard pressure	Ignatia, 184
Prostration with cold clammy sweat	Ant. Tart., 65
out of all pro-portion to physical ail-ment	Ars. Alb., 94, 95
with coldness, c o l l a p s e, c r a m p s, c y a n o s i s	Veratrum Alb., 350, 352

Rest

relieves	Anacardium, 55
worse	Silica, 298
Restlessness	
fear, anxiety, tension	Aconite, 49
as a result of bodily suffer-ing	Apis, 70
as a result of anxiety and fear (mental) *but with low tension*	Ars. Alb., 94, 98
anxiety with prostration	Ant. Tart., 66
restlessness	Ferrum Met., 173
restlessness due to physical symptoms	Rhus, 284
fidgety	Medorrhinum, 234

Sea-air
 aggravates Ars. Alb., 103
 Nat. Mur., 247
 seashore Lueticum, 218
 Tuberculinum,
 345
 amelioration Medorrhinum, 218,
 235
Sleep
 aggravates Apis, 75
 Arg. Met., 77, 86
 after sleep Lachesis, 201, 202
 Sepia, 296
 Sulphur, 314
 Tuberculinum,
 345
 ameliorates,
 even after a
 short sleep Phosph., 268
 wakes early —
 dreams falling
 from height Thuja, 323
Sweating
 ameliorates Bryonia, 128
Stimulants and
 drugs Chamomilla, 138
Sexual
 power
 diminished Lycopodium, 225
 increased desire,
 p o w e r
 diminished Phosphorus, 268
 hypersensitivity Platinum, 274
 apathy Sepia, 289
 aversion to
 coitus which
 is often pain-
 ful Sepia, 289
 indifferent to
 husband Sepia, 289
Side
 left Lachesis, 201, 202
 right Lycopodium, 221
 Phosphorus, 267
Time aggravations
 midnight, at Aconite, 53
 Ferrum Met., 173
 after Ars. Alb., 94
 Nux Vom., 259
 2–3 a.m. Calc. Carb., 134
 2–4 a.m. Kali Carb., 194
 3 a.m. Ant. Tart., 69
 Thuja, 328
 Bryonia, 122
 10 a.m. Nat. Mur., 247
 11 a.m. Sulphur, 313
 forenoon Sepia, 296
 (headache) noon Arg. Met., 83

Time aggravations—*contd.*
 late afternoon
 4–8 p.m. Lycopodium, 220
 3–5 p.m. Apis, 71
 3 p.m. Thuja, 328
 3–4 p.m. Belladonna, 120
 evening Sepia, 296
 9 p.m. Bryonia, 122
 9 p.m., maximum
 aggravation Chamomilla, 142
 twilight and dark-
 ness, mid-
 night Phosphorus, 266,
 267
 twilight — after
 midnight Puls., 281
 night
 amelioration
 after sunset Coca, 165
 aggravation,
 sunset to sun-
 rise Mercury, 241
 Lueticum, 210, 215
 sunrise to sun-
 set Medorrhinum, 232
 aggravation—
 night Rhus, 284
 Sulphur, 314
 Tuberculinum, 344
Touch
 aggravation Apis, 70
 Belladonna, 114
 tactile hypersen-
 sitivity Lachesis, 201
 light touch—
 aggravates Ignatia, 184
 amelioration Calc. Carb., 137
 Phosphorus, 266
 aversion to touch Chamomilla, 140
 from Medorrhinum,
 233
Thunder
 aggravates Gelsemium, 181
 Phosphorus, 266
 Sepia, 293
 Tuberculinum, 345
Waking
 aggravation of
 symptoms Apis, 75
 Baptisia, 107
 Lachesis, 201
 of emotional
 symptoms Lycopodium, 221
 Medorrhinum,
 232
Warmth in general
 aggravates Aconite, 53
 Apis, 70, 72
 Bryonia, 128

Winds
  aggravate,
    exposure   to
      cold   Aconite, 53
      dry winds   Bryonia, 122
      cold damp   Calc. Carb., 131
Weather
  aggravates   Arsenic, 103

Weather—aggravates—
  contd.   Mercury, 240
                    Rhus, 284
  ameliorates   Medorrhinum, 234
  damp   aggra-
    vates   Rhus Tox., 284
  cold winds aggra-
    vate   Rhus Tox., 284

DISTURBED EMOTIONAL REACTIONS

Anger   Anacardium, 56
                   Argentum. Metal-
                     lic, 83
                   Ars. Alb., 97
                   Bryonia, 123
                   Phosph., 266
                   Chamomilla, 139
  violent   Ferrum Phos., 174
                   Sepia, 289
  complaints from Chamomilla, 139
  complaints fol-
    ing *fear and
    fright*   Apis, 71
  in zealous, pre-
    cise *persons* Nux Vomica, 255
Anticipation   Anacardium, 58
                   Argent. Met., 83
                   Gelsemium, 177
                   Lycopodium, 219
                   Medorrhinum, 233
  better rest   Manganum, 229
Apathy   Apis, 71
                   Sepia, 288
                   Sulphur, 305
  alternating with
    irritability   Sepia, 290
  *alternating with
    emotional
    hypersen-
    sitivity*   China, 149
Anxiety   Aconite, 49
                   Apis, 71
  with restlessness Ars. Alb., 95
                   Cimicifuga, 152
                   Kali Carb., 195
  with prostration Ant. Tart., 66
Anxious tension   Aconite, 49
Bashful   Coca, 164
Capriciousness
  *wanting this or
    that*   Chamomilla, 140·
Company
  *aggravates symp-
    toms*   Anacardium, 56
                   Ant. Tart., 66
                   Bryonia, 123

Company—
  *Aggravates symp-
    toms—contd.*   China, 148
                   Ferrum Phos., 174
                   Natrum Mur., 247
                   Lycopodium, 219
  *prefers
    darkness*   Coca, 164
    solitude   Coca, 164
  ameliorates,   Pulsatilla, 274
Compulsion
  " *washing   the
    hands* "   Lueticum, 214
  " *fixed idea* " Silica, 214, 300
                   Thuja, 323
Concentration
  lack of   Calc. Carb., 134
                   Ferrum Phos., 174
  *and   shirking
    responsibility* Silica, 300
                   Sulphur, 305
Confidence
  *want   of   self-
    confidence*   Arg. Met., 77
Confusion
  *mind wanders,
    stuporous*   Baptisia, 107
Consolation
  aggravate   Argent. Met., 78
                   Natrum Mur.,
                     247
  amelioration   Chamomilla, 139
                   Pulsatilla, 277
                   Sepia, 289
  *contrasted with
    Pulsatilla*   Silica, 302
Control
  lack of   Chamomilla, 138
Day dreams   Sulphur, 312
Dulness
  *slow   mentally
    but painstaking* Calc. Carb., 131,
                     132, 133
Excitement   in
  fevers
  amelioration of Aconite, 51
  light food   Belladonna, 115

Difficulty of ex-
pression
answers slowly Medorrhinum, 233
enuresis in chil-
children   Rhus, 286
            Sepia, 294
Fastidiousness   Ars. Alb., 99
            Nux Vom., 256
Fear, fright and
anger
*complaints fol-
lowing*   Apis, 71
            Cimicifuga, 153
*following dis-
appointments
in affections* Cimicifuga, 152
            Gelsemium, 177
            Ignatia, 183
Fear   Sepia, 290
Fears,
of being alone   Ars. Alb., 95
            Kali Carb., 195
            Phosphorus, 266
of crowd   Ferrum Phos.,
            174
of darkness   Calc. Carb., 132
            Phosph., 266
of death   Aconite, 49
            Bryonia, 123
            Cimicifuga, 152
            Ferrum Phos., 174
            Phosphorus, 266
*of failure in
work, e.g.,
examination* Anacardium, 56,
            58
            Silica, 300
of insanity   Lueticum, 214
of misfortune Ferrum Phos., 174
of solitude   Lycopodium, 219
of thunder   Gelsemium, 181
            Nat. Mur., 247
            Phosphorus, 266
*of violent and
sudden onset* Aconite, 47
lying   down
ameliorates   Manganum, 229
*of something is
going to hap-
pen with rest-
lessness*   Ars. Alb., 98
better rest   Manganum, 229
Fixed ideas   Silica, 300
*melancholy and
depression
sion leading
to fixed ideas* Thuja, 323
Hopelessness   Lueticum, 214
Hopelessness   of
recovery   Ars. Alb., 97

Hypersensitivity
emotional   Chamomilla, 139,
            140
emotional hyper-
æsthesia   China, 148
*alternating with
apathy*   Coca, 149
alternating with
physical con-
ditions   Cimicifuga, 152
            Ignatia, 182
            Nux Vomica, 255
Hurry
*behaviour   is
hasty*   Mercury, 241
            Thuja, 323
*always   in   a
hurry*   Thuja, 323
talks hastily   Thuja, 323
Inferiority
*dislikes   being
laughed at*   Calc. Carb., 132
*disposition   to
consider him-
self ill-used*   China, 148
Ill-humour
better alone   Ant. Tart., 66
Irritability
*with dislike of
being   dis-
turbed*   Bryonia, 123
*dislike of com-
pany a n d
timidity*   Mercury, 238
with dejection Ant. Tart., 66
*peevishness i n
children*   Ant. Tart., 66
*peevishness i n
feeble consti-
tution*   Kali Carb., 195
Aversion to touch
in children   Ant. Tart., 66
            Chamomilla, 140
Impatient
rude to friends Chamomilla, 139
Indifference
to surroundings Phosphorus, 266
*alternating with
excitement*   Sepia, 289
Intellect
*intellectually
active, physi-
cally feeble*   Lycopodium, 219
Intuitive percep-
tion   Ignatia, 182
Jealousy   Lachesis, 204
Lazy   Sulphur, 312
Loquacity   Cimicifuga, 153
            Coca, 164
            Lachesis, 205

Megalomania Platinum, 273
arrogance with fear
with mental instability Platinum, 273
Memory
impaired for names Ferrum Phos., 174
Sulphur, 312
Mental
exertion aggravates Calc. Carb., 137
excitement accompanied by destructive and depraved and filthy habits Veratrum Alb., 351
Mental stress Anacardia, 106
Baptisia, 106
Music
aggravates Aconite, 50
Phosphorus, 268
Sepia, 289
Thuja, 323
Tuberculinum, 342
Moods
alternation of Ignatia, 182, 183
Phosphorus, 266
changeful disposition Pulsatilla, 276
alternation of mental and physical symptoms Platinum, 273

Moods—contd.
changefulness desires change of occupation and locality Tuberculinum, 336, 342
Sensibility of special senses increased Aconite, 50
Ars. Alb., 94
Belladonna, 113
China, 149, 152
Natrum Mur., 246
Nux Vom., 256
Phosphorus, 265
Sepia, 289
Sexual Disturbances associated with mental symptoms Platinum, 274
Tension
anxious tension Aconite, 49
irritable tension Nux Vom., 255
Unexpectedness of symptoms Ignatia, 183
Pulsatilla, 277
Vomiting
nausea and vomiting with thirstlessness Ant. Tart., 66
with prostration Ant. Tart., 66
Ars. Alb., 101
Weeping Ignatia, 182
Natrum Mur., 247
better sympathy Pulsatilla, 276
Sepia, 289

PECULIAR SYMPTOMS

As if an iron band round the head Tuberculinum, 342
As if a tight band round the forehead, drawn as it were Medorrhinum, 234
also
Ant. Tart.
Baptisia.
As if the body were brittle and would easily break Thuja, 323
As if he did not move the heart would stop Gelsemium, 180
As if he were going insane Lueticum, 214
c.f., Mancinella.

As if a nail is being driven into the head, headache pain Ignatia, 184
As if the stomach is hanging relaxed (stomach) Ipecac., 187
Wishes to throw herself from a height Gelsemium, 179
Imagines a living animal in the abdomen Thuja, 323
1. He feels there are two of him.
2. He is trying to get the two pieces together (mental confusion) Baptisia, 105

Time seems to pass quickly   Medorrhimum, 233

Time seems to pass slowly   Mercury, 241

Calcarea hand— *soft, moist, boneless, inclined to chap*   Calcarea, 131

Cheek flushed
  both   Belladonna, 140
  one   Chamomilla, 140
  (Compare *Moschus*—heat in one cheek, without redness while the other cheek is red without heat)

Cold in general relieves but sudden chill on a warm day aggravates   Pulsatilla, 279

Deafness
  difficulty to hear human voice, otherwise special senses acute   Phosphorus, 265

Dysuria
  if somebody be present   Nat. Mur., 249

Flatus
  rises from stomach as if œsophagus would be rent by force   Coca, 165

Spasm
  twitchings of muscles, e.g., Alœ Nasi   Lycopodium, 222

GENERAL INDEX

Aconite, 45
exciting causes indicating aconite, 48, 51, 52
general action on body, 45–47
homœopathic indications,
general indications, 48–53
modalities, 53
pneumonia, 51
Actæa spicata, 154
Acute disease, action of drugs in, 46–47
Alcohol, to allay craving for, 151, 211
Anacardium orientale, 54, 165–167
gastro-intestinal symptoms, 61
gross effects on body, 54
homœopathic indications,
mental symptoms, 55
respiratory tract, 62
skin, 61
Anæmia, use of china in, 148
use of ferrum in, 171
use of natrum mur. in, 246
use of pulsatilla in, 282
Antimonium tartrate, 62
general action on body, 63
homœopathic indications, 65–69
abdominal conditions, 66
backache, 69
modalities, 69
pneumonia, 68
respiratory tract, 67
skin, 68
use of, following anæsthesia, 65
Apis, 69
general action on body, 70
homœopathic indications, 70–75
alimentary tract, 72, 73
genito-urinary tract, 73
face, 72
modalities, 74, 75
skin and cellular tissues, 70, 74
Argentum metallicum, 75, 165–167
effect on cartilage, 85
effect on gonads, 80, 84
effect on nervous system, 77
homœopathic uses, 75
modalities, 86
Argentum nitricum, 58
Arndt's law, 7
Arsenicum album, 86
acute poisoning by arsenic, 87
chronic poisoning by arsenic, 87
homœopathic indications, 93
alimentary tract, 100, 101
cancer, 96, 98
face, 100

Arsenicum album—*contd.*
homœopathic indications—contd.
headache, 99
heart, 102
mental symptoms, 95, 97, 99
pain, 94
respiratory tract, 99, 102
skin, 103
time aggravation, 94
homœopathic uses, 93–104

Baptisia, 104
homœopathic indications,
febrile complaints, 104–106
influenza, 107
modalities, 109, 110
pharynx, 107
tongue, 107
typhoid fever, 108, 109
Belladonna, 110
general action on body, 110–113
homœopathic indications, 113–121
alimentary tract, 117; 118
dysmenorrhœa, 118
fevers, 121
headache, 116
mental symptoms, 115
mouth and throat, 117
pain, 114
respiratory tract, 119
scarlet fever, 114
skin, 120
Bryonia, 121
characteristics, movement, 122
secretions, 122
time aggravation, 122
weather reactions, 122
comparison with natrum mur., 128
with rhus tox., 125
homœopathic indications,
alimentary tract, 126
fevers, 124
headaches, 123
heart, 125
mental symptoms, 123
modalities, 128
pneumonia, 124
respiratory tract, 127

Calcerea carbonica, 128
general action on the body, 129–130
homœopathic indications,
alimentary tract, 136

Calcarea carbonica—*contd.*
  homœopathic indications—contd.
    genito-urinary tract, 134
    mental symptoms, 133
    modalities, 137
    respiratory tract, 135
    temperature reactions, 131
  indications for children, 131, 132
    for adults, 133
  lime starvation, 132
  pre-tubercular states, 136
Chamomilla, 138
  homœopathic indications,
    alimentary tract, 140
    dysmenorrhœa, 142
    mental characteristics, 139, 140
    otitis media, 142
    temperature reactions, 141
China, 143
  general action on the body, 143–148
  homœopathic indications,
    alimentary tract, 150
    debilitated states, 148
    headache, 149
    modalities, 151
    special senses, 149
  periodicity of, 149
  use in alcoholism, 151
  use in anæmia, 148
Chronic disease, 31, 32, 38
Cimifuga racemosa, 152
  general action on the body, 152
  homœopathic indications,
    alimentary tract, 154
    generative organs, 154
    headache, 153
    mental symptoms, 153
    pains, 153
    weather reactions, 153
Coca, 155
  general action on body, 162–163
  general considerations, 155–162
  homœopathic indications,
    genito-urinary tract, 164
    heart, 165
    mental symptoms, 164
    modalities, 165
    sensory nerves, 163
    special senses, 164
Crotalus, 200, 201–202

Dosage, homœopathic, 25
Drugs. *See* Remedy.

Elaps, 201, 202
Equisetum, 303
Erythropoiesis, function of iron in, 168

Ferrum metallicum, 168
  absorption, 169
  anæmia, use in, 168–171
  dosage of, 170
  general action on the body, 168–171
  homœopathic indications,
    alimentary tract, 172
    anæmia, 171
    general indications, 171
    genito-urinary tract, 172
    mental symptoms, 171, 172
    modalities, 173
Ferrum phosphoricum, 168, 173
  homœopathic indications,
    alimentary tract, 175
    genito-urinary tract, 176
    modalities, 176
    pleurisy, 175
    pneumonia, 175
    rheumatism, 176
Fever, 47, 48

Gelsemium, 176
  general action on the body, 176
  homœopathic indications,
    enteric fever, 180
    headache, 178
    influenza, 179
    mental symptoms, 177
    modalities, 180, 181
    neuritis, 180
    paralysis, 177–178
    respiratory tract, 179
Gonorrhœa, thuja in treatment of, 325–327

Homœopathic materia medica,
  dosage of drugs, 25
  pharmacy, 13
  potencies, preparation of, 14, 15
  sources of, 8, 13
  structure of, 8
Homœopathy, branch of therapeutics, 4, 7
  definition of, 3
  discovery of, 3
  experiment, the only test of the value of, 6
  methods of testing, 7
  principle of, 3, 7, 8
  " unconscious homœopathising," 5
Hypochromic anæmia, 169

Ignatia amara, 181
  homœopathic indications,
    alimentary tract, 185
    effects of grief, 183

Ignatia amara—*contd.*
 homœopathic indications—contd.
  general characteristics, 181,
   182, 184
  genito-urinary tract, 185
  headache, 184
  heart, 185
  mental symptoms, 182
  modalities, 185, 186
  nervous symptoms, 182
  relation to nux vomica, 181, 182,
   184
Ipecacuanha, 186
 general action on the body, 186–189
 homœopathic indications,
  alimentary tract, 189
  genito-urinary tract, 190
  mental symptoms, 191
  modalities, 191
  respiratory tract, 189, 190

Kali carbonicum, 192
 general action on the body, 192–
  194
 homœopathic indications,
  alimentary tract, 197, 198
  circulatory system, 195
  genito-urinary tract, 197
  mental symptoms, 194, 195
  modalities, 193, 199
  pains, 196, 197, 199
  respiratory system, 198, 199
  relation to arsenicum, 199
   to sepia, 195

Lachesis, 200
 effects on blood, 200
 homœopathic indications,
  alimentary tract, 206
  general characteristics, 201–
   204
  genito-urinary tract, 207
  headache, 206
  mental symptoms, 204
  respiratory tract, 207
  septicæmic states, 208
  skin, 209
 relation to lycopodium, 209
Lueticum, 209
 homœopathic indications,
  genito-urinary tract, 216
  joints, 216
  modalities, 211, 216, 217
  respiratory tract, 216
  syphilis, 210–218
 use in alcoholism, 211
Lycopodium, 218
 general characteristics, 218, 220–
  222

Lycopodium—*contd.*
 homœopathic indications,
  alimentary tract, 222, 224
  genito-urinary tract, 225
  heart, 226
  mental symptoms, 219, 221,
   224
  pains, 221
  respiratory tract, 225
  sleep, 227
  weather and temperature
   reactions, 221, 222

Macrotin, 155
Malaria, use of quinine in, 146–147
Manganum, 227
 general action on the body, 227–228
 homœopathic indications,
  alimentary tract, 230
  arthritis, 229
  mental symptoms, 229
  modalities, 230
  respiratory tract, 230
Materia medica, structure of, 8
Medorrhinum, 231
 general characteristics, 232
 homœopathic indications,
  headache, 234
  mental symptoms, 232, 233
  modalities, 232, 235
  rheumatism, 234
  teeth, 234
  temperature reactions, 235
Mercury, 236
 acute poisoning by, 236
 chronic poisoning by, 237–239
 homœopathic indications,
  alimentary tract, 242, 243
  general symptoms, 240
  genito-urinary tract, 243, 244
  joints, 245
  mental symptoms, 241
  mouth, 240
  respiratory tract, 244
  skin, 245
  special sense organs, 244
  sweat, 241, 244
  throat, 242
  tongue, 241
Mercury biniodide, 242
Mercury corrosivus, use in dysentery,
 243
Mercury cyanide, 243
Miasma, 30, 31, 309

Naja, 200, 202, 209
Natrum muriaticum, 245
 homœopathic indications,
  alimentary tract, 248

Natrum muriaticum—*contd.*
  homœopathic indications—contd.
    back, 249
    children, in, 247, 248
    eye symptoms, 248
    face, 248
    genito-urinary tract, 249
    headaches, 247
    heart, 249
    mental symptoms, 247, 250
    skin, 248, 249
    temperature reactions, 247
    time aggravation, 250
    tongue, 248
  relation to arg. nit., 251
    to bryonia, 250
    to quinine, 250
  use in anæmia, 246
Natrum sulph., 316
Nosodes, 328–333
Nux vomica, 251
  general actions on the body, 251–255
  homœopathic indications,
    alimentary tract, 256, 257, 258
    constipation, 256
    genito-urinary tract, 258
    mental symptoms, 255, 256
    respiratory tract, 258
    symptoms of spasm, 256, 257, 259
    temperature reactions, 255, 259
  tetanus, use in, 254

Pernicious anæmia, 171
Phosphorus, 260
  general action on the body, 260–264
  homœopathic indications,
    alimentary tract, 268–269
    bones, 268
    fever, 271
    general symptoms, 267, 268
    genito-urinary tract, 268
    hæmorrhages, 267, 268
    heart, 269–270
    mental symptoms, 265, 266
    organic nervous diseases, 266
    pains, 267
    respiratory tract, 270
    temperature reactions, 267, 271
    types indicating phosphorus, 265
Platinum, 271
  homœopathic indications,
    alimentary tract, 275
    genito-urinary tract, 274, 275

Platinum—*contd.*
  homœopathic indications—contd.
    headache, 274
    mental symptoms, 272, 273
    pains, 273
Potassium carbonate. *See* Kali carbonicum, 192
Potencies, experimental evidence of value of, 20
  possible action on the body of, 16–18, 21–25
Potentisation, insoluble substances, preparation of, 15
  method of preparation of potencies, 14, 15
Provings, value of clinical experience in, 10–13
Psychopathic symptoms, influence of homœopathic remedies on, 56
Pulsatilla, 276
  homœopathic indications,
    alimentary tract, 280, 281
    anæmia, 282
    ear, 281
    general reactions, 279, 281, 282
    genito-urinary tract, 278
    headache, 279
    joints, 280
    mental symptoms, 276–278
    mucous membranes, 280, 281
    temperature reactions, 279
    vertigo, 280
  relation to silica, 281

Radium bromide, 287
Remedy, acute disease, in, 37
  administration of, 35
  choice of, 26–44
  chronic disease, in, 32, 38
  given in alternation, 36
  preparation of remedies, 14
  repetition of the, 40, 41
Rhus toxicodendron, 282
  comparison with Anacardium orientale, 55
  homœopathic indications,
    alimentary tract, 286
    general symptoms, 283–284, 285
    joints, 285
    mental symptoms, 284, 285
    over-use of an organ, use of in, 285
    respiratory tract, 286
    skin, 285
    sleep, 287
  poisoning by, 282, 283
  relation to radium bromide, 287
Rhythm of life energies, 306–307

Sepia, 287
homœopathic indications,
  alimentary tract, 295
  children, use in, 290
  general symptoms, 287–289,
    290, 291, 296, 297
  genito-urinary tract, 291, 292,
    294
  headaches, 292
  mental symptoms, 288, 289
  respiratory tract, 296
  skin, 291, 297
Serpent poisons, 200
  in septicæmic states, 208
Silica, 297
homœopathic indications,
  alimentary tract, 302
  chronic inflammatory condi-
    tions, 302
  headache, 302
  mental symptoms, 300, 302
  reactions to temperature, 300,
    301
  suppuration, 301
  types indicating, 299
observations made by orthodox
  physicians on its actions, 297–
  299
relations to calcarea, 303
  to fluoric acid, 303
  to mercury, 303
  to pulsatilla, 281–303
Sodium chloride. *See* Natrum
  muriaticum, 245
Speransky, 255
Sulphur, 303
  general action on the body, 303–309
homœopathic indications,
  alimentary tract, 316
  general symptoms, 313–314
  genito-urinary tract, 317
  head, 315
  joints, fasciæ, 318
  mental symptoms, 311–312
  respiratory tract, 317
  skin, 311, 313, 319
  sleep, 319
  temperature reactions, 313
  types indicating, 311
Sycosis, 320, 322
Sycotic compound, similarity to
  medirrhinum, 236
Symptoms, aggravation of, following
  treatment, 20, 41
  complex in disease and drug
    symptoms, 34
  definition of symptoms, 2, 3

Symptoms—*contd.*
  drug symptoms, 3
  " general symptoms," 32
  " strange, rare and peculiar "
    symptoms, 33
  local, 32
  relative value, 27
  return of old, 41

Testing of drugs on the healthy, 7
Tetanus, 254
Thuja, 319
homœopathic indications,
  alimentary tract, 324, 325
  fasciæ, 327
  general symptoms, 320, 321
  genito-urinary tract, 325–327
  gonorrhœa, 325–327
  headaches, 323
  joints, 327
  mental symptoms, 323
  modalities, 328
  respiratory tract, 325
  skin, 328
  special senses, 324
  types, 323
relation to sycosis, 320, 322
Tonics, 148
Tuberculinum, 328
  dosage, 348
  general indications, 335
  gross effects on the body, 338
homœopathic indications,
  alimentary tract, 343
  genito-urinary tract, 343
  head, 342
  mental symptoms, 341
  modalities, 345
  pain, 344
  respiratory tract, 343
  skin, 344

Vaccination, 321, 322
Vaccinosis, 322
Veratrum album, 349
  general effects on the body, 349–
    350
homœopathic indications,
  coldness, 350
  collapse, 351
  mental symptoms, 351
  pain, 352
  profuse discharges, 350
  types, 352
Veratrum viride, 352